Frontiers of Artificial Intelligence in Medical Imaging

Online at: https://doi.org/10.1088/978-0-7503-4012-0

IOP Series in Artificial Intelligence in the Biomedical Sciences

Series Editor

Ge Wang, Clark and Crossan Endowed Chair Professor,
Rensselaer Polytechnic Institute, Troy New York, USA

About the Series

The *IOP Series in Artificial Intelligence in the Biomedical Sciences* aims to develop a library of key texts and reference works encompassing the broad range of artificial intelligence, machine learning, deep learning and neural networks within all applicable fields of biomedicine. There is now significant focus in using advancements in the field of AI to improve diagnosis, management, and better therapeutic options of various diseases. Some examples and applications incorporated would be AI in cancer diagnosis/prognosis, implementing artificial intelligence, data mining of electronic health records data, ambient intelligence in hospitals, AI in virus detection, AI in infectious diseases, biomarkers and genomics utilizing machine learning and clinical decision support with AR. These are just a few of the many applications that AI and related technologies can bring to the biomedical sciences. The series contains two broad types of approach. Those addressing a particular field of application and reviewing the numerous relevant artificial intelligence methods applicable to the field, and those that focus on a specific AI method which will permit a greater in-depth review of the theory and appropriate technology.

A full list of titles published in this series can be found here:
https://iopscience.iop.org/bookListInfo/iop-series-in-artificial-intelligence-in-the-biomedical-sciences#series.

Frontiers of Artificial Intelligence in Medical Imaging

Edited by
Navid Razmjooy
Department of Industrial Engineering, Ankara Yıldırım Beyazıt University (AYBU), 06010 Ankara, Turkey

Venkatesan Rajinikanth
Department of Computer Science and Engineering, Division of Research and Innovation, Saveetha School of Engineering, SIMATS, Chennai 602105, Tamil Nadu, India

IOP Publishing, Bristol, UK

ISBN 978-0-7503-4012-0 (ebook)
ISBN 978-0-7503-4010-6 (print)
ISBN 978-0-7503-4013-7 (myPrint)
ISBN 978-0-7503-4011-3 (mobi)

DOI 10.1088/978-0-7503-4012-0

Version: 20221201

IOP ebooks

British Library Cataloguing-in-Publication Data: A catalogue record for this book is available from the British Library.

Published by IOP Publishing, wholly owned by The Institute of Physics, London

IOP Publishing, No.2 The Distillery, Glassfields, Avon Street, Bristol, BS2 0GR, UK

US Office: IOP Publishing, Inc., 190 North Independence Mall West, Suite 601, Philadelphia, PA 19106, USA

Contents

Editor biographies

Navid Razmjooy

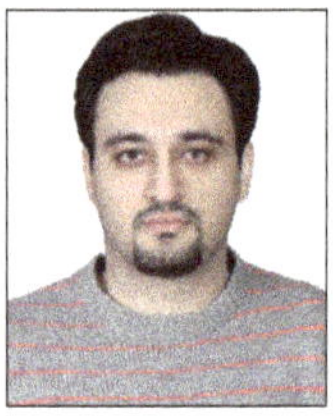

Dr Navid Razmjooy holds a PhD in Electrical Engineering (Control and Automation) from Tafresh University, Iran (2018), a BSc from the Ardabil branch of IAU University, Iran (2007), an MSc from the Isfahan branch of IAU University, Iran with honors in Mechatronics Engineering (2011), and a research opportunity internship at the Amirkabir University of Technology (2017–18). He was born in 1988. He is working in the following subjects: renewable energies, control, interval analysis, optimization, image processing, machine vision, soft computing, data mining, evolutionary algorithms and system control. He is a senior member of IEEE/USA and YRC in IAU/Iran. He has been ranked among the world's top 2% of scientists in the world based on the Stanford University/Scopus database. He has published more than 150 papers and six books in English and Farsi in peer-reviewed journals and conferences, and is now a reviewer in several national and international journals and conferences, which can be found at https://publons.com/researcher/1595287/navid-razmjooy/. More information can be found at https://www.researchgate.net/profile/Navid_Razmjooy.

Venkatesan Rajinikanth

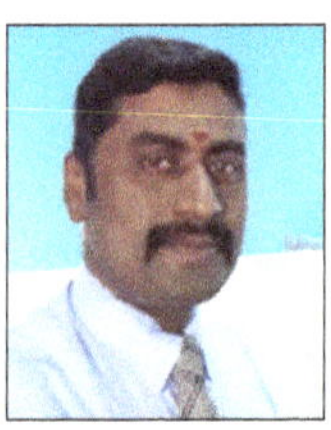

Dr Venkatesan Rajinikanth is a Professor in the Department of Electronics and Instrumentation Engineering at St. Joseph's College of Engineering, India. Recently, he has edited several books, *Advances in Artificial Intelligence Systems* (Nova Science, USA) and *Applications of Bat Algorithm and Its Variants* (Springer, Singapore). His main research interests include medical imaging, machine learning and computer aided diagnosis as well as data mining.

List of contributors

Ali Saud Al-Bimani

Dr Ali Saud Al-Bimani is a professor and Vice Chancellor at National University of Science and Technology, Sultanate of Oman. He has completed several funded projects and published more than 100 papers in peer reviewed high impact journals. He also received three international patent grants. His area of research includes, applications of AI, Data mining. Dr. Al-Bimani has a notable research background with numerous scientific publications, in international reputable journals, encyclopedia entries, conference proceedings, technical reports for various organizations in Oman and overseas, as well as other achievements.

Noradin Ghadimi

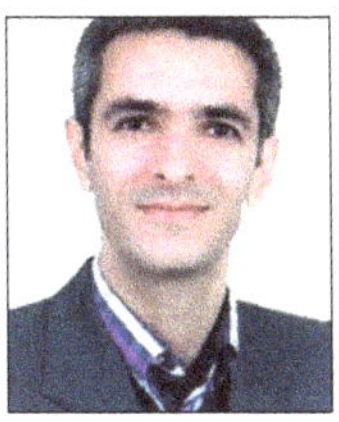

Dr Noradin Ghadimi is currently working as Head of Young Researchers and Elite Club, at the Islamic Azad University, Tehran, Iran. He completed his PhD in power systems from the same University. His main area of interest focuses on physical science engineering. His areas of expertise include power systems, energy management, energy systems, power market, electrical engineering and power engineering. He is author and co-author of 41 journal articles.

Seifedine Kadry

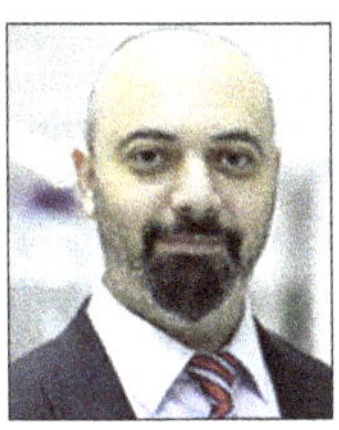

Dr Seifedine Kadry earned a Bachelor's degree in 1999 from Lebanese University, an MS degree in 2002 from Reims University, France and EPFL in Lausanne, a PhD in 2007 from Blaise Pascal University, France and a HDR degree in 2017 from Rouen University, France. At present his research focuses on data science, education using technology, system prognostics, stochastic systems and probability and reliability analysis. He is an ABET program evaluator for computing, and an ABET program evaluator for engineering tech.

Hong Lin

Dr Hong Lin received his PhD in Computer Science in 1997 at the University of Science and Technology of China. Before he joined the University of Houston-Downtown (UHD) in 2001, he was a postdoctoral research associate at Purdue University, USA, an assistant research officer at the National Research Council, Canada, and a software engineer at Nokia, Inc. Dr Lin is currently a professor in Computer Science with UHD. His research interests include cognitive intelligence, human-centered computing, parallel/distributed computing and big data analytics.

He is the supervisor of the Grid Computing Lab at UHD. He is also a senior member of the Association for Computing Machinery (ACM).

Suresh Manic

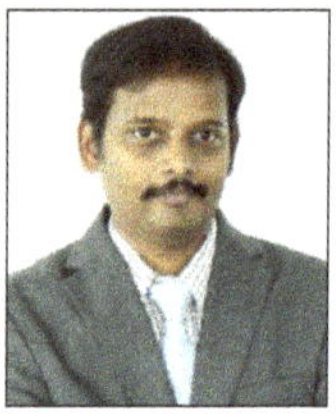

Dr K Suresh Manic is an Assistant Professor in the Department of Electrical and Communication Engineering at the College of Engineering, National University of Science and Technology, in the Sultanate of Oman. He has published more than 110 research articles and received research funding in value of over US$125 000. Recently, he has edited several books, *Medical Data Assessment Using Deep-Learning Schemes* and *Medical Image Evaluation with Joint Segmentation and Classification* (CRC Press, USA, Taylor and Francis Group). His main research interests include controller design, heuristic controllers, medical imaging, machine learning, and data mining.

Rajesh Kannan

Dr S Rajesh Kannan is an Associate Professor, Department of Electronics and Communication Engineering, St. Joseph's College of Engineering, Chennai. His areas of research includes Internet of things, sensor networks, medical imaging and data analytics.

J Sivakumar

Dr J Sivakumar is an Associate Professor, Department of Electronics and Communication Engineering, St. Joseph's College of Engineering, Chennai. His areas of research include image enhancement, medical imaging and data analytics.

Uma Suresh

Uma Suresh is currently a PHD scholar, doing research in the area of Artificial Intelligence at Anna University, Chennai. Her areas of expertise include Machine Learning and Deep learning approach for Medical Image Processing. She had masters in embedded system technology. She has a total of three patent grants and published many papers in peer reviewed journals.

Chapter 1

Health informatics system

Navid Razmjooy and Venkatesan Rajinikanth

In the current era, several facilities are employed in the health care domain to support the early diagnosis, appropriate treatment planning, and execution to treat and help the patient to recover from infectious and acute diseases. The traditional disease detection procedures are considerably enhanced by using a range of diagnostic hardware and software. Modern facilities in the health care domain provide the necessary support for humankind to have a disease-free life. Due to significant disease occurrence rates, several automatic disease detection systems are employed in hospitals to support faster disease detection. The traditional methods found in hospitals are still in use along with these methods; recent advancements, such as computerized patient screening, are also adopted to reduce the disease burden. An overview of the modern disease detection schemes present in hospitals is discussed in this chapter.

1.1 Introduction to health informatics

In the current era, many amenities have been developed and implemented to support the human community's safe and peaceful life irrespective of race, gender, and age. Over the years, many research works have been undertaken globally to develop ever more facilities to facilitate this living standard for humankind. After developing a facility, it will be tested before being recommended for practical use [1–5].

Even though many modern facilities exist, their access is limited due to various economic reasons. The available facilities in high-income and upper-middle-income countries are greater than those in lower-middle-income and low-income countries [6–8]. Irrespective of the country's economic condition, the incident rate of acute and infectious diseases in humans is rising globally due to various causes. The primary cause of most diseases are due to (i) heredity, (ii) immunodeficiency, (iii) age, and (iv) environmental conditions [9, 10]. The rapid increase in the disease occurrence rate in humans incurs various medical burdens from diagnosis to treatment, and this burden causes a severe impact on the country's economy and the people's health

doi:10.1088/978-0-7503-4012-0ch1

care. A report from the World Health Organisation stated that low-quality health care (LQH) is causing a considerable global impact, and further confirmed that LQH increases the burden of illness and its diagnostic cost [11].

The leading causes of LQH include (i) imprecise diagnosis, (ii) medication mistakes, (iii) unsuitable/unnecessary treatment, (iv) insufficient/unsafe medical amenities, and (v) unacceptable practices. LQH conditions cause various infectious diseases in hospitalized patients, particularly in low- and middle-income nations, and such conditions in turn increase the medical expenses and burden. Other infections due to LQH can be avoided by ensuring the appropriate treatment, superior hygiene, better infection-management practices and appropriate antimicrobials.

The primary motivation of the global health care system is to deliver quality health services (QHS) to patients in need by reducing the impacts of LQH, which cause extra expense and stress to families and local health systems.

Earlier research work confirms that a carefully designed health care system will help achieve a better QHS and reduce the impact of LQH considerably [8]. The design of an appropriate health care system involves (i) collecting complete information about the patient and disease information, (ii) employing all the possible tests to identify the disease accurately, (iii) sharing patient details with experts and receiving recommendation for appropriate treatment, and (iv) implementing the necessary treatment to help the patient recover from disease.

To ensure better patient treatment, present-day health care facilities employ a range of critical contemporary approaches to modernize the disease diagnosis, treatment, and monitoring procedures. Further, implementing a health informatics system (HIS) in hospitals improves their facilities through the various stages of care, such as patient admission, initial tests, disease diagnosis, treatment implementation, recovery monitoring, and follow-up of the patient after discharge [11–13].

Usually, a HIS is formed by uniting (i) health care data, (ii) information discipline, and (iii) computer science, which ensures complete automation of the health care system by implementing the necessary methods to provide a QHS. A HIS is generally arranged with medical information, diagnostic and treatment devices, resource optimization, data processing and storage, information retrieval, and implementation of collected data for the health and biomedical domains [14–16].

The recent literature relating to HISs confirms that theses facilities enhanced the medical domain application considerably and benefited from the united merits of various related domains, such as informatics systems, decision support schemes, remote monitoring, telemedicine, global health care schemes, translational exploration, and in-house patient care [17, 18].

Further, a carefully designed HIS will help to provide the necessary assistance for the following:

- *Complex medicinal assessment.* The appropriate diagnosis of severe infectious/acute disease needs various modern procedures to be followed. If a hospital is associated with a HIS facility, then the necessary diagnosis and timely treatment can cure the patient.

- *Evidence-based medicine.* This technique helps employ the best modern disease detection and treatment procedures for the patient. This approach supports access to state-of-the-art schemes to implement the appropriate treatment for the patient.
- *Illness supervision.* Monitoring the recovery rate is essential to confirm any improvement in the patient's health condition. When a HIS facility is employed, it supports the in-house and remote patient monitoring with the help of modern communication facilities, known as the Internet of Medical Things (IoMT) [19, 20].
- *Population health supervision.* The monitoring of the health condition of a population during the spread of infectious diseases can easily be achieved with HISs. Further, the employed HIS will lend support in the appropriate suggestion of treatment with the help of experts available in various parts of the country. This supports the complete monitoring and control of the infectious disease in a human population group.

1.2 Traditional scheme

The various stages involved in the detection and treatment of a disease depend on the nature of the disease and the availability of medical facilities. Figure 1.1 depicts the detailed methodology followed by the traditional disease detection and treatment scheme. When a patient experiences a disease symptom or abnormality, they will visit the doctor for an assessment and confirmation. If the symptom is mild and the disease in the patient is mild/moderate, the doctor will suggest appropriate medicine to be taken to get relief from the disease. Per the doctor's suggestion, the patient will complete a course of medication and inform the doctor of the recovery.

When the disease symptoms are harsh, an experienced doctor will perform an initial test(s) to identify and confirm the illness rate of the patient. During the initial test, information such as age, gender, weight, body temperature, blood pressure,

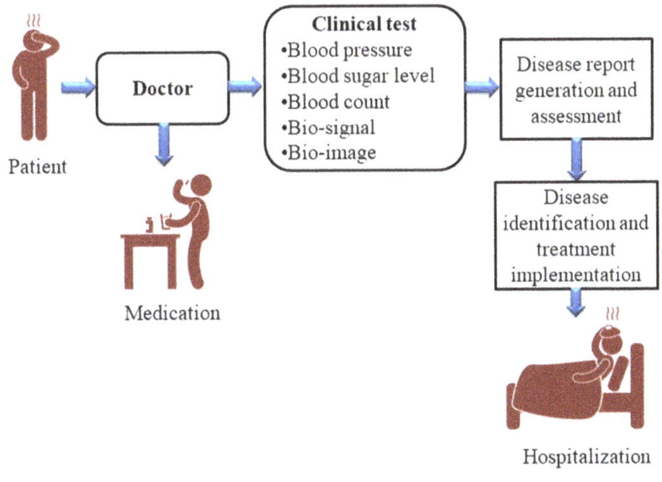

Figure 1.1. Traditional disease detection and treatment scheme.

sugar level, and related parameters are initially recorded. Suppose the rate of illness is high, along with the above regular patient data. In that case, the doctor will also recommend a pathology test to confirm the disease's reason, origin, and nature. If the pathology test fails to provide the necessary information, then biosignal- and bioimage-assisted techniques help the doctor to reach a diagnosis. After collecting the essential disease report for the patient, the doctor will decide on the treatment to be implemented to cure the patient. Based on the severity of the disease, the patient may be admitted into the hospital under a general care unit (GCU) or intensive care unit (ICU) until their condition returns to normal.

Figure 1.1 depicts the traditional disease detection and treatment schemes widely followed in hospitals in low- and middle-income countries. Most of these works are performed manually, and the treatment for the patient is implemented based on the experience or the suggestion obtained from an experienced doctor. In the traditional scheme, only a few processes are done automatically. Most of the work depends on the human operators involved in patient registration, disease identification, medication, and patient discharge.

Even though up-to-date medicines are provided for the patient, this scheme has its demerits, such as (i) prolonged diagnostic time, (ii) waiting for the arrival of an expert member of staff to make a decision regarding the disease, (iii) delayed treatment, and (iv) not maintaining the essential record about the patient/disease for the future use. The limitations of the traditional scheme can be overcome by automating the necessary sections in hospitals and employing current technology to maintain efficient monitoring during treatment.

1.3 Recent advancements

Recent advancements in science and technology have helped to enhance facilities in hospitals, as well as helped to improve the quality of traditional hospitals. As a result, every hospital in high-income countries and multispecialty hospitals in low/middle-income countries can employ all possible inventions to facilitate a better overall health care system.

Recent facilities implemented in hospital involve (i) mobile-application-based appointment booking, (ii) advance scheduling the time for disease diagnosis, (iii) early primary treatment, (iv) automated diagnosis and treatment, (v) automated monitoring of patient conditions, and (vi) follow-up after treatment.

In such an updated scenario, every hospital available in the locality/state is centralized using a web application, and the patient/user has access to facilities such as (i) viewing the availability of doctors for the appointment, (ii) seeing the diagnostic facilities available, (iii) the number of beds available/occupied, (iv) the number of patients under treatment (general/intensive care), and (v) existing follow-up procedures [21–24]. In modern hospitals, every task is thoroughly monitored using a dedicated computer, which will keep a complete record of information about the patient, such as the patient's personal details, diagnostic procedures employed and their outcome, various drugs and the dosages given, condition of the patient before and after reatment, medical expenses, and so on [14–16]. A modern hospital

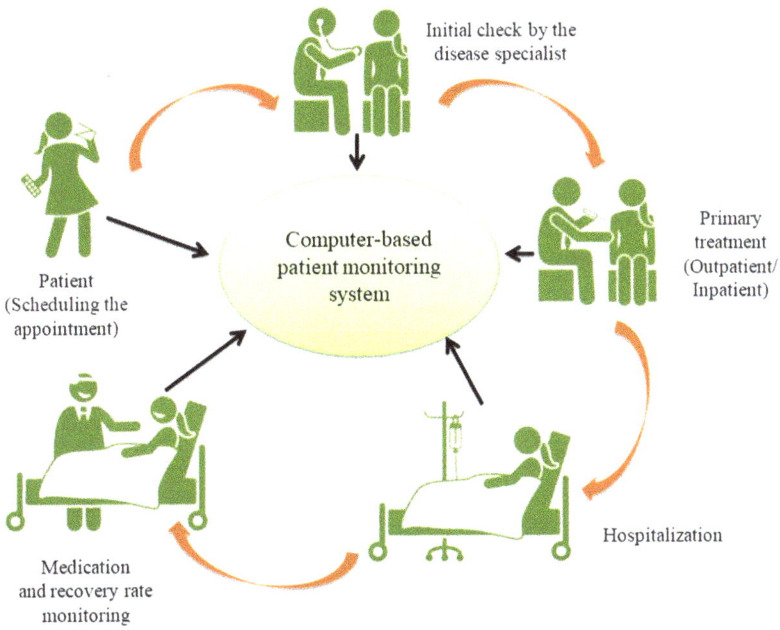

Figure 1.2. Modern disease detection and treatment scheme.

system is patient-friendly and provides all the necessary facilities to take care of patients admitted to the hospital.

Figure 1.2 depicts a block diagram of the facilities existing in modern hospitals. When a patient experiences any indication(s) of disease, they can directly book a doctor's appointment via phone or mobile application and schedule a convenient time to visit. Through the phone/mobile application, the patient can register their personal information as well as any notes on the disease's symptoms, which will help the doctor reduce the time for the diagnosis. When the patient reaches the hospital as per the scheduled time, the doctor will perform an initial check to confirm the type and harshness of the disease. The doctor also will suggest any additional test(s) to be done to identify the severity of the disease. When the patient is diagnosed with the additional test, the test report will be immediately shared with the doctor. The doctor will convey the treatment-related information to the patient. When the patient agrees to the treatment, a primary treatment process is initiated, and the treatment information is automatically recorded on the computer. When the disease is harsh, the patient is admitted to the hospital, where every treatment implemented for the patient is continuously recorded using a computer. The patient's record is maintained until the patient leaves the hospital after the treatment. When the patient is completely cured and discharged from the hospital, a scheduled follow-up will be maintained by the hospital to confirm the health condition of the patient.

In modern hospitals, every patient is assigned a registration number. Based on this number, a patient database is created and maintained, which forms a prime part of a patient monitoring system. The hospital maintains the collected data, and the necessary treatment information is shared with the patient based on request. The modern scheme's main merit is its transparency and automated patient monitoring. This scheme has been successfully deployed in modern hospitals; hence, more and more hospitals are adopting modern approaches to eliminate the demerits inherent in the traditional hospital scheme.

1.4 Artificial intelligence schemes

The limitations in the traditional disease detection and treatment schemes existing in hospitals are rectified by modernizing the hospitals [25–28]. In modern hospitals, most processes, such as patient admission, disease diagnosis, prediction of the disease recovery process, treatment execution, and helping the patient to recover in time from the disease, are organized, and every process is monitored using a dedicated computer algorithm.

The availability of high-speed computing facilities and related software have helped to automate every industrial sector, and the health care domain has adopted its methodologies in turn, as discussed in the literature [29, 30]. The automation of the hospital not only reduces the burden on doctors and staff but also provides hope for the patient since every action is pre-organized and based on stored instructions, the stages of the disease treatment are implemented accordingly, and the recovery rate of the patient is verified. Furthermore, this scheme maintains scheduled patient monitoring and helps provide all the necessary support to the patient until the disease is completely cured.

The computerization of the hospital automates the actions executed in the hospitals. Currently, this job is enhanced by employing the necessary computer software, which schedules the medication procedure for each patient and supports the complete supervision of patients with the assistance of appropriate monitoring equipment. The current works in the literature substantiate that artificial intelligence schemes (AIS) are extensively adopted in modern hospitals to computerize the whole tasks of illness analysis, decision-making, treatment implementation, and recovery monitoring. The conventional configuration of an AIS-assisted patient monitoring scheme is depicted in figure 1.3. This figure validates that AIS-based techniques help to accomplish the following.

(i) *Early disease detection.* Every modern hospital is equipped with AIS-method-based disease detection. Usually, the monitoring computer employed in the AIS scheme is already trained with a considerable quantity of disease data, and this scheme is also associated with the necessary disease models. When a new patient is admitted for treatment, the necessary disease information is then collected from the patient. This information is then compared against the existing data/model in the AIS to get a faster disease prediction and treatment execution. The AIS also collects the following information from the patient: disease symptoms, harshness, treatment procedures, medication to be implemented, and recovery time. The collected data is then utilized for disease detection more efficiently than in a traditional scheme. The existing AIS is already

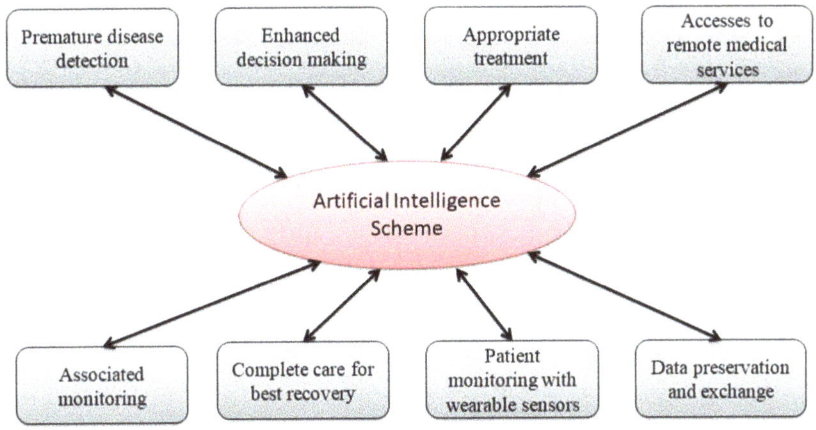

Figure 1.3. Artificial intelligence supported patient monitoring system.

trained with the necessary disease information. When it receives the information/symptoms from the patient, it will immediately predict the disease and instruct the doctor regarding any other tests to be performed to confirm the disease [31, 32]. AIS-supported early disease diagnosis can help to identify classes of infectious diseases and acute diseases [33, 34] in their early phases, which will avoid any delay in treatment.

(ii) *Enhanced decision-making*. Most hospitals in low/middle-income countries have a lower doctor-to-patient ratio, and hence a considerable delay occurs in disease diagnosis and the decision-making process. Most recent hospitals are equipped with an automated disease detection system to avoid this limitation, which can act as a supporting tool for doctors. A computer algorithm performs an initial level of the disease detection and decision-making process, and generates a report that is sent to a doctor for further verification and approval [51–53]. The various stages involved in this pipeline include (i) collection of the necessary information from the patient, (ii) collection of the clinical information, (iii) comparing the collected information with the similar existing information/models in the AIS, (iv) confirming the disease and generating a report for further analysis, and (v) getting approval from the doctor and treatment implementation. Figure 1.4 demonstrates the AI-supported decision-making process for the chosen case study of COVID-19 diagnosis [26–28]. Let us consider the case of patients visiting a hospital with the disease's symptoms. Every patient is initially verified with a reverse transcription polymerase chain reaction (RT-PCR) test and, based on the test outcome, further diagnosis is performed [35–37]. As in figure 1.4, it is diagnosed as harmful when a patient receives a positive result. This information is then sent to the AIS, which verifies the RT-PCR result with other RT-PCR results in the medical cloud and suggests the necessary imaging scheme to be employed to confirm the COVID-19 and

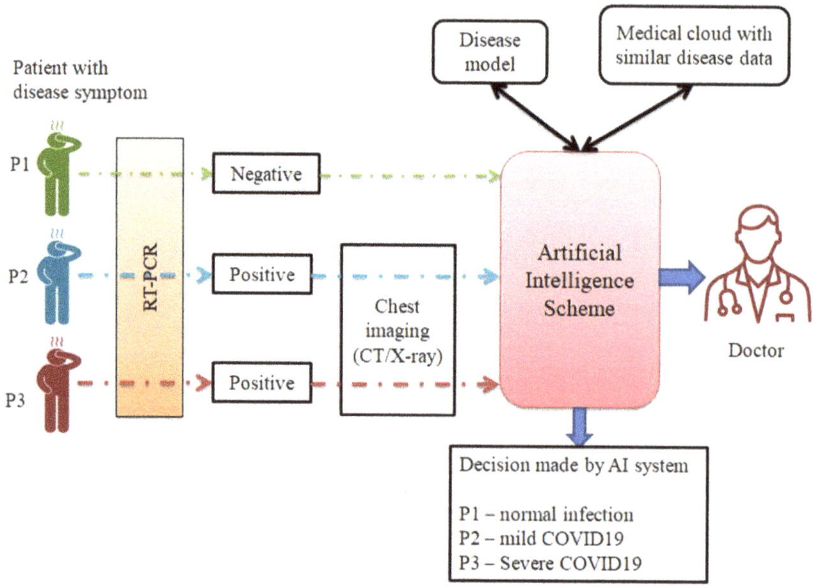

Figure 1.4. Artificial intelligence supported data assessment and decision-making.

its harshness. Based on the suggestion by the AIS or the doctor, the infected lung section is examined using a recommended imaging procedure. Usually, the lung image obtained with computed tomography or x-ray is considered adequate to confirm the disease score. A necessary treatment procedure is suggested based on its score to cure the patient. The employed AIS helps to analyze the disease information, make a decision, and suggest treatment to be implemented to help the patient recover from COVID-19.

(iii) *Appropriate treatment implementation.* The merit of AI-supported disease diagnosis is efficient detection of the disease with lesser time and timely treatment implementation. As depicted in figure 1.4, the AIS can enable remote expert monitoring and decision-making, enhancing the treatment implementation and recovery process.

(iv) *Facility to access remote medical services.* The AIS is linked with a medical cloud, which can support facilities in remote diagnosis, decision-making, medication assistance, and monitoring [38–40].

(v) *Associated monitoring.* When the entire hospital is automated and connected to the medical cloud, then the patient under treatment can be monitored with the help of a doctor resident in the hospital (i.e. in-house monitoring); further, additional work can be facilitated by a remote doctor who might be an expert in the disease. Usually, a critical patient will be taken by the in-house and remote doctors, and this associated monitoring and treatment will confirm better patient monitoring.

(vi) *Through care for a speedy recovery.* Every hospital aims to provide the best treatment facilities to its patient and to provide every measure necessary to help patients recover disease. In multispecialty and modern hospitals, every patient is continuously monitored with the help of medical software, which is designed to monitor the patient's condition and bioelectric signals continuously with the help of wearable sensors. A dedicated computer examines the data obtained using these sensors and, based on the decision by the computer, any necessary drugs can be provided to hence improve the recovery rate of the patients. Further, AIS schemes will also have the facility to predict the patient's recovery rate based on the monitored conditions, which will help reduce the medical expense and treatment time.

(vii) *Monitoring of patient with all possible sensors.* When a patient is admitted to an ICU, the patient's condition must be monitored thoroughly. Usually, this task is completed using a dedicated computer associated with the necessary AIS. Every patient's information is shared with the computer through a wired/wireless sensor unit, and this computer will continuously monitor the patient's condition and alert the medical assistant(s) if any abnormality arises. In some critical cases, this facility also supports automated drug delivery to the patient whenever necessary. The patient's actual condition is monitored with the help of necessary sensors/electrodes, which provide the essential information to confirm the patient's recovery.

(viii) *Disease information preservation and exchange.* The principal merit of a computerized disease monitoring scheme is automated disease diagnosis with the help of an AIS. Every patient admitted to hospital is assigned an identification number, and the patient details are stored in computer memory based on this number. The employed AIS will help to achieve the following tasks: (i) patient personal information registration, (ii) assessment of disease information through clinical reports, (iii) automated analysis of biosignals/bioimages of the patient, (iv) identification of disease and treatment suggestion, (v) preserving the disease information for future use, and (vi) sharing the preserved information through the medical cloud to solicit remote experts' opinion regarding treatment planning and execution. Furthermore, when a complete record of the disease information of the patient is available, it will help create a model for the disease, and this disease model can be considered to identify similar disease cases.

1.5 Deep-learning schemes

Human disease incident rates are gradually rising worldwide due to various causes, and every disease needs to be precisely recognized for the implementation of appropriate treatment. In most low- and middle-income countries, the shortage of doctors will cause a considerable disease diagnostic burden. Hence, most hospitals are now employing computerized disease screening procedures. The outcome achieved from the computerized system can be verified and confirmed by a doctor, and this decision is then considered to implement the appropriate treatment.

Usually, every hospital has a sufficient number of experienced doctors in a particular field and ample awareness about treating the disease. The possible limitations with the actual doctors is due to their individual prejudice, significant deviation in illness conditions, doctors' accessibility, and fatigue that will influence the delay in disease diagnosis and treatment. Further, when the number of patients visiting the hospital for disease screening rises, the available information to be examined will also rise, leading to so-called big medical data (BMD). The examination of BMD is challenging and time consuming; hence, most hospitals employ AIS to evaluate this information automatically [54–56]. The recent medical literature confirms the employment of several machine-learning (ML) and deep-learning (DL) systems to examine BMD. These techniques help reduce the doctor's data-assessment burden. BMD in hospitals includes vital information such as patient information, initial screening reports, biosignals collected from the patients, and bioimages recorded using a chosen modality. Patient data handling and assessment are challenging: most modern hospitals are thus equipped with automatic disease evaluation systems using ML/DL schemes. The DL schemes have considerable merit compared to ML techniques; when a database of BMD is to be examined, existing DL systems can be considered to examine any information, such as text data, one-dimensional (1D) physiological signals, and two/three-dimensional (2D/3D) medical images [41, 42]. The DL schemes are able to learn continuously from the medical data and help to offer reliable disease detection compared to other existing methods in hospitals.

The existing DL methods can extract and evaluate abnormal sections from 1D/2D/3D medical data or to segregate the existing BMD into various classes, such as healthy, mild, moderate, and harsh diseases. When the data is segregated appropriately, patients with harsh disease symptoms will receive a higher priority for treatment than those with mild and moderate illnesses. Moreover, in most disease cases, an existing DL scheme can reliably predict the harshness of the illness, drug discovery, treatment procedure to be employed, and the recovery rate prediction. This will considerably reduce the doctor's work and ensure the implementation of quality treatment.

The literature shows that several pre-trained and conventional DL methods exist that can support disease information segmentation and classification. However, the choice in selecting the appropriate DL procedure depends on (i) the volume of the BMD, (ii) recommended diagnostic accuracy, and (iii) complexity during implementation, training, and testing of the model [43]. Further, a DL scheme employed for a given disease cannot necessarily be directly considered to detect another disease (i.e. DL schemes are disease specific), and consequently each time, based on the disease data, the system has to be trained and validated.

Typically, DL architecture is built using various layers of a neural network (convolutional neuronal network), consisting of different layers with a given task, such as convolution, maxpool, fully connected, and classification. For a chosen disease case, the DL architecture has to be developed from scratch, and every section of this architecture needs to be appropriately optimized with a chosen procedure in order to improve the learning capability of the disease detection system. Further, a carefully designed DL scheme will also help achieve better disease detection with lesser CPU run time. The added merit of DL schemes is that they can be employed in standalone monitoring computers and modern hospitals, and that such schemes can be accessed from a remote server with the help of the medical cloud. Even though a DL scheme's installation and maintenance cost is higher than with traditional approaches, they exhibit considerable merits. Hence, most recent hospitals have adopted a DL scheme to supported disease diagnosis, decision-making, and treatment [44, 45].

1.6 The Internet of Medical Things in health informatics

In earlier days, to be availed of a medical facility, the patient would have to personally visit the hospital to meet a doctor, and the doctor would do all the necessary tests to identify the illness. However, the traditional method of illness detection is time consuming and can delay the treatment process. This delay can further cause various problems; some patients may die if they do not receive timely treatment [46, 47].

Hence, most modern hospitals adopt remote disease diagnosis and monitoring facilities to reduce the delay in treatment. Most modern hospitals have adopted the concept of a digitally enhanced telemonitoring scheme with the help of a high-speed communication network which connects the patient directly to the doctor/computer to monitor the illness. Recent advancement in communications, known as the Internet of Things (IoT), have helped to support remote-monitoring facilities with the help of a high-speed sensing system and dedicated communication network. The IoT employed in health care is known as the Internet of Medical Things (IoMT), which has considerably reduced the gap between the patient and doctor.

When we are interested in monitoring patients' health with a health-monitoring system or telemedicine, the IoMT can provide the appropriate facility. In the current era, many wearable sensors have been developed to monitor the health condition of ill/older adults. Every person has a smartphone that can be associated with the necessary health-monitoring applications. This facility helps to connect every patient to the hospital through the IoMT. Furthermore, IoMT expertise helps with information gathering and examination from remote locations to ensure timely treatment.

Figure 1.5 depicts an IoMT-supported automated patient monitoring system typically employed in modern hospitals [48]. Every patient admitted in the ambulance/hospital is provided with a wearable radio frequency identification (RFID) band, which will continuously transmit their essential information, such as body temperature, blood pressure, and oxygen saturation level, to the RFID reader; this information is then relayed to a monitoring computer through a dedicated communication network. This monitoring computer is connected with other necessary facilities, such as a clinical database, health cloud, earlier disease

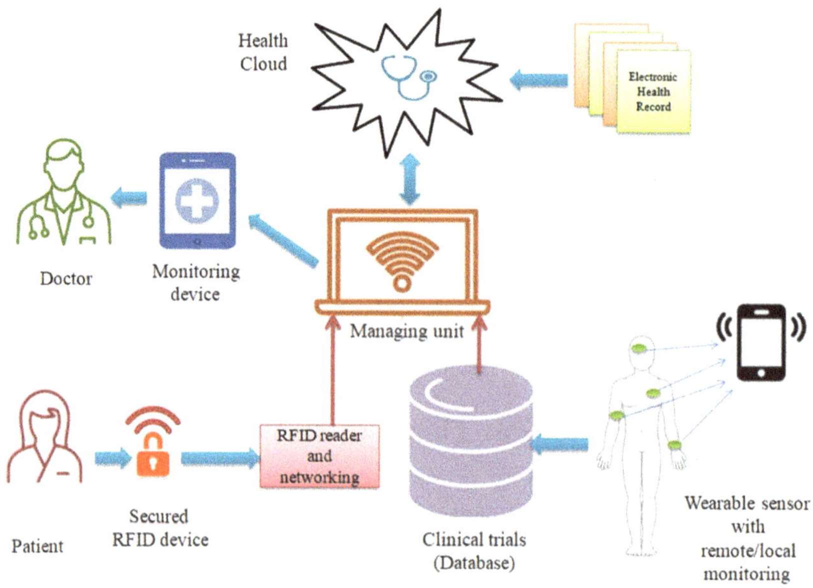

Figure 1.5. IoMT-based automated patient monitoring scheme.

record, and a handheld monitoring device carried by the doctor. Further, this system also collects the necessary information with the help of wearable sensors and transmits this information to the doctor through the IoMT network. The doctor is able to monitor the patient's condition remotely and send treatment-related instruction to the medical attendants. This procedure is continued till the patient's health condition becomes stable. This procedure is a recommended approach; hence, most hospitals employ this facility to support the timely delivery of medical services to the patient.

A traditional HIS supports the following practices: information collection, evaluation, and supervising health information, and, finally, implementation of medical concepts using a suitable technique. In the current era, HISs play a significant role in hospitals since they guarantee that everyone is provided with the finest quality health care. Further, a HIS will help integrate cutting-edge facilities, such as computer algorithms, BMD, IoMT, and related technologies, to provide quality treatment to patients suffering from illness.

1.7 Health-band-supported patient monitoring

Earlier approaches to patient condition monitoring involve taking care of the patient by hospital health workers. In this system, every patient is initially diagnosed by a doctor, and, based on the patient's disease severity, the patient is treated as an outpatient or inpatient. After an initial check, the patient is allowed to continue the treatment at home when the patient's condition is acceptable. During this procedure, the patient is advised to take the proper medication prescribed by the doctor. In this case, the patient is referred to as an outpatient and visits the doctor based on a predefined schedule. This procedure is suitable for mild disease conditions.

When the patient's condition is severe and they are infected with an acute disease, then, as per the doctor's advice, the patient is admitted to the hospital, and continuous treatment is executed until the patient recovers from the disease. This patient is known as an inpatient (in-house patient). Usually, the treatment expenses of inpatients is greater than outpatients, and the doctor makes the decision based on the diagnosis report.

Most older adults are infected with various diseases due to their age, and each time visiting the hospital will be a challenging task. Hence, current research in science and technology has helped to provide a possible solution to the problem, which involves remote patient monitoring and the employment of a so-called body area network to monitor the health condition of the elderly continuously. One of the advanced monitoring schemes developed and practically implemented is a wireless-network-connected wearable health-monitoring System (WHS). Most WHSs today help enhance the health care structure by using remote supervising services. The arrival of WHS in health care engineering has brought a remarkable transformation in care delivery. The tangible benefits can be observed much more quickly with a WHS compared to traditional health-monitoring procedures. This makes them a perfect fit for emergencies and triage circumstances. Further, the data acquired is of clinical grade [49, 50].

Current versions of WHSs engage the patients in self-monitoring their health using monitoring gadgets such as mobile phones or laptops. For example, a WHS connected with a mobile phone helps in the early recognition of abnormality, leading to a better prognosis. In addition, it provides real-time access to patients' health records, enabling quick diagnosis and better treatment outcomes—wearable technology in health care that is also user-friendly and unobtrusive.

This enables the recently discharged patient to self-monitor their health and thus reduce the length of their hospital stay. The wireless data transmission and alerting mechanisms present also help in immediate care delivery during emergencies. The data derived from medical-grade wearables are reliable and consistent, and can reliably be used to diagnose, treat, or manage health conditions. This technology has attracted a sizeable user base, and most individuals are currently using these systems. The most commonly found WHS is a smart watch (wristband), which helps acquire the necessary information, such as blood pressure, body temperature, sleep pattern, and the number of walking steps completed by the person. Dedicated software installed in a mobile phone along with blue-tooth connectivity is sufficient to exchange the information from the wristband to the smartphone's monitoring screen. Further, this scheme supports setting a threshold to alert the individual when an abnormality in the collected signal is found.

The implementation of WHSs helps in self-monitoring biological signals and warning users if any abnormalities arise. This will help reach the hospital in time to diagnose the abnormality using clinical-grade equipment. Further, continuous monitoring schemes employed for the elderly are capable of supporting health condition monitoring from a remote location, which can connect the doctor with the patient virtually. The doctor can monitor the patient's vital biosignal-related data through a dedicated monitoring device. Such a solution helps implement a low-cost remote-monitoring scheme and also supports the detection of abnormalities in good time.

Because of its merits, several health care companies are concentrating on developing various health bands to monitor patients with complete care. A recently developed solution includes heart rate monitoring, respiration monitoring, brain condition monitoring, and walking stress monitoring. When an appropriate WHS is employed, every patient can be ideally monitored from a remote location, and, whenever necessary, a suitable suggestion can be transferred from the doctor to the patient.

1.8 Accurate disease diagnosis

Modern hospitals are equipped with advanced diagnostic and treatment facilities. Most developed countries are equipped with modern hospitals with state-of-the-art facilities. Modern hospitals are associated with (i) latest diagnostic equipment, (ii) recent laboratory facilities with appropriate signal/image-capturing devices, (iii) well-trained health care workers, (iv) ICUs with complete monitoring facilities, (v) remote disease diagnosis and report generation, and (vi) treatment implementation and suggested medication to support speedy recovery.

The availability of medical facilities and state-of-the-art treatment will attract many medical tourists. When a patient needs treatment from these modern hospitals, the patient and any attendant caretaker will visit the hospital to receive the recommended treatment.

In order to improve the diagnostic facilities, most hospitals are equipped with computerized diagnostic methods, which help in delivering faster disease assessment and decision-making using the aforementioned recently developed machine-learning methods (MLMs) and deep-learning methods (DLMs). When AI is combined with traditional procedures, accurate disease detection is achieved.

Recent articles confirm that the employment of MLMs and DLMs helped diagnose COVID-19 with recommended accuracy. Hence, still, the detection of COVID-19 is usually achieved using computer algorithms. The combined MLM/DLM, along with the traditional data collection, helps diagnose a variety of acute and communicable diseases with better precision. Most of these algorithms also suggest the treatment procedure to be implemented to cure the disease. When AI schemes are employed along with the traditional disease detection scheme, every patient is efficiently diagnosed with the proposed scheme, which will reduce the diagnostic burden on doctors.

1.9 Summary

This chapter of the book has highlighted clinical-level disease diagnosis with traditional and recently developed AI schemes. In earlier days, disease in an individual was detected using traditional procedures with a prescribed medical protocol, such as a personal check by an experienced doctor, clinical-level tests to confirm the disease, biomedical signal/image recording to confirm the location and severity of the disease, followed by decision-making and treatment implementation. The procedures followed in the traditional technique are uncomplicated, which helps to identify several diseases. However, the major limitation of the traditional process is its diagnostic time. This drawback is rectified by replacing the manually performed diagnostic methods with suitable computer algorithms. Further, modern health care facilities can support IoMT-based patient monitoring and WHS schemes. This further reduces the risk of the wrong identification of the disease; whenever an expert's opinion is necessary, the electronic data (signal/image) is then shared with an experienced doctor, who will decide the disease's severity, location, and treatment.

Current methods help to quickly decide patient treatment and deliver a speedy recovery, in comparison to previous, slower methods. Along with the IoMT, wearable sensor networks and other advancements will always help achieve a better result when a patient is examined. Recent advancements in the health care industry help toward better disease identification for further assessment and treatment implementation.

References

[1] Shen Y and Tao Y 2022 Associations between spatial access to medical facilities and health-seeking behaviors: a mixed geographically weighted regression analysis in Shanghai, China *Appl. Geogr.* **139** 102644

[2] Chiu H Y R, Hwang C K, Chen S Y, Shih F Y, Han H C, King C C and Oyang Y J 2022 Machine learning for emerging infectious disease field responses *Sci. Rep.* **12** 328

[3] Batko K and Ślęzak A 2022 The use of big data analytics in healthcare *J. Big Data* **9** 3

[4] Aman A H M, Hassan W H, Sameen S, Attarbashi Z S, Alizadeh M and Latiff L A 2021 IoMT amid COVID-19 pandemic: application, architecture, technology, and security *J. Netw. Comput. Appl.* **174** 102886

[5] Rajinikanth V and Dey N 2022 *Magnetic Resonance Imaging: Recording, Reconstruction and Assessment* (Amsterdam: Elsevier)

[6] Fernandes G, Hassan I and Sridhar D 2022 Building resilient health-care supply chains to manage pandemics in low-and middle-income countries *Bul. World Health Org.* **100** 174

[7] Warman P I, Seas A, Satyadev N, Adil S M, Kolls B J, Haglund M M and Fuller A T 2022 Machine learning for predicting in-hospital mortality after traumatic brain injury in both high-income and low-and middle-income countries *Neurosurgery* **90** 605–12

[8] Dombou C, Omonaiye O, Fraser S, Cénat J M and Yaya S 2022 Barriers and facilitators associated with the use of mental health services among immigrant students in high-income countries: a scoping review protocol *System. Rev.* **11** 22

[9] Tsao C W *et al* 2022 Heart disease and stroke statistics—2022 update: a report from the american heart association *Circulation* **145** e153–639

[10] Sharma A E, Lyson H C, Cherian R, Somsouk M, Schillinger D and Sarkar U 2022 A root cause analysis of barriers to timely colonoscopy in california safety-net health systems *J. Patient Safety* **18** e163–171

[11] https://who.int/news/item/05–07-2018-low-quality-healthcare-is-increasing-the-burden-of-illness-and-health-costs-globally

[12] Qu J 2022 Blockchain in medical informatics *J. Indust. Inf. Int.* **25** 100258

[13] Joseph A L, Stringer E, Borycki E M and Kushniruk A W 2022 Evaluative frameworks and models for health information systems (HIS) and health information technologies (HIT) *Stud. Health Technol. Inform.* **289** 280–5

[14] London S D, Fontelo P, Boroumand S and Dye B A 2022 COVID-19 provides an opportunity for integration of dentistry into the health informatics system *J. Am. Dental Assoc.* **153** 3–8
[15] Kaspar M, Fette G, Hanke M, Ertl M, Puppe F and Störk S 2022 Automated provision of clinical routine data for a complex clinical follow-up study: a data warehouse solution *Health Inform. J.* **28** 1
[16] Christopoulou S C 2022 Impacts on context aware systems in evidence-based health informatics: a review *Healthcare* vol 10 (Basel: MDPI) p 685
[17] Ayyoubzadeh S M, Shirkhoda M, Kalhori S R N, Mohammadzadeh N and Zakerabasali S 2022 A smartphone remote monitoring app to follow up colorectal cancer survivors: requirement analysis *JMIR Cancer* **8** e18083
[18] Mutanu L, Gupta K and Gohil J 2022 Leveraging IoT solutions for enhanced health information exchange *Technology in Society* **68** 101882
[19] Hossen M N, Panneerselvam V, Koundal D, Ahmed K, Bui F M and Ibrahim S M 2022 Federated machine learning for detection of skin diseases and enhancement of internet of medical things (IoMT) security *IEEE J. Biomed. Health Inf.* https://doi.org/10.1109/JBHI.2022.3149288
[20] Rahmani M K I, Shuaib M, Alam S, Siddiqui S T, Ahmad S, Bhatia S and Mashat A 2022 Blockchain-based trust management framework for cloud computing-based internet of medical things (IoMT): a systematic review *Comput. Intel. Neurosci.* **2022** 9766844
[21] Parmar P, Ryu J, Pandya S, Sedoc J and Agarwal S 2022 Health-focused conversational agents in person-centered care: a review of apps *NPJ Digital Medicine* **5** 21
[22] O'Sullivan B, Couch D and Naik I 2022 Using mobile phone apps to deliver rural general practitioner services: critical review using the walkthrough method *JMIR Formative Research* **6** e30387
[23] Alharbi N S, AlGhanmi A S and Fahlevi M 2022 Adoption of health mobile apps during the COVID-19 lockdown: a health belief model approach *Int. J. Environ. Res. Public Health* **19** 4179
[24] McCool J, Dobson R, Whittaker R and Paton C 2022 Mobile health (mhealth) in low-and middle-income countries *Ann. Rev. Public Health* **43** 525–39
[25] Sabir Z, Botmart T, Raja M A Z, Sadat R, Ali M R, Alsulami A A and Alghamdi A 2022 Artificial neural network scheme to solve the nonlinear influenza disease model *Biomed. Signal Process. Control* **75** 103594
[26] Kadry S, Rajinikanth V, González Crespo R and Verdú E 2022 Automated detection of age-related macular degeneration using a pre-trained deep-learning scheme *J. Supercomput.* **78** 7321–40
[27] Kadry S, Rajinikanth V, Taniar D, Damaševičius R and Valencia X P B 2022 Automated segmentation of leukocyte from hematological images—a study using various CNN schemes *J. Supercomput.* **78** 6974–94
[28] Vijayakumar K, Rajinikanth V and Kirubakaran M K 2022 Automatic detection of breast cancer in ultrasound images using mayfly algorithm optimized handcrafted features *J. X-Ray Sci. Technol.* **30** 751–66
[29] Rajinikanth V, Aslam S M and Kadry S 2021 Deep learning framework to detect ischemic stroke lesion in brain MRI slices of flair/DW/T1 modalities *Symmetry* **13** 2080
[30] Cheong K H, Tang K J W, Zhao X, Koh J E W, Faust O, Gururajan R and Acharya U R 2021 An automated skin melanoma detection system with melanoma-index based on entropy features *Biocyber. Biomed. Eng.* **41** 997–1012

[31] Mehta N and Shukla S 2022 Pandemic analytics: how countries are leveraging big data analytics and artificial intelligence to fight COVID-19? *SN Computer Science* **3** 54
[32] Larie D, An G and Cockrell C 2022 Preparing for the next COVID: deep reinforcement learning trained artificial intelligence discovery of multi-modal immunomodulatory control of systemic inflammation in the absence of effective anti-microbials *bioRxiv* 480940
[33] Zaizen Y, Kanahori Y, Ishijima S, Kitamura Y, Yoon H S, Ozasa M and Fukuoka J 2022 Deep-learning-aided detection of mycobacteria in pathology specimens increases the sensitivity in early diagnosis of pulmonary tuberculosis compared with bacteriology tests *Diagnostics* **12** 709
[34] Habib A R, Kajbafzadeh M, Hasan Z, Wong E, Gunasekera H, Perry C and Singh N 2022 Artificial intelligence to classify ear disease from otoscopy: a systematic review and meta-analysis *Clinical Otolaryngology* **47** 401–13
[35] Hildebrandt M, Mapara M Y, Körner I J, Bargou R C, Moldenhauer G and Dörken B 1997 Reverse transcriptase-polymerase chain reaction (RT-PCR)-controlled immunomagnetic purging of breast cancer cells using the magnetic cell separation (MACS) system: a sensitive method for monitoring purging efficiency *Exp. Hematol.* **25** 57–65
[36] Kendall L V and Riley L K 2000 Reverse transcriptase polymerase chain reaction (RT-PCR) *J. Am. Assoc. Lab. Animal Sci.* **39** 42
[37] Saad Menezes M C, Santinelli Pestana D V, Ferreira J C, Ribeiro de Carvalho C R, Felix M C and Marcilio I OHCFMUSP COVID-19 Study Group 2022 Distinct outcomes in COVID-19 patients with positive or negative RT-PCR test *Viruses* **14** 175
[38] DeGrave A J, Janizek J D and Lee S I 2021 AI for radiographic COVID-19 detection selects shortcuts over signal *Nature Mach. Intel.* **3** 610–9
[39] Nguyen D C, Ding M, Pathirana P N and Seneviratne A 2021 Blockchain and AI-based solutions to combat coronavirus (COVID-19)-like epidemics: a survey *IEEE Access* **9** 95730–53
[40] Teboulbi S, Messaoud S, Hajjaji M A and Mtibaa A 2021 Real-time implementation of AI-based face mask detection and social distancing measuring system for COVID-19 prevention *Sci. Program.* **2021** 8340779
[41] Rajinikanth V, Kadry S, Taniar D, Kamalanand K, Elaziz M A and Thanaraj K P 2022 Detecting epilepsy in EEG signals using synchro-extracting-transform (SET) supported classification technique *J. Amb. Intel. Humanized Comput.* https://doi.org/10.1007/s12652-021-03676-x
[42] Abdi Alkareem Alyasseri Z, Alomari O A, Al-Betar M A, Awadallah M A, Hameed Abdulkareem K, Abed Mohammed M and Rho S 2022 EEG channel selection using multiobjective cuckoo search for person identification as protection system in healthcare applications *Comput. Intel. Neurosci.* **2022** 5974634
[43] Noor M B T, Zenia N Z, Kaiser M S, Mahmud M and Mamun S A 2019 Detecting neurodegenerative disease from MRI: a brief review on a deep learning perspective *Brain Informatics* vol 11976 (Cham: Springer) pp 115–25
[44] Khan M A, Muhammad K, Wang S H, Alsubai S, Binbusayyis A, Alqahtani A, Majumdar A and Thinnukool O 2022 Gastrointestinal diseases recognition: a framework of deep neural network and improved moth-crow optimization with DCCA fusion *Human-Centric Comput. Inf. Sci.* **12** 25

[45] Nawaz M, Nazir T, Masood M, Ali F, Khan M A, Tariq U, Sahar N and Damaševičius R 2022 Melanoma segmentation: a framework of improved DenseNet77 and UNET convolutional neural network *Int. J. Imaging Syst. Technol.* **32** 2137–53

[46] Ahmed J, Nguyen T N, Ali B, Javed A and Mirza J 2022 On the physical layer security of federated learning based IoMT networks *IEEE J. Biomed. Health Inform.* https://doi.org/10.1109/JBHI.2022.3173947

[47] Samuel O, Omojo A B, Onuja A M, Sunday Y, Tiwari P, Gupta D and Shamshirband S 2022 IoMT: a COVID-19 healthcare system driven by federated learning and blockchain *IEEE J. Biomed. Health Inform.* https://doi.org/10.1109/JBHI.2022.3143576

[48] Rajinikanth V and Kadry S 2021 Development of a framework for preserving the disease-evidence-information to support efficient disease diagnosis *Int. J. Data Warehousing Mining* **17** 63–84

[49] Samuel O, Omojo A B, Mohsin S M, Tiwari P, Gupta D and Band S S 2022 An anonymous IoT-based E-health monitoring system using blockchain technology *IEEE Syst. J.* https://doi.org/10.1109/JSYST.2022.3170406

[50] Agrawal R, Faujdar N, Kumar P and Kumar A 2022 Security and privacy of blockchain-based single-bit cache memory architecture for IoT systems *IEEE Access* **10** 35273–86

[51] Estrela V V, Monteiro A C B, França R P, Iano Y, Khelassi A and Razmjooy N 2018 Health 4.0: applications, management, technologies and review *Med. Tech. J.* **2** 262–76

[52] Estrela V V, Khelassi A, Monteiro A C B, Iano Y, Razmjooy N, Martins D and Rocha D T 2019 Why software-defined radio (SDR) matters in healthcare? *Med. Tech. J.* **3** 421–29

[53] Abreu L M, Hora H R M D, Rangel J J A, Erthal M, Navid, Estrela V V and Iano Y 2020 A multi-criteria modelling for ranking CO_2 emitting G20 countries from the Kaya identity and their impacts on elderly health *Brazilian Technology Symp.* pp 477–87

[54] Alferaidi A, Yadav K, Alharbi Y, Navid R, Viriyasitavat W, Gulati K, Kautish S and Dhiman G 2022 Distributed deep CNN-LSTM model for intrusion detection method in IoT-based vehicles *Math. Problems Eng.* **2022** 3424819

[55] Ranjbarzadeh R, Dorosti S, Jafarzadeh Ghoushchi S, Safavi S, Razmjooy N, Tataei Sarshar N and Bendechache M 2022 Nerve optic segmentation in CT images using a deep learning model and a texture descriptor *Complex Intel. Syst.* **8** 3543–57

[56] Alferaidi A, Yadav K, Alharbi Y, Navid R, Viriyasitavat W, Gulati K, Kautish S and Dhiman G 2022 Distributed deep CNN-LSTM model for intrusion detection method in IoT-based vehicles *Math. Problems Eng.* **2022** 3424819

Chapter 2

Medical-imaging-supported disease diagnosis

Navid Razmjooy and Venkatesan Rajinikanth

Diseases in internal/external organs can be effectively diagnosed using biosignaling/bioimaging-supported methods. Compared to biosignals, bioimages recorded with different imaging modalities are widely employed in hospitals to examine disease. Further, bioimages are available in various forms, such as in grayscale, red–green–blue (RGB), two-dimensional (2D) and three-dimensional (3D) form. Based on the need, they can be examined using an experienced doctor or with the help of a dedicated computer algorithm. The accessibility of clinical images for academic/scientific research is limited and hence benchmark images are widely considered by researchers to test any proposed methodology/algorithm to diagnose the disease automatically. This work presents an overview of the medical imaging techniques considered in the literature and their applied locations. These images can be considered by the researchers to test and evaluate the proposed methodology and the achieved outcome can be validated against the existing results in the literature.

2.1 Introduction

Due to a variety of causes, the incidence rate of diseases in mankind is gradually rising. Appropriate detection and treatment is essential to detect disease, plan the appropriate treatment procedure, and to cure the disease with necessary treatment.

A 2020 report of the World Health Organisation (WHO) confirmed that the occurrence of cancer is increasing in humans due to various conditions, such as heredity and environmental conditions, as well as other unpredicted reasons [1]. Normally, cancer is a common expression for a huge collection of abnormalities which can affect any division of human physiology. The main difficulty of a cancer is that it will cause severe illness and, left untreated, can lead to death. When a cancer develops, abnormal cell growth in the affected area rapidly increases; uncontrolled/untreated cell growth will cause very serious conditions. Further, the abnormal cells which are released to the bloodstream will spread the cancer to other body parts.

doi:10.1088/978-0-7503-4012-0ch2

Hence, appropriate diagnosis and treatment is necessary to cure the affected individual from the cancer. The release of cancer cells to blood cells, leading to further growths, is technically known as metastases, which is the prime cause of death in cancer patients. When the cancer is diagnosed in its premature phase, it is possible to control/cure its severity using recommended procedures, such as medicines, chemotherapy, radiotherapy, and surgery [2–5].

The report of the WHO stated that, compared to other diseases, global deaths due to cancer are gradually rising: in 2020 alone, nearly 10 million deaths were reported due to cancer, worldwide. This confirms that cancer is one of the major medical emergencies confronting humankind and that the detection and treatment of cancer causes a huge burden to the medical industry. Due to this reason, a considerable number of awareness programs are being conducted worldwide to inform the populace about the major causes of cancer and its methods of prevention. Further, a considerable number of anti-cancer drugs are discovered and still the research works are happening to develop appropriate procedure to cure the cancer in its early phase.

The 2020 report of the WHO listed the major causes of cancer in mankind and the organs which are regularly affected by it due to various reasons. The most common types of cancer are normally found in the following organs:

- Breast: which commonly affects women; in 2020 alone, there were 2.26 million reported cases.
- Lung: this type of cancer is commonly found in elderly people and causes severe breathing issues; untreated cancer will lead to death. In 2020, this cancer affected around 2.26 million individuals, globally.
- Colorectal: this category of cancer normally begins in the digestive system; it is the third-leading type in mankind globally, and in 2020, 1.93 million cases were reported worldwide.
- Prostate: this is one of the common cancers widely found in men; its reported rate in 2020 was around 1.41 million reported cases.
- Skin: skin cancer is an abnormality, widely found in Caucasians; increased exposure of skin to ultraviolet (UV) rays and sunburn are the leading causes for such cancer. Globally, skin cancer affected 1.20 million individuals in 2020.
- Stomach: this is also one of the leading cancers worldwide, affecting 1.09 million individuals in 2020.

The above discussed information discloses the major organs which are frequently affected due to cancer. Appropriate care and handling of these organs will reduce the occurrence rate of the cancer. The 2020 report of the WHO also disclosed the death rates of individuals due to these cancers:

(i) Lung cancer caused a global death toll of 1.80 million.
(ii) Colon/rectum cancer caused a global death toll of 935000.
(iii) Liver cancer caused a global death toll of 830000.
(iv) Stomach cancer caused a global death toll of 769000.
(v) Breast cancer caused a global death toll of 685000.

The above depicted results confirm that cancers of the lung, colon/rectum, liver, digestive system, and breast causes major death in mankind compared to other infectious and acute diseases.

Normally, cancer occurs due to the alteration of healthy cells into infected/tumor cells due to a multiphase progression, which normally advances from a pre-cancerous (benign) lesion to a malignant tumor. A cancer in an individual is the outcome of interactions among a person's hereditary causes along with other causes, such as physical carcinogens (exposure to UV and other ionizing radiation), chemical carcinogens (inhaling of asbestos particles, consumption of tobacco in any form, intake of aflatoxin-contaminant food and arsenic-contaminant water), and biological carcinogens (untreated viruses, bacteria, or parasite infectious). Along with the abovementioned causes, aging is also a prime contributor to most cancers. In elderly people, the cellular repair mechanisms become increasingly weakened and, hence, the growth rate of abnormal cells can easily be initiated; this is a common cause of cancer in the various organs of the human body [6–10].

2.2 Cancer prevention

Cancer in mankind causes a very heavy diagnostic burden in hospitals and, in most of cases, prevention is possible. Nearly 30%–50% of cancers can easily be prevented by avoiding the risk factors [11, 12]. Further, implementation of evidence-based prevention strategies as recommended by the doctor/hospital can reduce the occurrence rates of cancer. Further, early screening and treatment will further reduce the cancer burden in individuals and appropriate treatment will help the patient toward a complete recovery.

The following considerations may help to reduce the risk of cancer:

- Avoiding tobacco of any form (smoke, chewing, etc).
- Maintaining an appropriate body mass index (BMI) and having a healthy body with recommended weight.
- Consuming more fruits and vegetables, and maintaining a healthy diet.
- Practicing regular exercise to maintain good fitness.
- Avoiding the heavy consumption of alcohol.
- Getting recommended vaccinations to avoid infectious diseases.
- Avoiding frequent exposure to UV and other ionizing radiations.

Along with the above recommendations, a scheduled health checkup also will help to detect cancer in its early phases, and if any symptom is identified, it will help the doctor to monitor the patient to reduce the occurrence of cancer.

2.3 Early detection

Early detection of cancer is essential for appropriate treatment planning and implementation. Hence, a number of clinical-level detection procedures have been widely adopted and implemented [53, 54]. The detection of a cancer involves blood collection and testing (the number of white blood cells, WBCs, is one of the measure

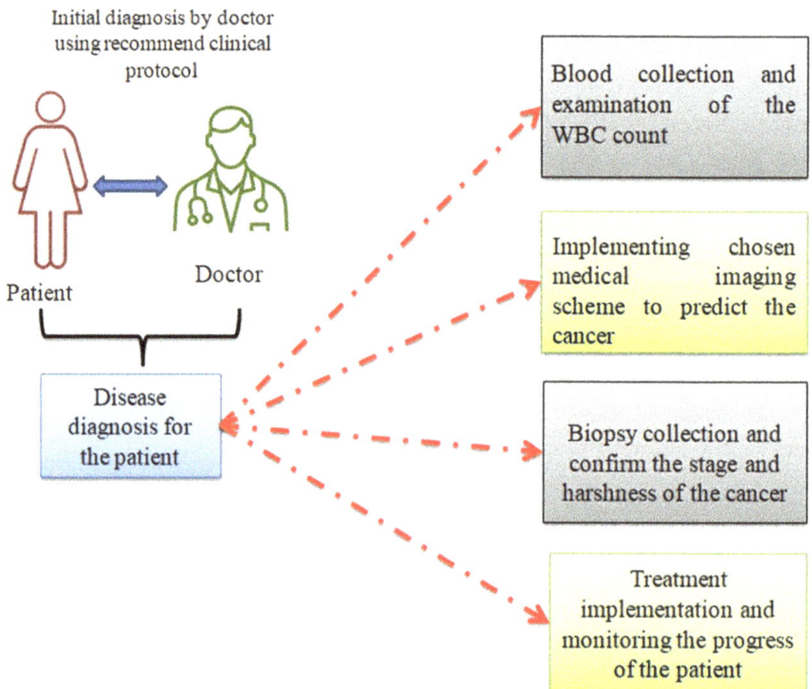

Figure 2.1. Common cancer detection procedure followed in hospital.

which helps to predict cancer in an individual), medical-imaging-supported diagnosis and needle biopsy implementation, and confirmation of the cancer and its stage using a clinical-level detection modality [13, 14].

The different stages of the cancer detection procedure are depicted in figure 2.1.

Medical imaging is one of the commonly adopted noninvasive procedures, which can be implemented using various methods ranging from simple camera-supported methods to radiation-supported imaging schemes [55]. The selection of a recommended imaging technique relies mainly on (i) the body organ to be inspected, (ii) the physical/mental condition of the patient, and (iii) the knowledge of the doctor performing the diagnosis. After collecting the necessary information from the patient, an appropriate procedure needs to be implemented to evaluate the collected information from the patient, the outcome of which will help the doctor to perform further analysis, which will give necessary insight about the disease to be cured. In earlier years, every operation (collection of information, separation of information, analysis and decision-making) was performed manually, hence a considerable delay existed between diagnosis and treatment. In recent years, the availability of computing facilities and appropriate diagnostic software has considerably improved the cancer detection process [56]. The existing literature confirms that computerized (automatic) procedures are now common in hospitals from patient preparation to treatment, and this improvement considerably reduces the diagnostic burden. Further, these procedures help to administer appropriate and timely treatment to patients. This section of

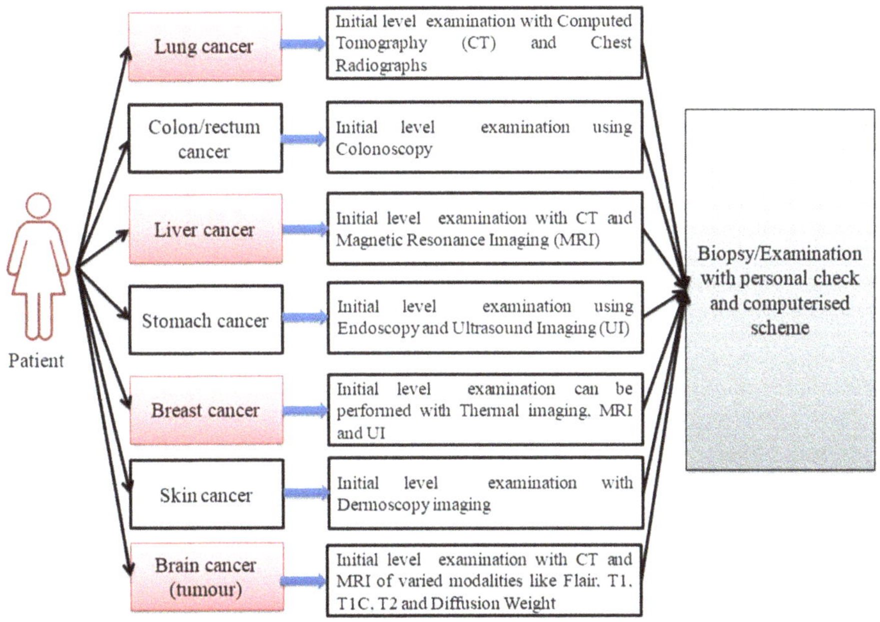

Figure 2.2. Various cancers and their screening methods.

the book aims to present an overview of the computerized disease-screening methods followed in hospitals for a chosen organ abnormality. The diseases considered in this section include (i) cancers in organs, (ii) infectious diseases, and (iii) age-related issues found in the elderly. This section presents the necessary information about the invasive/noninvasive imaging procedures considered to collect disease information from the patients, initial enhancement procedures implemented to convert the collected data into usable form, diagnosis of the disease with a chosen computer algorithm, and decision-making and treatment implementation.

Further, earlier works in medical imaging confirm that infection/disease found in the exterior parts of the body are simple to distinguish and treat when compared to infection/disease in internal organs. Further, disease in every organ needs to be identified using a recommended clinical protocol and imaging scheme. The commonly employed disease detection schemes along with the corresponding organs are depicted in figure 2.2.

This figure confirms that cancer in the organs of the body needs to be detected using an appropriate clinical protocol along with a recommended medical imaging scheme (MIS). In most of cases, patient preparation plays a vital role during the cancer screening. When a patient experiences any cancerous symptoms, a doctor will perform a thorough preliminary examination. After a personal check by the doctor, a chosen MIS is recommended to detect the cancer in the organ. The choice of a particular MIS depends mainly on the organ region to be inspected [57]. In some cases, the consideration of more than one medical imaging technique is also recommended.

When the imaging needs to be done using a radiological procedure, as in computed tomography (CT) and magnetic resonance imaging (MRI), then it is advisable to consider the inclusion of a contrast agent (e.g. gadolinium) to acquire clear imaging. During this operation, the contrast agent is injected into patient's body and, after sufficient spread of the agent, the abnormal region is recorded and evaluated. The injection of the contrast agent may create mild/moderate side effects to the patient; this type of procedure is unavoidable during the examination of the cancers in the lungs, liver, and brain. This contrast agent also plays a vital role during the recording of a magnetic resonance angiogram [15, 16].

After recording the image using the chosen scheme, necessary pre-processing and post-processing methods need to be implemented to evaluate the image to find the afflicted section. Normally, the raw image collected during the clinical evaluation may have some associated artifacts, as well as capturing other sections along with the section under examination. Hence, in order to acquire a better diagnosis, a considerable number of image-processing schemes are employed to convert the raw medical image into a legible image and after verifying the abnormality in the initial imaging scheme. The harshness and the stage of the cancer need to be confirmed using a clinically proven procedure called a biopsy.

During a biopsy, a sample of suspicious tissue/cell region from the cancer-affected organ is extracted and clinical-level assessment is undertaken. This assessment helps to confirm the cancer and its stage. Normally, a biopsy can be considered to implement cell/tissue-level examination using a digital microscope and related clinical tests. After confirming the stage of the cancer, it is then treated using the following recommended procedures: appropriate drugs, chemo/radiotherapy, and surgery [58]. Surgery can be used to completely remove the infected cells from the body to avoid the spread of the cancer cells into the bloodstream and further metastases. Chemo/radiotherapy can be initiated to reduce the growth rate of the cancerous cells. In most cases, all the above said methods are followed under the guidance of an experienced radiologist and doctor. These procedures deliver better results when the cancer is diagnosed in its early phases; the success rate of the above said procedures is lower for patients diagnosed with stage 3 or 4 cancer, which have malignant cancerous cells.

Examination of the medical imaging obtained using a chosen modality can be performed by an experienced doctor or an appropriate computer algorithm. The initial examination with a chosen computer algorithm is widely preferred, and hence a number of segmentation and classification methods have been developed and implemented by researchers [17–20].

2.4 Internal organs and medical imaging

This section of the chapter presents information regarding the chosen body organ and its image-collection procedure. In this work, diseases/cancers relating to the vital organs, such as lungs, colon/rectum, liver, breast, skin and brain are considered for assessment. Along with cancer diagnosis, this section also discusses medical-imaging-supported assessment of the recently discovered pandemic disease COVID-19.

2.4.1 Lung abnormality examination

The lungs are associated with the respiratory system and are critical to the exchange of air between the atmosphere and the bloodstream. Disease/cancer in the lungs will severely disturb this process, and untreated lung abnormalities may lead to other respiratory-related issues, sometimes causing death. The 2020 WHO report confirmed that lung cancer caused the most deaths globally and stated that this rate can be reduced when the lung disease is diagnosed in its early phase.

The detection of lung abnormalities, including lung cancer, is detected with a chosen imaging modality followed by a biopsy, as shown in figure 2.3. The choice of the medical imaging modality depends on the doctor and the harshness of the disease. Lung cancer occurs due to irregular cell growth in the lungs region and, according to the cells affected, it is classified as either small-cell or non-small-cell lung cancer. Clinical-level diagnosis can be performed using radiological imaging procedures such as CT scans and chest radiographs. A CT scan can be performed with either a low or high dose; every approach aims to detect the suspicious (cancerous) section from the image with better accuracy. The recording procedure

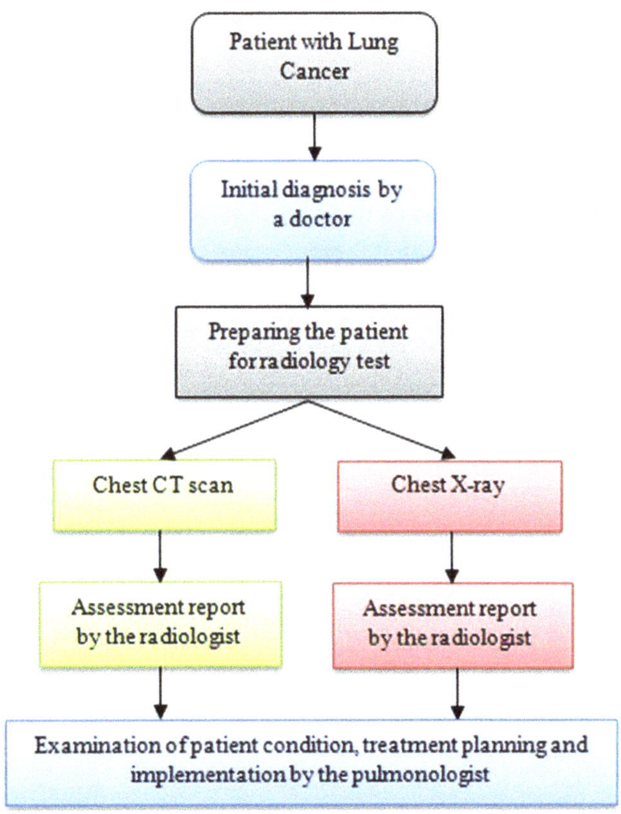

Figure 2.3. Various steps of lung cancer detection methods.

for a CT is depicted in figure 2.4. This methodology helps to generate a reconstructed 3D image, which can be examined in 3D or 2D form.

This approach scans and records an intersection of the chosen body parts with better visibility. CT is normally performed with an x-ray taken from various angles, and then a computer-software-supported procedure helps to reconstruct the image from the information obtained from the varied-angle x-ray. These images help to provide highly visible and highly informative scans compared to traditional x-ray images and, hence, lung cancer examination is normally examined using CT scan images (3D/2D).

Usually, patient preparation for a CT scan is one of the necessary processes, and a similar methodology is considered during both MRI and x-ray scans:

- Arrival for scanning: the patients are requested to arrive early as per the direction by the doctor.
- Diet: taking of food and drinking of water is to be done as per the suggestion by the doctor, and must be completed a minimum 4 hr before the scan.
- Medications: the necessary medication must be avoided as per the instruction of the doctor to avoid any allergic reaction.
- Comfort: during the scan, metal ornaments/jewels must be removed and it is necessary to wear comfortable clothes. Normally, a hospital gown is provided during the CT scan.

During the scan, the contrast agent can be given to the patient after a systematic check by the doctor. The type of contrast agent and its dosage will be decided by the doctor after a discussion with the radiologist. The main purpose of the contrast agent is to help gain a clear view of the suspicious section of the organ under study. This agent can be adminstered as follows:

- Through mouth: if the stomach and its related section need to be scanned, then the contrast agent is applied via the mouth as a liquid; the patient is requested to swallow this liquid as per the guidance of the doctor.

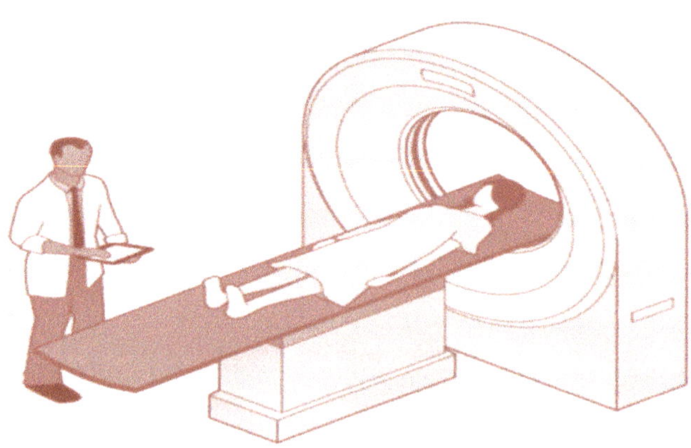

Figure 2.4. Computed-tomography-supported lung section examination.

- Through injection: in most cases, the contrast medium can be injected into the bloodstream through a vein and will spread to the whole body and accumulate close to the section when the abnormality exists.

After preparing the patient for the scan, it is then executed as per the clinical protocol. This scan helps to get a reconstructed 3D image. Examination of the 3D image is quite complex and it needs more computation effort. Further, the doctor cannot necessarily understand the information existing in the 3D image, and hence 3D to 2D conversion is performed and the abnormal section is printed in a specialized medical film. The doctor will then evaluate the medical image printed in a film, and this assessment helps the doctor to plan for treatment to cure the disease. The 3D to 2D conversion process helps to generate axial plane, coronal plane, and sagittal plane images, and one or all of these planes is then verified by the doctor.

The conversion of a 3D lung CT into 2D slices is depicted in figure 2.5. This procedure demonstrates that the extracted 2D slices are quite easy to examine compared to its original 3D structure. The ITK-Snap tool [21, 22] is an open source software widely considered to convert 3D to 2D images. Such an image demonstrates 2D slices of the axial, coronal, and sagittal planes, and every image is associated with a lung mass (tumor) section. When this tumor dimension is small, it is considered to be noncancerous (benign); when the dimension is large, then it can be considered as a malignant (cancerous) tumor. An appropriate assessment with a doctor/computer algorithm will help to categorize the tumor. Based on the identified tumor category, appropriate treatment is then implemented.

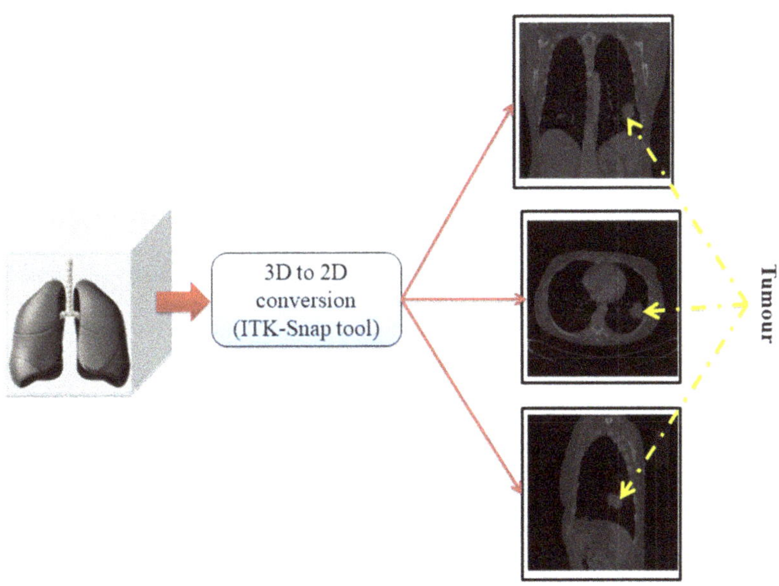

Figure 2.5. ITK-Snap-tool-based conversion of 3D CT into 2D slices.

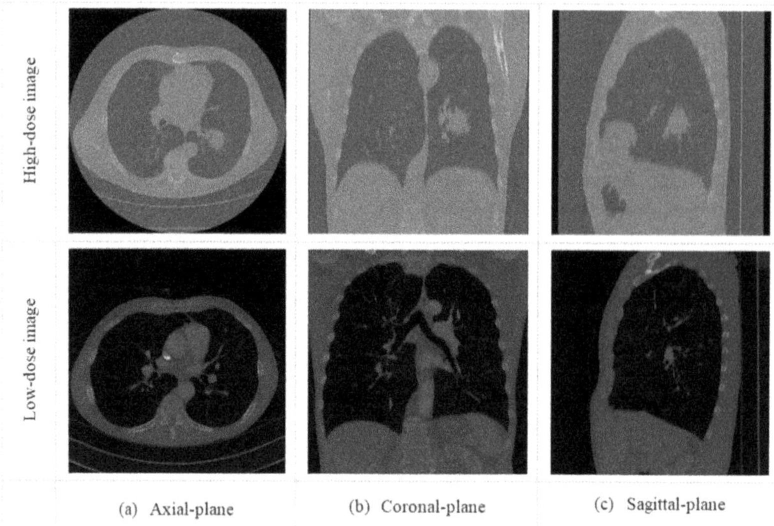

Figure 2.6. Sample test images of lung CT with different 2D planes.

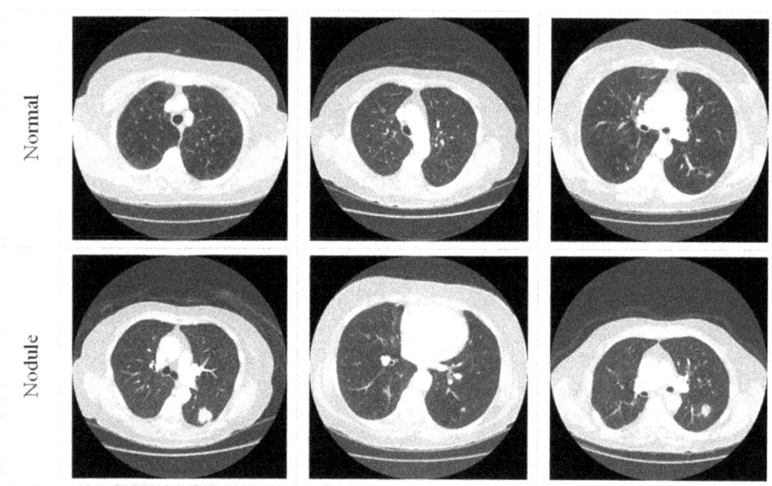

Figure 2.7. Lung CT slices depicting normal/nodule class axial plane pictures.

Figure 2.6 shows high/low-dose CT images collected from The Cancer Imaging Archive (TCIA) database [23]. Normally, for the purposes of experimental demonstration, axial plane images are widely considered compared to the coronal and sagittal planes. Figure 2.7 demonstrates normal/nodule class images of the Lung Image Database Consortium image collection (LIDC-IDRI) [24, 25] data set, which is one of the widely considered image databases for benign/malignant class lung nodule assessment tasks.

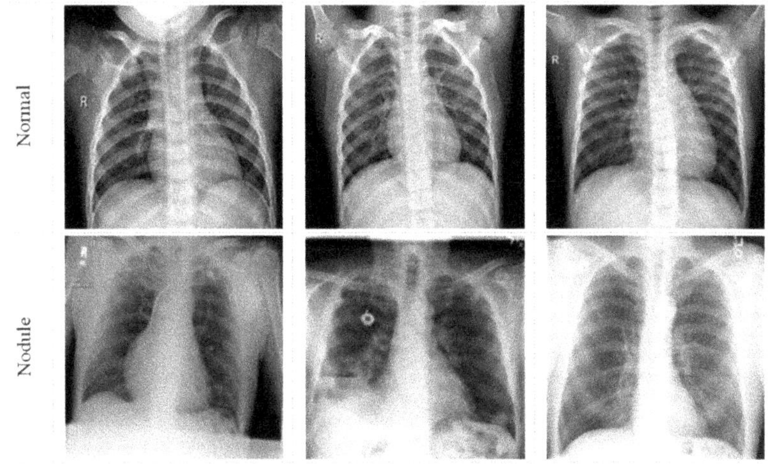

Figure 2.8. Chest x-rays depicting normal/nodule class images.

Advantages: Lung CTs are one of the most extensively considered procedures to examine a variety of internal body organs. A lung CT helps to register imagery with/without a contrast agent, and the reconstructed image supplies a 3D picture of the lung region to be examined. The visibility of the lung cancer is extremely precise in CT compared to other methods.

Disadvantages: The estimation of the 3D CT is complex and therefore a 2D conversion is necessary. It is a complicated radiological practice and should be executed in a controlled environment under the supervision of a knowledgeable radiologist. In this scheme, the injection of a contrast agent is sometimes recommended to gain an improved visibility of any cancerous division and this contrast agent may generate a number of side effects.

Similar to lung CT images, traditional chest x-ray images are also widely considered in hospitals to evaluate lung abnormalities. X-ray images are considered due to their simplicity, low cost, and relatively low radiation. Figure 2.8 shows chest x-ray images of normal/nodule class images collected from the benchmark data set [26].

Advantages: Chest radiographs are one of the most simple and low-cost imaging techniques commonly considered to examine lung abnormalities. They are one of the oldest and most commonly adopted methods in hospitals. The x-ray images printed on x-ray film are easy to examine and, hence, this imaging procedure is still widely employed in hospitals.

Disadvantages: The visibility of abnormalities in x-ray images is much impaired in comparison to CT. Further, the clarity of the image is considerably lower and, hence, in most cases the detection accuracy achieved with x-ray images is comparatively lower than with CT.

2.4.2 Colon/rectum abnormality examination

Abnormalities in the digestive tract severely influence the health of affected individuals. An infection/cancer in the digestive tract (colon/rectum) is a medical

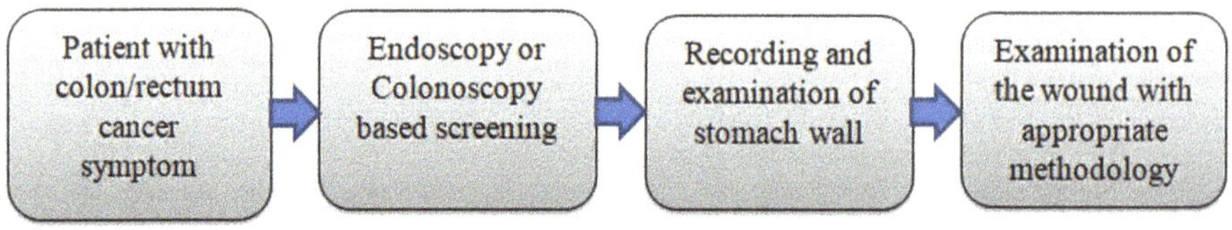

Figure 2.9. Methodology implemented for clinical-level colon/rectum cancer screening.

emergency and appropriate detection and treatment of these ailments is essential. The WHO 2020 report confirmed that cancer of the colon/rectum are considered to be second most severe cancer globally.

The detection of a cancerous region (gastric polyp) in the colon/rectum can be detected with the help of a wired/wireless endoscopic procedure, which provides a clear picture or video footage of the stomach wall. Figure 2.9 demonstrates a clinical-level screening of a gastric polyp and the appropriate detection procedure necessary to evaluate the abnormal section. After verifying the abnormal section, the cancer's stage is then identified using a needle biopsy procedure. During this process, a tissue group of the gastric polyp is extracted and then clinically evaluated to confirm the cancer and its stage. A sample test image of the digestive tract is depicted in figure 2.10 and its histology image (biopsy) is depicted in figure 2.11. After collecting the necessary image from the patient, an appropriate computerized methodology is then implemented to confirm the disease and its harshness, as discussed in earlier research works [27, 28].

Figure 2.10 shows sample test images from the Kvasir database [29], which depict the various classes of colonoscopy images such as normal, polyp, dry polyp, dry resection, and cancerous cases. A wet/dry polyp is less harmful compared to the dry and the bleeding case. During assessment, the recorded images are examined by doctor/computer algorithm. These images can be considered for the initial screening; after confirming any abnormality, a biopsy is then performed and the extracted section is then examined using digital microscopy. Figure 2.11 depicts microscopy images of a biopsy; by evaluating the cell structure and its texture, the abnormality and its harshness are computed using an appropriate computer algorithm. Earlier works performed with these database can be found in [30, 31].

Advantages: A colonoscopy is a simple and effective procedure to record and analyze the digestive system and its abnormalities. Normally, this approach is inserted into the digestive system, which collects an image/video of the colon/rectum region; the recorded image can then be examined by an experienced doctor. After the assessment, a treatment is employed to cure the disease with an appropriate methodology.

Disadvantages: To record these images, the endoscopy/colonoscopy needs to be inserted into the digestive system. This procedure will cause more damage to the cell group infected with the cancer. Further, this imaging procedure will increase bleeding and may cause much pain for the patient who is already infected with the cancer.

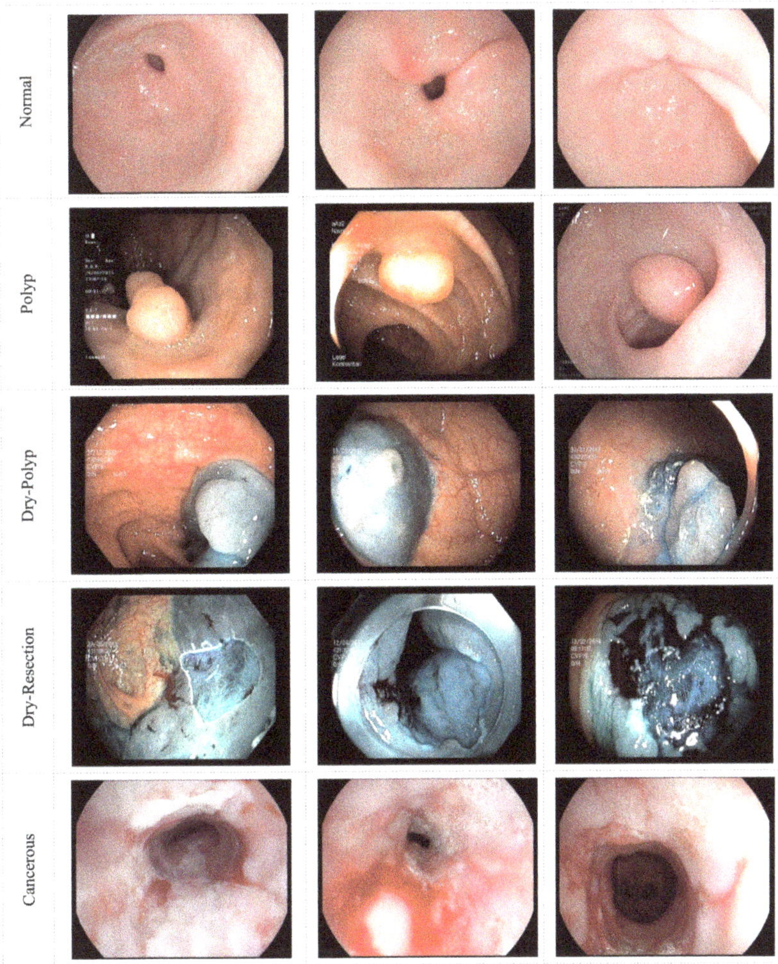

Figure 2.10. Colonoscopy test images of different sample classes.

After analyzing the colon abnormality using the endoscopy pictures, the stage of the cancer needs to be confirmed in order to plan for treatment. The common treatments involved are medication, chemotherapy, and surgery. Confirmation of the cancer's stage is achieved only with biopsy and microscopy analysis. Collected sample images of a colon biopsy are depicted in figure 2.11, and this image needs to be examined using an appropriate procedure to confirm the stage [32, 33].

Advantages: This methodology helps to perform cell-level assessment of the cancer. In this method, the collected tissue/cell is examined using a digital microscope, and this assessment will help to identify any cancerous cells and the stage of growth. Normally, this procedure is employed to gain complete information about the cancer and its stage with better accuracy.

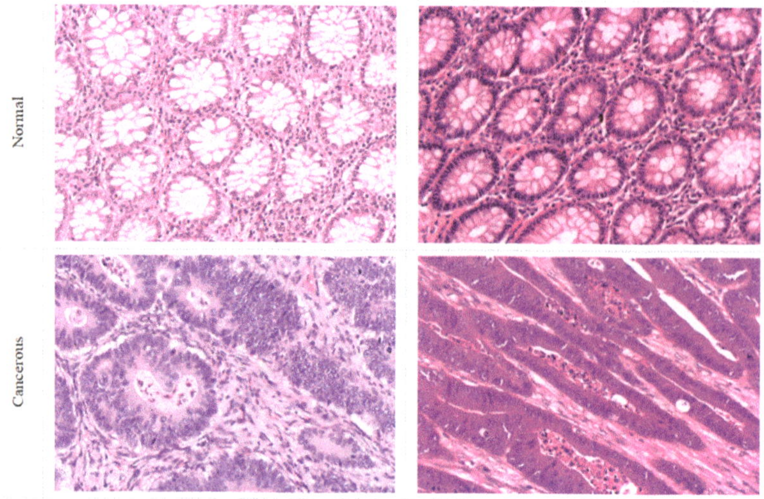

Figure 2.11. Sample biopsy images of colon cancer.

Disadvantages: Collection of the biopsy from the infected section is difficult, and it is a harsh and invasive procedure. This procedure may further increase the wound due to the cancer and, if the level of the cancer is severe, the possibility of the cancer spreading.

2.4.3 Liver abnormality examination

Liver abnormalities are the third largest cause for death globally, as per the WHO report, and such cancers must be detected and treated with an appropriate methodology. In human physiology, the liver is one of the chief solid organs, which is responsible for eliminating contaminants from the body's bloodstream, regulating blood sugar values, regulating clotting of blood, and managing all other functions including the digestion of food. Any abnormality in the liver can severely affect these operations.

Further, obesity and heavy alcohol consumption also cause severe problem in liver, and causes fatty liver disease. Abnormalities in the liver can be clinically assessed with medical imaging procedures such as CT scans and ultrasound imaging. Liver cancer is normally assessed with the help of CT scan slices; clinical-grade CT images collected from the TCIA database can be found in figure 2.12, in which the axial plane is widely adopted to examine the liver sections [34]. The considered data set is made available along with the expert's annotations, known as ground truth (GT). Figure 2.13 shows sample test images of the axial plane along with its GT. The GT is available in grayscale and binary versions. During the evaluation, a chosen computer algorithm is considered to extract and evaluate the liver section, and the outcome is compared with the GT for the assessment [35].

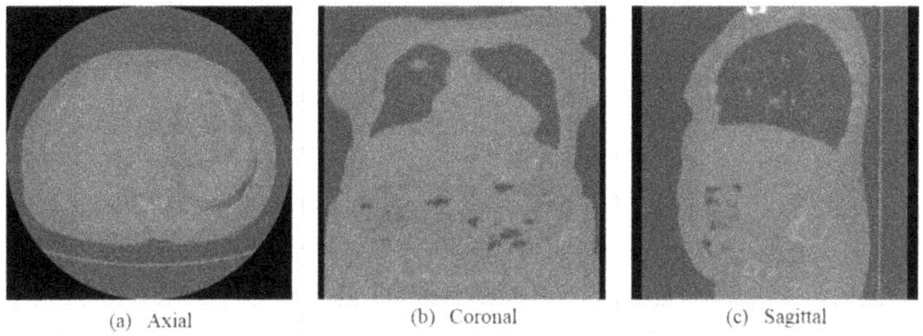

Figure 2.12. Different 2D planes of liver CT imaging obtained with 3D to 2D conversion using ITK-Snap.

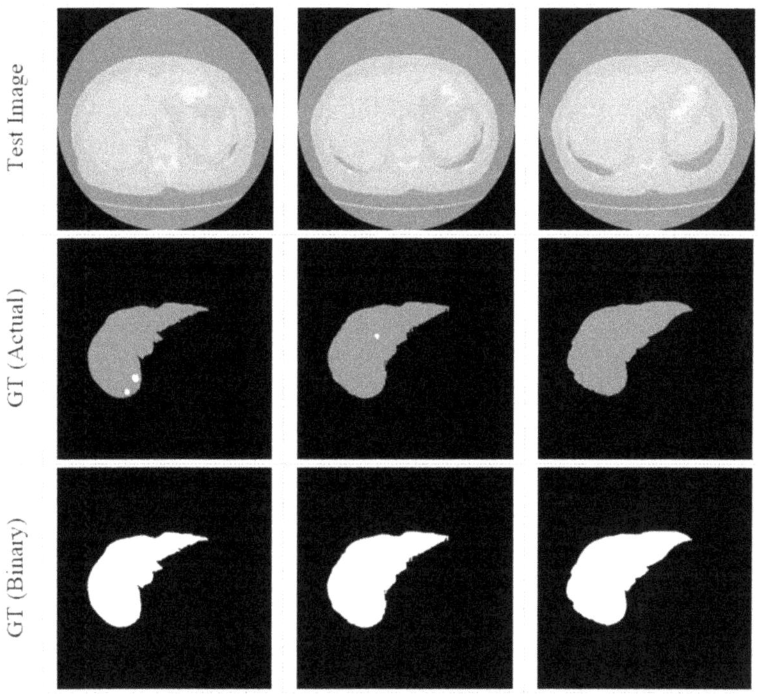

Figure 2.13. Sample liver CT images along with ground truth (GT) pictures.

Advantages: Liver CT scans are one of the most widely adopted techniques to inspect the liver. A liver CT scan helps to record imagery with/without a contrast agent, and the reconstructed image supplies a 3D picture of the liver section to be examined. The visibility of the liver abnormality is exceptionally accurate in CT compared to other images.

Disadvantages: The assessment of the 3D CT is complex and hence a 2D modification is essential. In this method, the addition of a contrast medium is occasionally suggested to help acquire an enhanced visibility of any cancerous section(s), and this contrast medium might produce a number of side effects.

2.4.4 Breast abnormality examination

The WHO statement substantiated that breast cancer in women is one of the harshest diseases afflicting that group, and that early screening will help to detect the disease in its premature phase. The report also confirmed that, in 2020, about 2.3 million women were diagnosed with breast cancer, with 685000 reported deaths globally. Breast cancer usually develops in women due to a variety of causes, including aging. When a woman is affected with a developing breast cancer, then the phase and the harshness of the disease can be analyzed with the help of a clinical biopsy, which helps to inspect the breast tissues and cells. In addition, imaging-supported methods in modalities such as MRI, ultrasound, mammograms, thermal imaging, elastography, and histopathology are also considered to inspect any breast abnormalities with better detection accuracy. Compared to a needle biopsy, imaging methods are noninvasive techniques and help to identify any illness with a visual examination by a doctor or with the help of a chosen computer algorithm. Figure 2.14 depicts the clinical-level procedures considered to diagnose breast cancer and sample images collected from the data set depicted in this subsection.

Breast cancer is one of the illnesses in women which afflicts a huge number of individuals each year. The accessibility of current therapeutic potential can assist

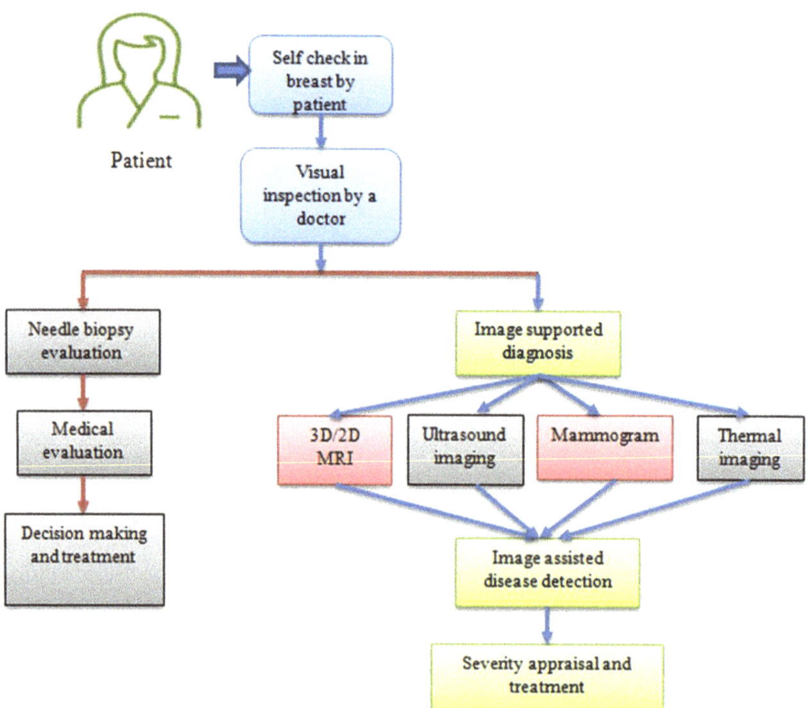

Figure 2.14. Block diagram to demonstrate clinical-level breast cancer assessment.

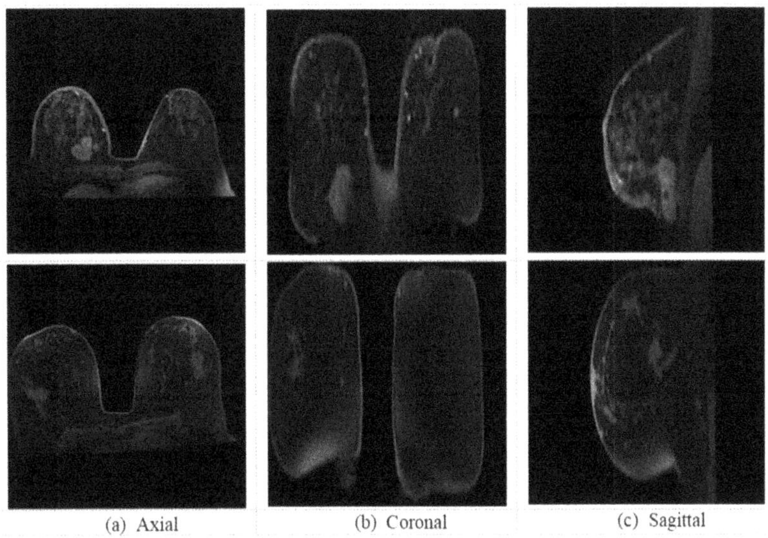

Figure 2.15. Breast cancer recorded with MRI scheme.

women in society to understand uneven cell growth in the breast segment through clinical-level screening procedures. When a breast irregularity is recognized, it is possible to suggest suitable handling to heal the illness. Breast cancer typically begins in breast cells and forms in either the lobules or the ducts in the breast. The preliminary stages of breast cancer can be analyzed with the help of an irregularity called a ductal carcinoma *in situ* (DCIS), which happens due to the presence of irregular cells inside a milk duct of the breast. DCIS can be considered as an initial variety of breast cancer. Medical-stage recognition of the DCIS and breast cancer is frequently executed by means of common imaging schemes.

Primarily breast cancer is due to uneven swelling in the breast tissue, which is called a tumor. Mammograms and MRI are the most common radiological practices considered to observe grown tumors. However, these procedures on rare occasion may fail to notice the breast disease when the cancer is in a premature stage. Hence, thermal imaging, ultrasound imaging, and elastography are extensively considered to record and analyze the breast malignancy.

- Breast MRI

Figure 2.15 depicts trial breast MRI slices of a variety of planes mined from a 3D breast MRI, obtainable from the Reference Image Database to Evaluate Therapy Response (RIDER) of the TCIA data set [36]. The RIDER-TCIA is one of the well-established standard databases widely adopted by researchers to test and examine computerized algorithms in development for breast cancer recognition. The assessment of a 3D MRI is computationally complex, and hence 3D to 2D conversion is employed using ITK-Snap. The assessment of a 2D MRI help to detect a tumor with enhanced accuracy by means of any one or all of the 2D planes, such as the axial, coronal, and sagittal planes.

Advantages: MRI is an extensively considered imaging method to evaluate an assortment of interior organs. Breast MRI supports classification of images with a diverse set of modalities and provides a 3D view of abnormal breast cell division. The visibility of the breast cancer is extremely precise in MRI compared to other imagining practices.

Disadvantages: The appraisal of the 3D MRI is complex and therefore a 2D conversion is necessary. It is a radiological practice and should be performed in controlled surroundings under the supervision of an experienced radiologist. This work sometimes necessitates the injection of a contrast agent to gain an improved visibility of any cancerous division, and this contrast medium can generate some side effects.

- Mammograms

Mammograms are an approved imaging practice, extensively used to authenticate breast division. During this imaging practice, an especially selected x-ray is used to record the breast division with the assistance of a conventional film-based practice or digital practice. Due to the accessibility of current x-ray schemes, digital mammogram recording is extensively accomplished. The recorded mammogram is then appraised by a doctor to distinguish any irregularities.

Figure 2.16 shows sample examination images of the mini-Mammographic Image Analysis Society data set, available at [37]. This is one of the most commonly considered mammogram databases to assess breast irregularities [38]. This imagery consists of a class of mammogram slices of size $1024 \times 1024 \times 1$ pixels; throughout the appraisal, it can be resized to a desired dimension to reduce the computation

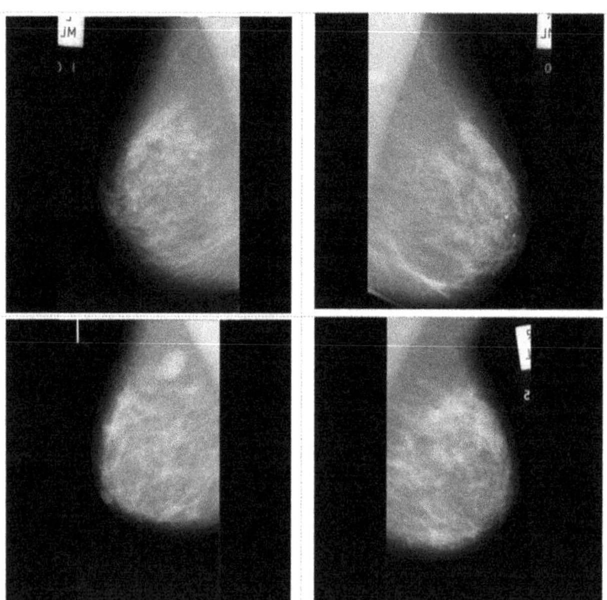

Figure 2.16. Breast irregularity recorded with mammogram.

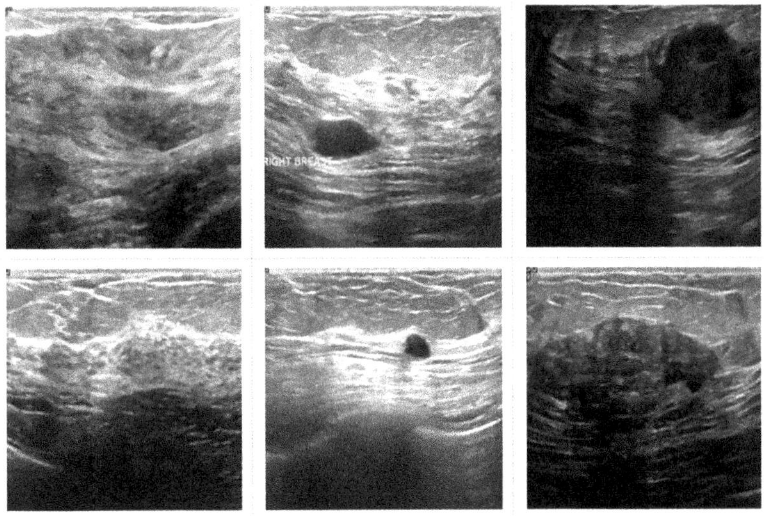

(a) Normal (b) Benign (c) Malignant

Figure 2.17. Breast section recorded using ultrasound imaging.

difficulty of the picture assessment scheme employed to identify the breast irregularity.

Advantages: Mammograms are one of the most straightforward and extensively chosen low-cost practices for breast cancer estimation.

Disadvantages: The process of documenting the mammogram requires radiation, and it might bring a mild irritation. Further, the execution of the mammogram may incur a mild/moderate pain throughout the recording.

- Ultrasound imaging

Over the last two decades, ultrasound imaging has been considered in the medical domain to acquire information on the action of interior organs, tissues, and blood flow. This practice uses high-frequency sound waves (sonography) to record the necessary picture [39, 40]. Compared to other modalities, it is proved to be extremely secure and will not make any tissue-level harm. Recently, this imaging method has been widely adopted to monitor a selection of diseases including breast irregularities.

An ultrasound image of a breast segment is represented in figure 2.17. This presents various classes of breast cancer image section, such as normal, benign, and malignant. These images are then assessed with a selected practice [41]. Figure 2.18 depicts an elastography recording, which is widely adopted in medical imaging along with ultrasound pictures. It helps to detect any abnormal sections using red-green-blue (RGB) scale images by transforming the abnormal section into a chosen color map.

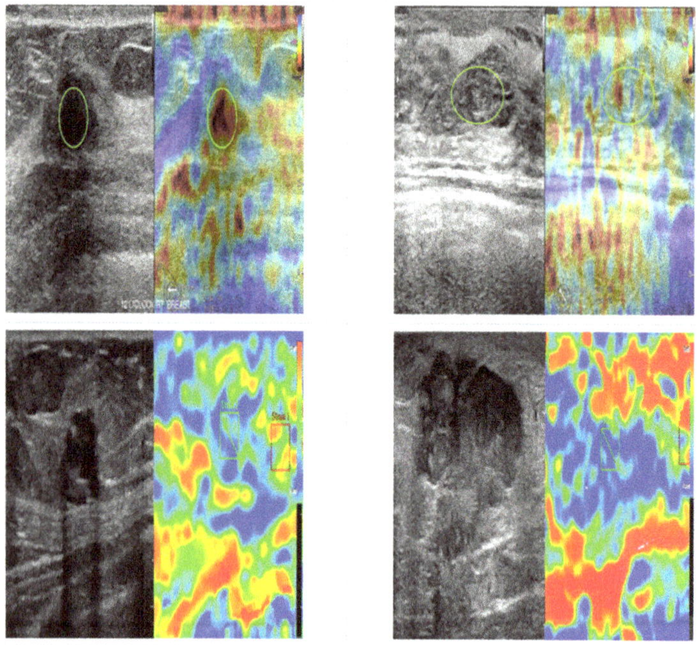

Figure 2.18. Breast section recorded using elastography.

Advantages: Ultrasound presents a simple and efficient technique to assess the activity of and any abnormalities within the organs with noninvasive and simple imaging procedures.

Disadvantages: The quality of the image is very poor compared to MRI and requires a special diagnostic procedure during the abnormality detection.

- Thermal imaging

Thermal imaging is a recent imaging technique in which infrared radiation (IR) is recorded using a chosen technique to construct an image of the section to be examined. Digital infrared thermal imaging (DITI) is a type of thermography widely used to record abnormal breast sections for further evaluation. The level of the IR wave being emitted from the organ under examination mainly depends on its condition; a thermal camera can be used to capture this radiation and convert it into image patterns using a dedicated software unit. The recorded thermal image will have a varied image pattern based on the level of the IR wave, and by simply analyzing its pattern it is possible to detect any abnormality in the image.

Figure 2.19 presents thermal images recorded using a chosen imaging modality, available in [42]. Figures 2.19(a) and (b) depict the grayscale version of the thermal imaging and figures 2.19(c) and (d) depict the RGB scale version. Figures 2.19(e) and (f) depict the grayscale and RGB scale image of a chosen patient with a breast abnormality. These images confirm that the thermal imaging modality is a non-invasive technique that can be considered to record essential images from an affected

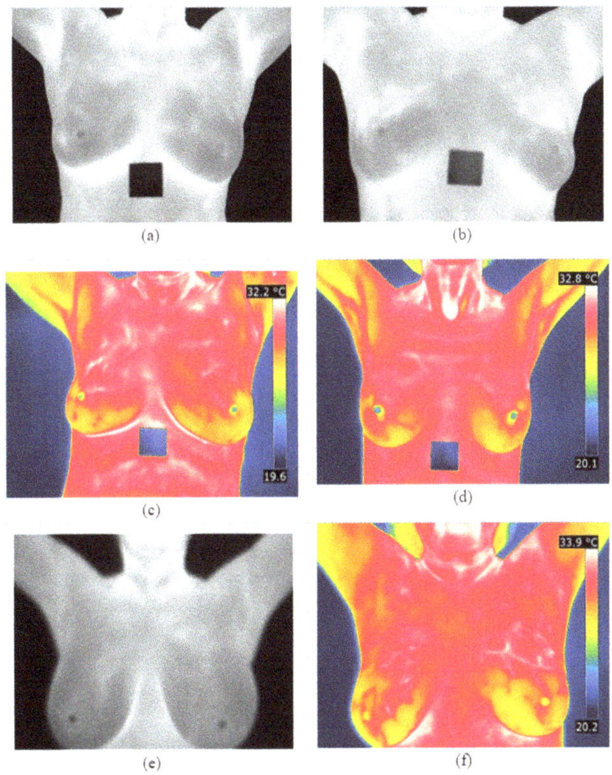

Figure 2.19. Breast abnormalities recorded using thermal imaging technique.

patient in order to diagnose any abnormalities. Earlier works on breast thermogram analysis of DCIS and cancer can be found in [43, 44].

Advantages: Thermal imaging is one of the most recent noncontact imaging systems to be widely adopted in a number of hospitals and scan centers. It is a handy system in which a special digital camera is used to detect and convert the IR radiation into a picture.

Disadvantages: Assessment of the thermal imaging needs special procedures, since it is constructed using thermal patterns.

- Histology

Histology is a branch of study in which the microanatomy of various cells, tissues, and organs are examined using digital microscopic images. This technique inspects the associations among the arrangement and functional differences between healthy and diseased samples collected from patients. Normally, histology-based assessment is used to confirm the condition of a disease using biopsy samples [45, 46].

In order to confirm breast cancer, a needle biopsy is implemented to collect the breast tissue, and then its cell and tissue structure is examined using digital microscopic images. Figure 2.20 depicts histological images of breast cancer

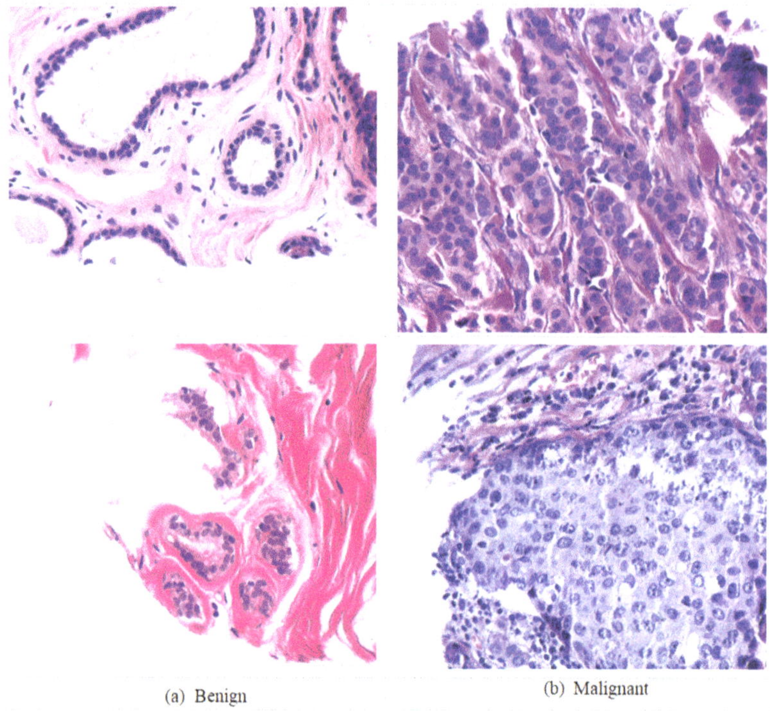

Figure 2.20. Microscopic image of breast tissues with cancer cells.

samples, in which figures 2.20(a) and (b) depict the benign and malignant class, respectively. Histological analysis will normally offer a better insight with regards to the breast cancer to be evaluated and treated.

Advantages: Using histology, tissue-level diagnosis of the disease is possible, which helps to implement accurate treatment to cure the disease.

Disadvantages: This technique requires sample tissues collected using a needle biopsy. The biopsy will create pain and the preparation of the histological slide needs special care. It can only be diagnosed with the help of an experienced doctor.

This subsection has presented various image modalities available to assess breast abnormalities. Every imaging modality has its own merits and demerits, and the choice of a particular imaging procedure depends on the doctor's expertise. If the breast cancer is less visible in the image-based analysis, the doctor will suggest a biopsy-assisted examination to confirm the condition (benign/malignant) of the breast cancer, which helps to implement the essential treatment procedure. The imaging techniques, such as breast thermograms and sonography, are relatively harmless in comparison to mammograms and breast MRI.

2.4.5 Skin cancer examination

Skin cancer initiates in the external layer (epidermis) of skin due to transformations occurring in the DNA of skin cells. Regular and extended exposure to UV radiation

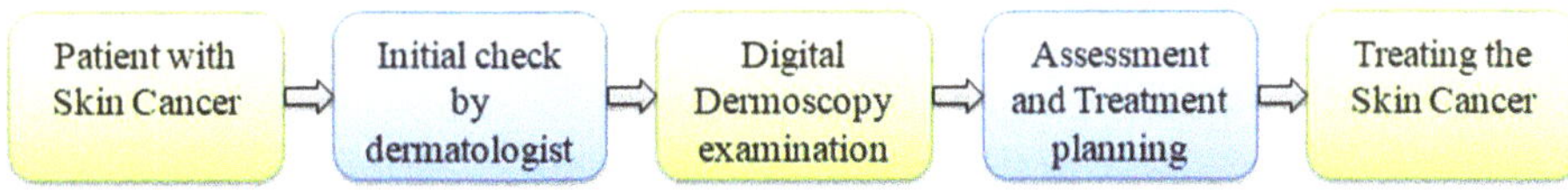

Figure 2.21. Skin cancer detection procedures in clinics.

is a chief reason for the occurrence of skin cancer. Along with the UV radiation, other aspects, such as lack of melanin (fair skin), sunburn, gradually growing moles, pre-cancerous lesions, and heredity also contribute to the occurrence rate of skin cancer in mankind.

Due to its impact, a number of research works are projected in the literature to support clinical-level screening of skin cancer. Common skin cancer screening involves (i) personal checkups, (ii) examination by dermatologists, (iii) clinical-level inspection using digital dermoscopy images (DDI), and (iv) grading of the skin cancer management.

Usually, the medical-stage discovery of the skin cancer is performed by dermatologists using DDI collected from patients. After collecting the necessary images, an ABCD/ABCDE rule is implemented to confirm the skin cancer. This rule states that the evaluation of cerain parameters, such as asymmetry (A), border (B), colour (C), and diameter (D), plays a vital role for the direct detection of the disease. The other parameter, evolving (E), is considered during the long-term follow-up for the suspicious skin section.

Figure 2.21 depicts the various stages involved in the clinical-level assessment of a skin section. This procedure involves (i) patient preparation, (ii) recording the DDI, (iii) evaluating the DDI, and (iv) planning the treatment to control/cure the disease.

Figure 2.22 shows benchmark dermoscopy images from the DermIs database [47]. Figures 2.22(a) and (b) denote nevus and malignant class images. Figure 2.23 presents ISIC2016 images collected from [48]. These images present examples of nevus, benign, and malignant class DDI. After collecting the necessary images from the patient, they are then examined by a dermatologist or a chosen image-processing method.

2.4.6 Brain cancer examination

The brain is one of the vital organs in human physiology and responsible for processing information, storing information, and taking necessary control and decision-making. Abnormalities in the brain severely affect the whole system, and untreated brain abnormalities lead to various physical and mental problems. Figure 2.24 depicts the various phases involved in the clinical-level assessment of a brain abnormality. Examination of the brain's condition can be done with signal-based methods (electroencephalogram, EEG) and image-supported techniques (MRI/CT). Examination with the latter brain imaging techniques is a quite simple and widely employed procedure compared to an EEG.

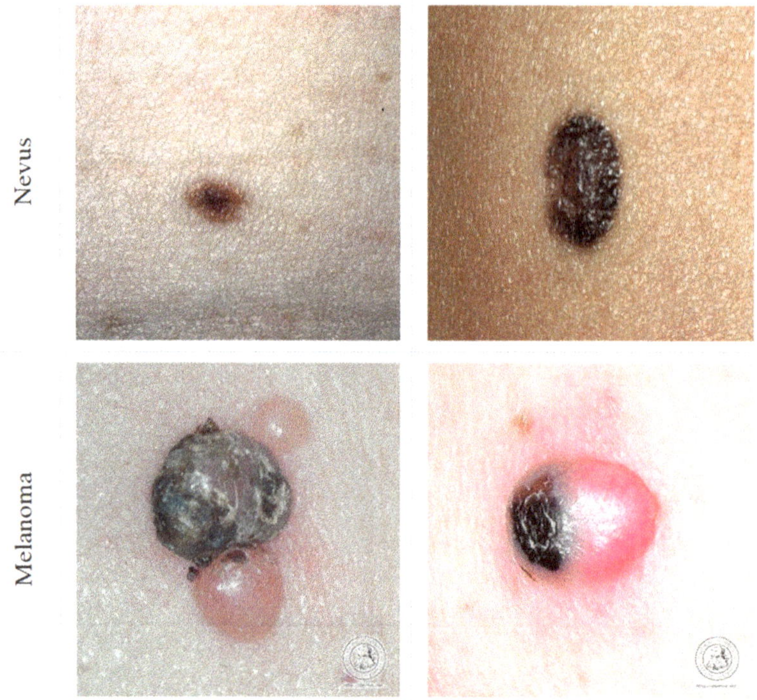

Figure 2.22. Sample test images collected from DermIs database. Reprinted with permission from [47].

Brain cancer (tumor) is one of the most severe conditions and, untreated, will lead to death. Based on its severity, a brain tumor is classified into different stages, and early screening and treatment will help to save the patient from the disease. Glioma (low/high grade) and glioblastoma is one of the most severe brain tumor stages and appropriate detection and treatment is essential.

In the literature, a number of procedures are employed to examine brain MRI using various machine-learning and deep-learning methods. Figure 2.25 depicts the BRaTS2015 data set, and demonstrates a low-grade glioma (LGG) and high-grade glioma (HGG) with various modalities such as Flair, T1c, and T2, along with the GT pictures. The assessment of the LGG/HGG can be performed using an appropriate methodology and, based on the tumor grade, the necessary treatment needs to be implemented to cure the patient [49, 50].

2.4.7 COVID-19 examination

From the literature, it can be recognized that the increase of communicable sickness in humanity is more widespread and increasing. If this increase affects a large proportion of mankind globally, then it is referred to as a pandemic. Even though a substantial amount of communicable sicknesses are extensively found

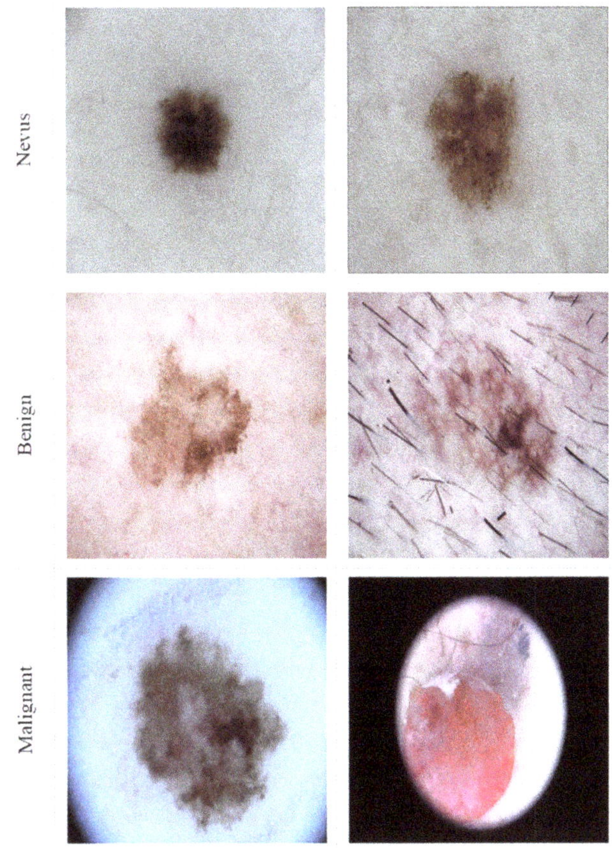

Figure 2.23. Sample test images collected from ISIC2016. Reprinted from [48].

worldwide in endemic levels, the infection and death rate due to the novel coronavirus disease (COVID-19) reached globally significant levels in 2020, and hence it was declared as a pandemic in 2020 by the WHO. The common procedure followed to detect COVID-19 in individuals includes (i) symptom examination, (ii) RT-PCR test, (iii) image-supported disease severity confirmation, and (iv) treatment implementation.

Previous investigations into COVID-19 substantiate that it can cause a harsh pneumonia in humans; any ignored or untreated pneumonia will lead to casualty. Hence, a number of anticipatory and defensive methods are recommended and have been implemented worldwide to manage the occurrence and spread of the illness. Frequently adopted COVID-19 discovery methods include radiological procedures, such as CT and chest radiographs (x-ray). The radiological imagery, recorded by means of a preferred method, is appraised by a knowledgeable radiologist and a

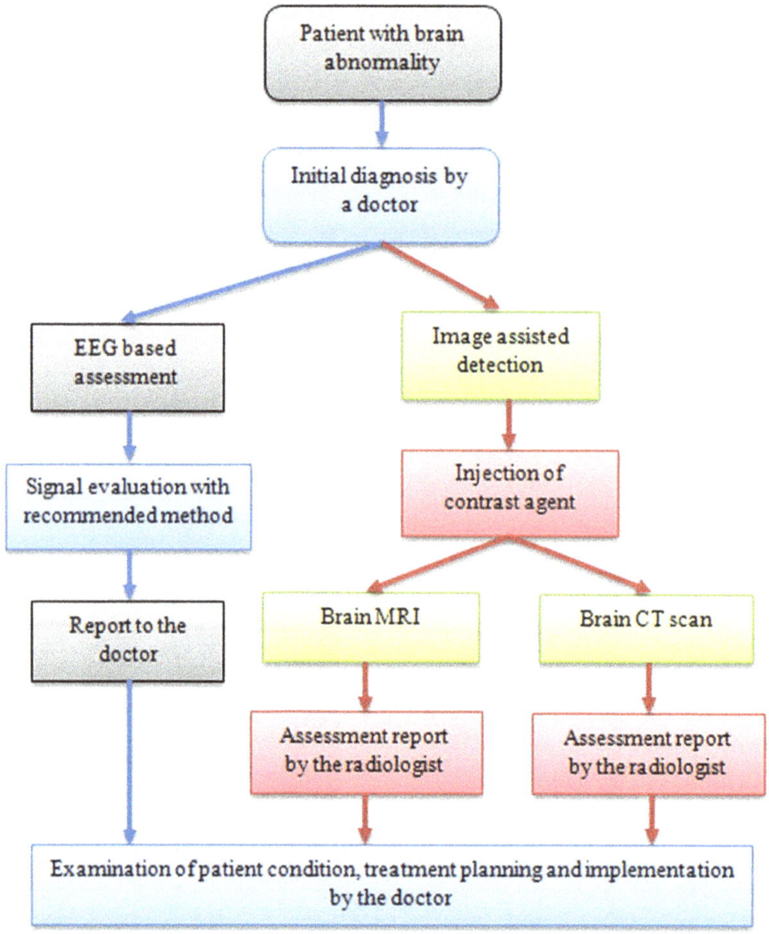

Figure 2.24. Stages in clinical-level detection of a brain abnormality.

doctor by means of a personal checkup as well as using computer-assisted imaging methods. Based on the report and its suggestions, a treatment procedure is planned and implemented to cure the patient.

Figure 2.26 depicts the methodology employed in clinics to detect COVID-19. A CT scan helps to acquire 3D images; figure 2.27 presents 3D to 2D converted images. Figures 2.27(a)–(c) present the axial, coronal, and sagittal planes of from a benchmark data set [51, 52]. Figure 2.28 depicts normal/COVID-19 class images widely considered in research work. Along with CT, x-ray images are also considered to detect COVID-19 infection in humans; figure 2.29 presents sample x-ray images of normal/COVID-19 class images found in the literature.

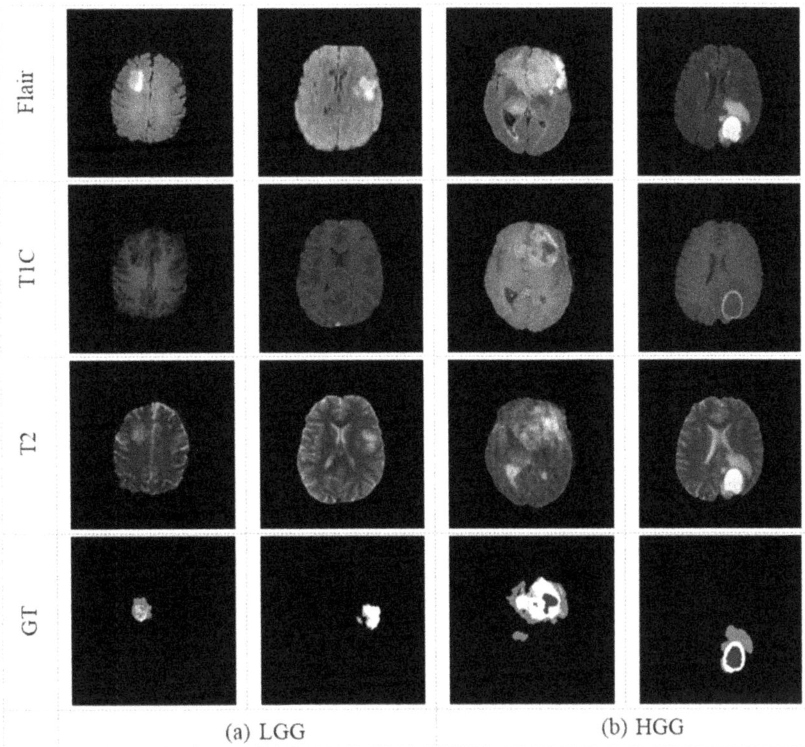

Figure 2.25. Sample test images from the BRaTS database. Reprinted with permisison from [49].

2.5 Summary

This chapter of the book gave a broad summary with sufficient information regarding the occurrence of cancer in humans and its causes. Further, this section also delineated the major organs affected by cancer and its global impact. Along with the organ overview, it also presented the various available biomedical imaging modalities which help to detect cancer in vital organs with appropriate accuracy. For each organ, a selected imaging practice needs to be utilized to record a picture of the organ with improved visibility under controlled medical surroundings. Further, this chapter demonstrates the different processes used to record and inspect the images. From this section, it can be seen that a number of imaging methods are available for disease-screening procedures based on the organs; the choice of a particular method depends on the knowledge of the doctor or medical practitioner. The recorded imagery can be converted into a digital format that can be scrutinized by means of computer algorithms, which help doctors to reduce the diagnostic burden. The joint result of this computerized practice as well as observation by a doctor will enable capable treatment planning and implementation to control and cure the cancer.

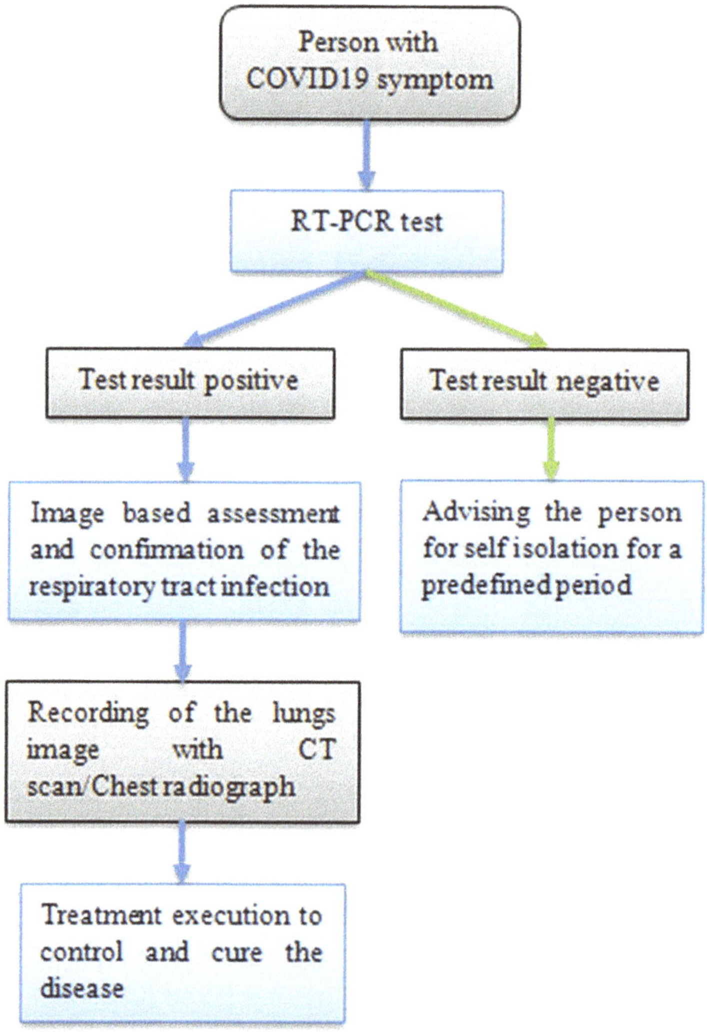

Figure 2.26. Block diagram depicting clinical-level detection of COVID-19.

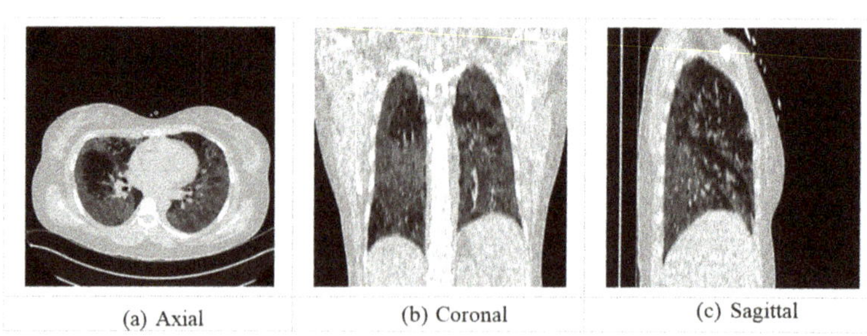

Figure 2.27. Sample CT slices with various 2D planes.

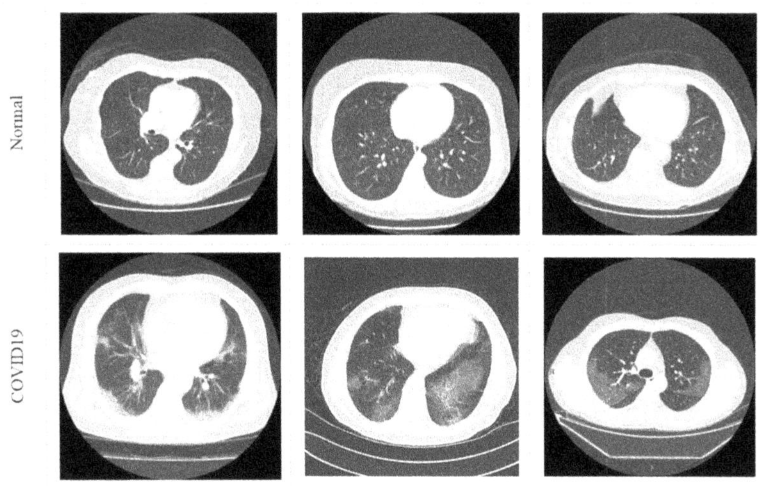

Figure 2.28. Sample CT slices of normal/COVID-19 class.

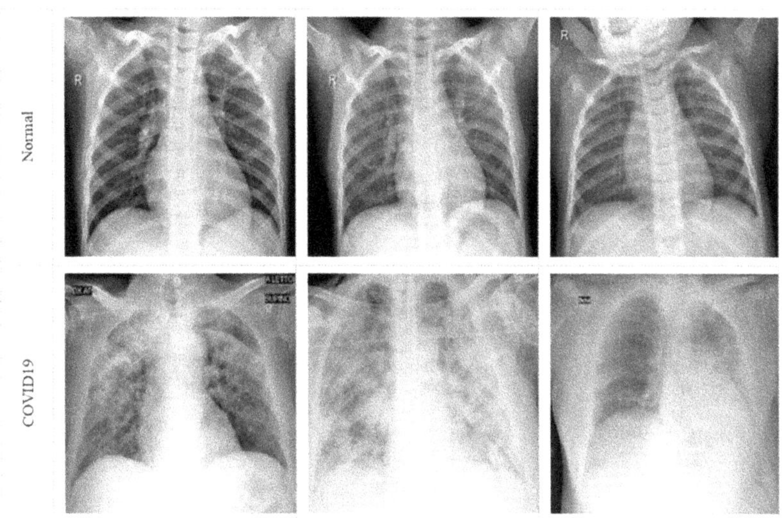

Figure 2.29. Sample x-ray images of normal/COVID-19 class.

References

[1] WHO 2020 Fact sheet: Cancer https://www.who.int/news-room/fact-sheets/detail/cancer

[2] Sarfati D, Koczwara B and Jackson C 2016 The impact of comorbidity on cancer and its treatment *Cancer J. Clinicians* **66** 337–50

[3] Mitchell S A, Beck S, Hood L E, Moore K and Tanner E R 2007 Putting evidence into practice: evidence-based interventions for fatigue during and following cancer and its treatment *Clin. J. Oncol. Nursing* **11** 99–113

[4] Siegel R L, Miller K D, Fuchs H E and Jemal A 2021 Cancer statistics, 2021 *Cancer J. Clinicians* **71** 7–33

[5] Cleeland C S 2021 Pain assessment in cancer *Effect of Cancer on Quality of Life* (Boca Raton, FL: CRC Press) pp 293–305

[6] Kim Y, Je Y and Giovannucci E L 2021 Association between dietary fat intake and mortality from all-causes, cardiovascular disease, and cancer: a systematic review and meta-analysis of prospective cohort studies *Clinical Nutrition* **40** 1060–70

[7] Lees B, Hampton J M, Trentham-Dietz A, Newcomb P and Spencer R 2021 A population-based study of causes of death after endometrial cancer according to major risk factors *Gynecol. Oncol.* **160** 655–9

[8] Ramos A, Sadeghi S and Tabatabaeian H 2021 Battling chemoresistance in cancer: root causes and strategies to uproot them *Int. J. Mol. Sci.* **22** 9451

[9] Sencan S, Tanriover M, Ulasli M, Karakas D and Ozpolat B 2021 UV radiation resistance-associated gene (UVRAG) promotes cell proliferation, migration, invasion by regulating cyclin-dependent kinases (CDK) and integrin-β/Src signaling in breast cancer cells *Mol. Cell. Biochem.* **476** 2075–84

[10] Ilic M and Ilic I 2022 Epidemiology of stomach cancer *World J. Gastroenterology* **28** 1187

[11] Śliżewska K, Markowiak-Kopeć P and Śliżewska W 2020 The role of probiotics in cancer prevention *Cancers* **13** 20

[12] Zare M, Norouzi Roshan Z, Assadpour E and Jafari S M 2021 Improving the cancer prevention/treatment role of carotenoids through various nano-delivery systems *Crit. Rev. Food Sci. Nutr.* **61** 522–34

[13] Hubbell E, Clarke C A, Aravanis A M and Berg C D 2021 Modeled reductions in late-stage cancer with a multi-cancer early detection test *Cancer Epidemiol. Prevent. Biomark.* **30** 460–8

[14] Rocca A, Brunese M C, Santone A, Avella P, Bianco P, Scacchi A and Brunese L 2021 Early diagnosis of liver metastases from colorectal cancer through CT radiomics and formal methods: a pilot study *J. Clinical Medicine* **11** 31

[15] Raja N, Fernandes S L, Dey N, Satapathy S C and Rajinikanth V 2018 Contrast enhanced medical MRI evaluation using Tsallis entropy and region growing segmentation *J. Amb. Intel. Humanized Comput.* https://doi.org/10.1007/S12652-018-0854-8

[16] Rajinikanth V and Dey N 2022 *Magnetic Resonance Imaging: Recording, Reconstruction and Assessment* (Amsterdam: Elsevier)

[17] Khan M A, Muhammad K, Wang S H, Alsubai S, Binbusayyis A, Alqahtani A and Thinnukool O 2022 Gastrointestinal diseases recognition: a framework of deep neural network and improved moth-crow optimization with DCCA fusion *Human-Centric Comput. Inf. Sci.* **12** 25

[18] Rajinikanth V, Aslam S M, Kadry S and Thinnukool O 2022 Semi/fully-automated segmentation of gastric-polyp using aquila-optimization-algorithm enhanced images *Computers Materials and Continua* **70** 4087–105

[19] Bibi A, Khan M A, Javed M Y, Tariq U, Kang B G, Nam Y and Sakr R H 2022 Skin lesion segmentation and classification using conventional and deep learning based framework *CMC-Comp. Mater. Cont.* **71** 2477–95

[20] Cheong K H, Tang K J W, Zhao X, Koh J E W, Faust O, Gururajan R and Acharya U R 2021 An automated skin melanoma detection system with melanoma-index based on entropy features *Biocyber. Biomed. Eng.* **41** 997–1012

[21] itk-SNAP 2018 ITK-SNAP software application www.itksnap.org/pmwiki/pmwiki.php

[22] Yushkevich P A, Piven J, Hazlett H C, Smith R G, Ho S, Gee J C and Gerig G 2006 User-guided 3D active contour segmentation of anatomical structures: significantly improved efficiency and reliability *Neuroimage* **31** 1116–28

[23] Clark K, Vendt B, Smith K, Freymann J, Kirby J, Koppel P and Prior F 2013 The cancer imaging archive (TCIA): maintaining and operating a public information repository *J. Digital Imaging* **26** 1045–57

[24] https://wiki.cancerimagingarchive.net/display/Public/LIDC-IDRI#1966254a2b592e6fba14f94 9f6e23bb1b7804cc

[25] Jacobs C, van Rikxoort E M, Murphy K, Prokop M, Schaefer-Prokop C M and van Ginneken B 2016 Computer-aided detection of pulmonary nodules: a comparative study using the public LIDC/IDRI database *European Radiology* **26** 2139–47

[26] Mooney P 2017 Chest X-Ray Images (Pneumonia) *Data Set* https://kaggle.com/datasets/paultimothymooney/chest-xray-pneumonia

[27] Pogorelov K *et al* 2017 KVASIR: a multi-class image dataset for computer aided gastro-intestinal disease detection *Proc. 8th ACM on Multimedia Systems Conference (Taipei, Taiwan)* pp 164–9

[28] https://endocv2021.grand-challenge.org/

[29] Pogorelov K, Randel K R, Griwodz C, Eskeland S L, de Lange T, Johansen D and Halvorsen P 2017 Kvasir: a multi-class image dataset for computer aided gastrointestinal disease detection *Proc. 8th ACM on Multimedia Systems Conf* **2017** 164–9

[30] Dey N, Shi F and Rajinikanth V 2020 Image examination system to detect gastric polyps from endoscopy images *Information Technology and Intelligent Transportation Systems Frontiers in Artificial Intelligence and Applications* vol 323 (Amsterdam: IOS) pp 107–16

[31] Khan M A, Kadry S, Alhaisoni M, Nam Y, Zhang Y, Rajinikanth V and Sarfraz M S 2020 Computer-aided gastrointestinal diseases analysis from wireless capsule endoscopy: a framework of best features selection *IEEE Access* **8** 132850–9

[32] Sirinukunwattana K, Pluim J P, Chen H, Qi X, Heng P A, Guo Y B and Rajpoot N M 2017 Gland segmentation in colon histology images: the glas challenge contest *Med. Image Anal.* **35** 489–502

[33] https://paperswithcode.com/dataset/glas

[34] Erickson B J, Kirk S, Lee Y, Bathe O, Kearns M, Gerdes C and Lemmerman J 2016 The Cancer Imaging Archive: Radiology data from the cancer genome atlas liver hepatocellular carcinoma [TCGA-LIHC] collection

[35] https://kaggle.com/datasets/andrewmvd/liver-tumor-segmentation/version/1

[36] Meyer C R, Chenevert T L, Galbán C J, Johnson T D, Hamstra D A, Rehemtulla A and Ross B D 2015 The Cancer Imaging Archive: Data from RIDER_breast_MRI

[37] http://peipa.essex.ac.uk/info/mias.html

[38] https://kaggle.com/datasets/kmader/mias-mammography

[39] Al-Dhabyani W, Gomaa M, Khaled H and Fahmy A 2020 Dataset of breast ultrasound images *Data in Brief* **28** 104863

[40] https://scholar.cu.edu.eg/?q=afahmy/pages/dataset

[41] http://onlinemedicalimages.com/index.php/en/

[42] https://visual.ic.uff.br/dmi/

[43] Rajinikanth V, Raja N S M, Satapathy S C, Dey N and Devadhas G G 2017 Thermogram assisted detection and analysis of ductal carcinoma *in situ* (DCIS) *Int. Conf. on Intelligent Computing, Instrumentation and Control Technologies (ICICICT)* pp 1641–6

[44] Rajinikanth V, Kadry S, Taniar D, Damaševičius R and Rauf H T 2021 Breast-cancer detection using thermal images with marine-predators-algorithm selected features *7th Int. Conf. on Bio Signals, Images, and Instrumentation (ICBSII)* pp 1–6
[45] https://kaggle.com/paultimothymooney/breast-histopathology-images
[46] Li X and Plataniotis K N 2015 Color model comparative analysis for breast cancer diagnosis using H and E stained images *Proc. SPIE* **9420** 94200L
[47] https://uwaterloo.ca/vision-image-processing-lab/research-demos/skin-cancer-detection
[48] https://challenge.isic-archive.com/data/
[49] https://med.upenn.edu/sbia/brats2018/data.html
[50] Pedano N, Flanders A E, Scarpace L, Mikkelsen T, Eschbacher J M, Hermes B and Ostrom Q 2016 The Cancer Imaging Archive: Radiology data from the cancer genome atlas low grade glioma [TCGA-LGG] collection
[51] https://ieee-dataport.org/aopen-access/covid-19-low-dose-and-ultra-low-dose-ct-scans
[52] https://ieee-dataport.org/open-access/bimcv-covid-19-large-annotated-dataset-rx-and-ct-images-covid-19-patients
[53] Estrela V V, Monteiro A C B, França R P, Iano Y, Khelassi A and Razmjooy N 2018 Health 4.0: applications, management, technologies and review *Med. Tech. J.* **2** 262–76
[54] Estrela V V, Khelassi A, Monteiro A C B, Iano Y, Razmjooy N, Martins D and Rocha D T 2019 Why software-defined radio (SDR) matters in healthcare? *Med. Tech. J.* **3** 421–29
[55] Abreu L M, Hora H R M D, Rangel J J A, Erthal M, Navid, Estrela V V and Iano Y 2020 A multi-criteria modelling for ranking CO_2 emitting G20 countries from the Kaya identity and their impacts on elderly health *Brazilian Technology Symp.* pp 477–87
[56] Alferaidi A, Yadav K, Alharbi Y, Navid R, Viriyasitavat W, Gulati K and Dhiman G 2022 Distributed deep CNN-LSTM model for intrusion detection method in IoT-based vehicles *Math. Problems Eng.* **2022** 3424819
[57] Ranjbarzadeh R, Dorosti S, Jafarzadeh Ghoushchi S, Safavi S, Razmjooy N, Tataei Sarshar N and Bendechache M 2022 Nerve optic segmentation in CT images using a deep learning model and a texture descriptor *Complex Intel. Syst.* **8** 3543–57
[58] Alferaidi A, Yadav K, Alharbi Y, Navid R, Viriyasitavat W, Gulati K and Dhiman G 2022 Distributed deep CNN-LSTM model for intrusion detection method in IoT-based vehicles *Math. Problems Eng.* **2022** 3424819

IOP Publishing

Frontiers of Artificial Intelligence in Medical Imaging

Navid Razmjooy and Venkatesan Rajinikanth

Chapter 3

Traditional and AI-based data enhancement

Navid Razmjooy and Venkatesan Rajinikanth

Cancer/communicable disease in humankind are successfully detected using a selected bioimaging method. Universal disease screening methods adopted in clinics include (i) personal checkup by a skilled doctor and (ii) assessment of the illness and its severity by a suitable computerized algorithm. In common disease cases, imaging techniques have been comprehensively adopted to record sickness in the internal/external organs of the body with the aid of a chosen imaging scheme. The initial stage of a disease registered using an imaging technique is known as the raw or untreated picture. However, due to various causes, this raw image is associated with artifacts in the disease sections to be inspected. In order to remove these artifacts and improve the picture segment for assessment, it is crucial to apply a preferred pre-processing technique to improve the image condition. This chapter elaborates on the commonly employed image-enhancement practices to pre-process the raw test images adopted in most computerized evaluation procedures, such as segmentation, machine learning, and deep learning. This section presents an analysis of the various image-processing methods, such as enhancements, filtering, feature improvements, and segmentation procedures, and each technique is presented using appropriate results.

3.1 Clinical image improvement practices

When a disease is identified, then the necessary medical images are collected from the patient using a chosen imaging scheme. After collecting pictures by means of a favored scheme, their condition (visibility, dimension, and disease section enhancement) needs to be improved using various methods, such as picture development, pre-processing, post-processing, and assessment. This part of the book demonstrates the picture development methods extensively used in the literature to pre-process medical imagery.

Frequently, an image of a favored measurement and particular modality is considered to supply information in terms of its pixel contribution, which supplies

doi:10.1088/978-0-7503-4012-0ch3

particulars as to the form of its method of visual representation. According to the registration, the image is categorized as being two-dimensional (2D) or multidimensional (3D); the enhancement activities implemented for 2D images are reasonably straightforward compared with 3D processes. Furthermore, this imagery is additionally classified into customary images (recorded with grayscale/red-green-blue, RGB, pixels) and binary pictures [1, 2].

In a variety of fields, imagery recorded by means of a chosen format with a favored pixel configuration can be used to assign and store important information. In some situations, the information found in raw images is hard to distinguish, and therefore a range of pre-processing and post-processing steps are implemented by researchers [3]. Such image-processing schemes can help to increase the state of the unrefined picture with an assortment of methodologies, such as contrast enhancement, edge detection, noise removal, filtering, fusion, thresholding, segmentation, and saliency detection.

Most of the available intensification methods work fine for grayscale images compared to RGB-scale images. In the literature, a range of image-evaluation measures are available to pre-process trial imagery, and these procedures help to transform raw images into images satisfactory for use. The needs of image augmentation and their practical implications are clearly discussed in the forthcoming subsections for both grayscale and RGB images.

3.2 Significance of image enrichment

Usually, the initial images recorded by means of a selected modality are referred to as raw images. Based on requirements, this raw imagery may be treated with preferred image alteration or enrichment practices. Digital imagery recorded with the well-known imaging methodologies may be linked with a variety of problems. Before beginning evaluation, it is necessary to improve the information existing in the picture. In recent years, digital imagery has been modified and stored with digital electronic devices; in this process, in order to guarantee fidelity and quality, a selected image modification practice is needed to change the raw image into a processed image. Enhancement procedures, such as (i) artifact removal, (ii) filtering, (iii) contrast enrichment, (iv) edge detection, (v) thresholding, and (vi) smoothing are some frequent actions which are extensively employed in the literature to translate the raw image into a processed image. Picture improvement is necessary to augment the visibility of any disease information, and mining this information from an enhanced picture is quite easy compared to an unprocessed image [4–6].

3.3 Common image improvement methods

Most modern medical imaging systems are computer-controlled systems, and every imaging procedure is operated and controlled with an appropriate computer algorithm. Thus, the imagery achieved with such imaging procedures is digital in nature and can easily be stored and processed using a range of methods [7–9]. The potential superiority of the picture is validated based on the visibility of the region of interest (ROI) and the dissimilarities linking the background and ROI. As aforementioned, the image recorded with a chosen imaging scheme is called a raw image, which then is examined by means of a selected picture processing practice to convert the raw picture into a working picture. This practice is a necessary though potentially complex task when the ROI is linked with superfluous noise and artifacts [10–12].

Hence, in recent years a range of image-enhancement practices have been developed and adopted by researchers. Some of the frequently employed techniques are discussed in the following.

3.3.1 Artifact elimination

Artifact elimination is necessary to separate the image into a number of subsections based on a selected threshold. Artifact removal methods regularly utilize a threshold filter along with a grouping scheme, in order to cluster and mine the image pixels into a selection of separations based on said preferred threshold level. This technique is extensively employed in medical image assessment applications to eliminate any artifacts existing in 2D slices of computed tomography (CT) and magnetic resonance imaging (MRI) scans. This section considers a 2D CT slice and 2D brain MRI slice to demonstrate the performance of a chosen threshold filter [13–15].

Figure 3.1 demonstrates a threshold-filter-based separation of an artifact and ROI from a test image. During this process, a threshold value is selected based on the pixel level of the image: the area of the threshold over a chosen value is the artifact and the area of the threshold under a chosen value is the ROI. This process is clearly demonstrated using a lung CT image, as depicted in figures 3.2(a)–(c), which gives the scans along with the threshold values. This methodology is applicable only for grayscale images. A similar procedure is demonstrated with a brain MRI and its outcome is depicted in figure 3.3.

Advantages: This approach splits the test image into a ROI and artifact region, and this process reduces the complexity of the test picture to be examined.

Limitations: The main limitation of this technique is the selection of the finest threshold which will separate the test image into its two regions. In many cases, the threshold selection has to be completed manually with a trial and error approach. This approach is a time-consuming process; further, this practice works only on grayscale pictures.

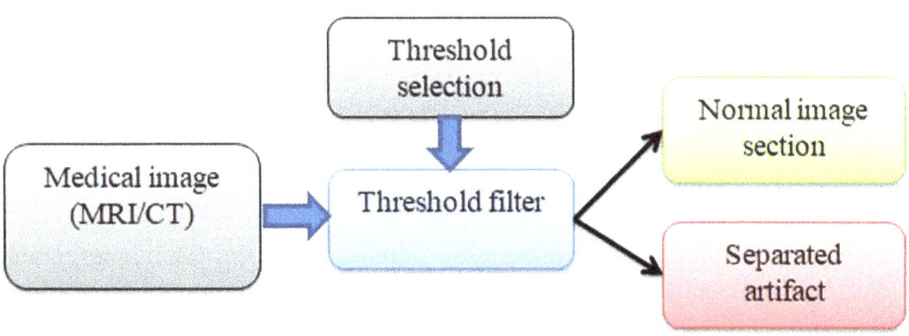

Figure 3.1. Implementation of threshold filter to separate MRI/CT scans into two sections.

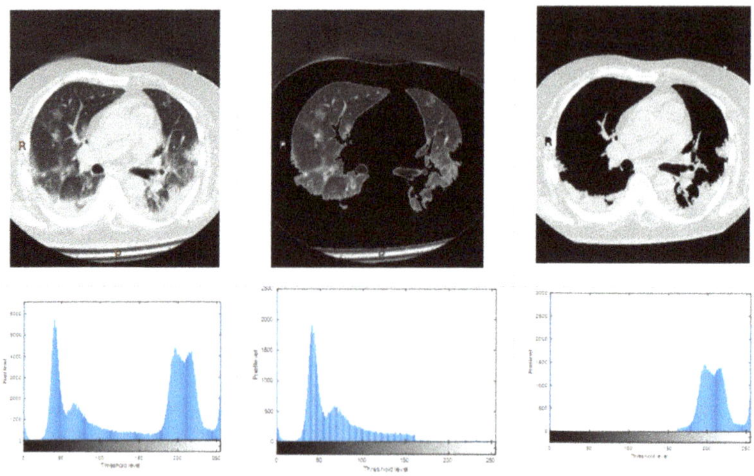

(a) Original image (b) ROI to be examined (c) Artifact

Figure 3.2. Threshold filter implementation for a lung CT image.

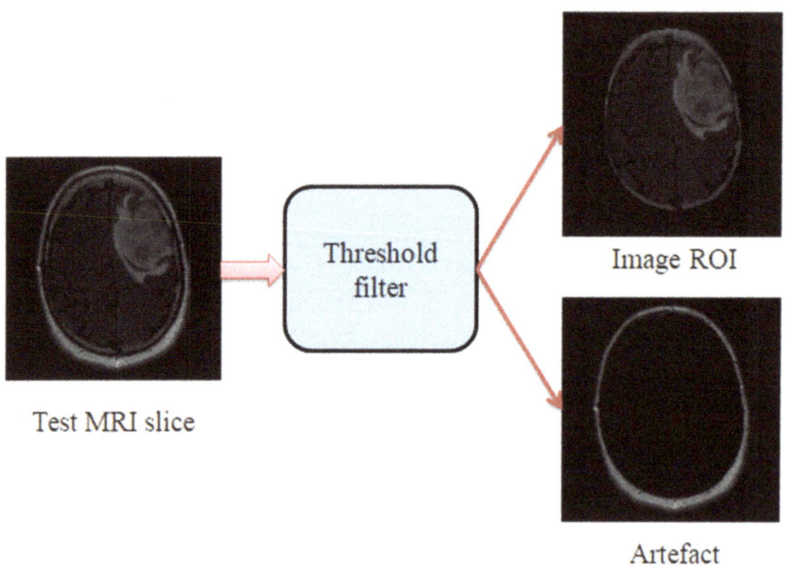

Figure 3.3. Threshold filter implementation and segmentation of brain MRI.

3.3.2 Noise elimination

In the traditional digital signal processing domain, a digital filter is implemented with a carefully selected method and a chosen filter order is used to permit/stop signal values based on their frequency. Similar to this process, superfluous pixels present in a digital image can be removed/blocked with a favored pixel filter.

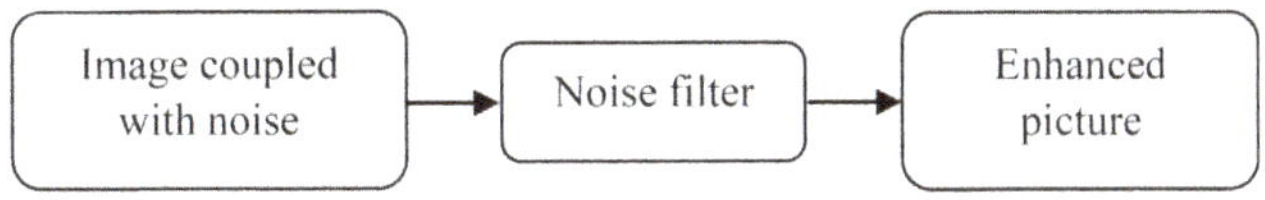

Figure 3.4. Digital filter to eliminate noise.

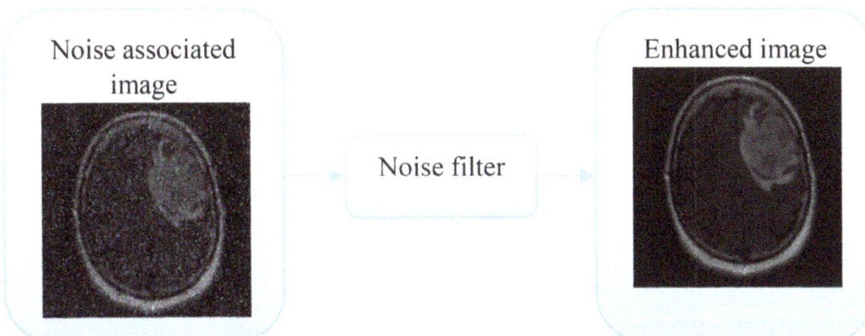

Figure 3.5. Removal of salt-and-pepper noise from brain MRI slice.

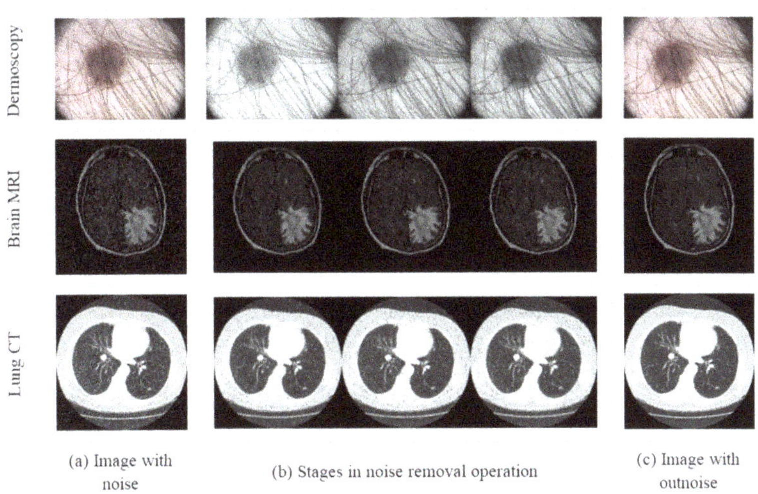

Figure 3.6. Removal of noise in grayscale/RGB pictures.

Figure 3.4 shows the scheme of a conventional filter which eliminates the noise in a grayscale/RGB digital picture. Figure 3.5 shows the results achieved for a 2D brain MRI. The noise filter is implemented to remove the salt-and-pepper noise existing in the test picture [16]. After eliminating the noise, a fine image with finest pixel resolution is obtained, which can then be considered for supplementary enhancement by means of a selected image-enhancement method to extract and evaluate any irregularites in the image. Other results achieved for selected grayscale/RGB images are depicted in figure 3.6. It can be seen that it works only for grayscale images.

Hence, RGB to grayscale conversion is necessary to process these images by means of a noise-elimination filter [17–20].

Advantages: An image filter eliminates the excess unwanted noise pixels in the selected digital image, and this procedure can be adopted as a necessary pre-processing scheme for medical images of different modalities.

Limitations: Execution of a preferred and effective image filter to eradicate noise is more multifaceted. Further, the presently developed image-processing proposals will work fine even if the images are associated with noise.

3.3.3 Contrast enhancement

Frequently, the information available in grayscale pictures is relatively poor compared to RGB pictures. In a grayscale image, enhancing the ROI with reference to the background is a challenging task, and therefore a number of image-enhancement methods have been developed and used by laboratory professionals [21]. Contrast improvement is one such of these extensively used methods in medical imaging evaluation tasks. Some of the procedures utilized in the contrast enhancement of grayscale images are histogram equalization, color-map tuning, and contrast limited adaptive histogram equalization [22–24].

Figures 3.7 and 3.8 present the various image-enhancement methods and their respective outcomes. From these images, it can be noted that the outcomes of these methods can assist in improving the visibility of the ROI. The investigational scheme with the presented result confirms that these procedures will help in improving medical images of various modalities. Figure 3.9 depicts the various imaging modalities treated with contrast enhancement.

Image-enhancement schemes are necessary during personal examination, traditional computer assessment, and machine-learning-based examination. These methods will not provide any improvement when a deep-learning-supported examination is implemented. The main task is to improve the visibility of the image by adjusting the pixel distribution.

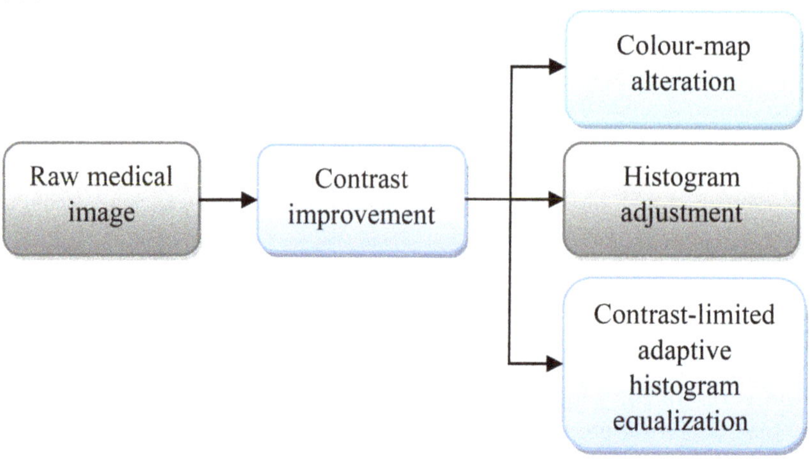

Figure 3.7. Commonly implemented contrast improvement schemes.

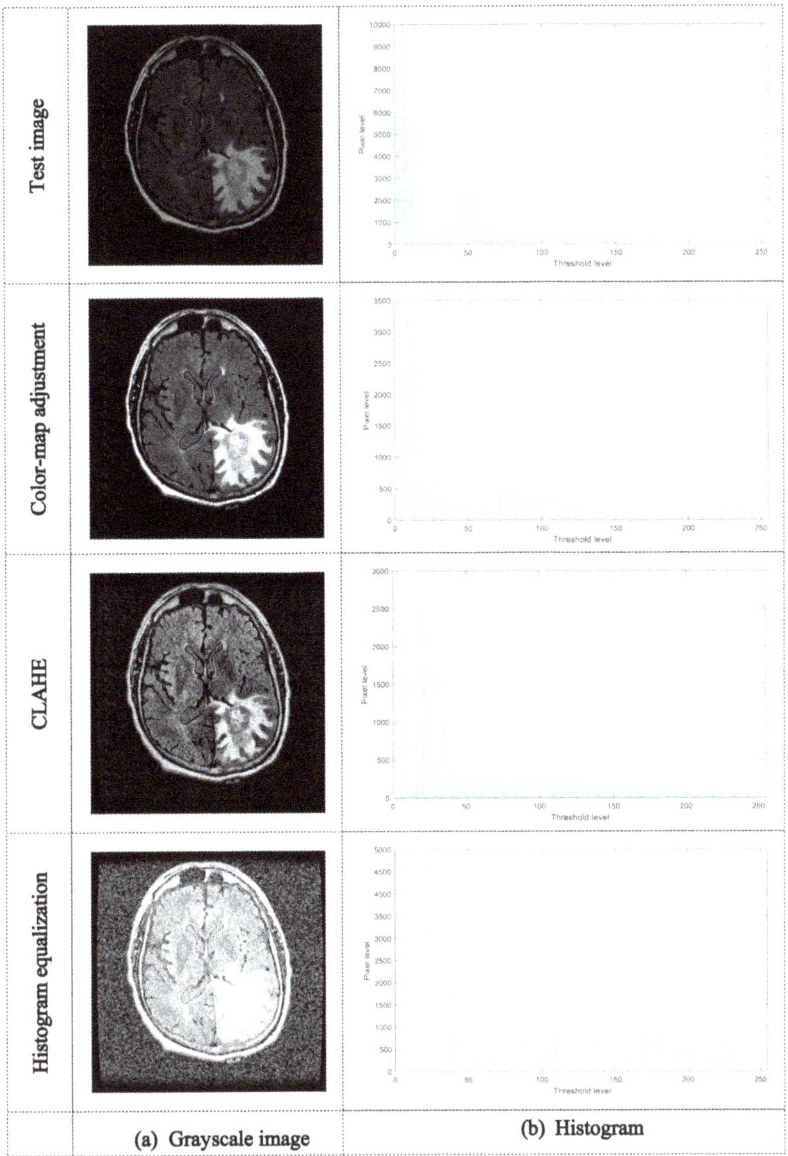

Figure 3.8. Enhanced grayscale images and their corresponding histograms.

Image improvement schemes employed on a raw trial picture can facilitate improvements to the ROI region by altering its pixel sharing (regulating the histogram), based in executed practice. A variety of modified forms of a grayscale histogram of a brain MRI are presented in figure 3.8. Figure 3.8(a) shows the resulting images and figure 3.8(b) presents their histograms. A similar procedure executed on other imaging modalities, such as MRI, ultrasound, CT and a

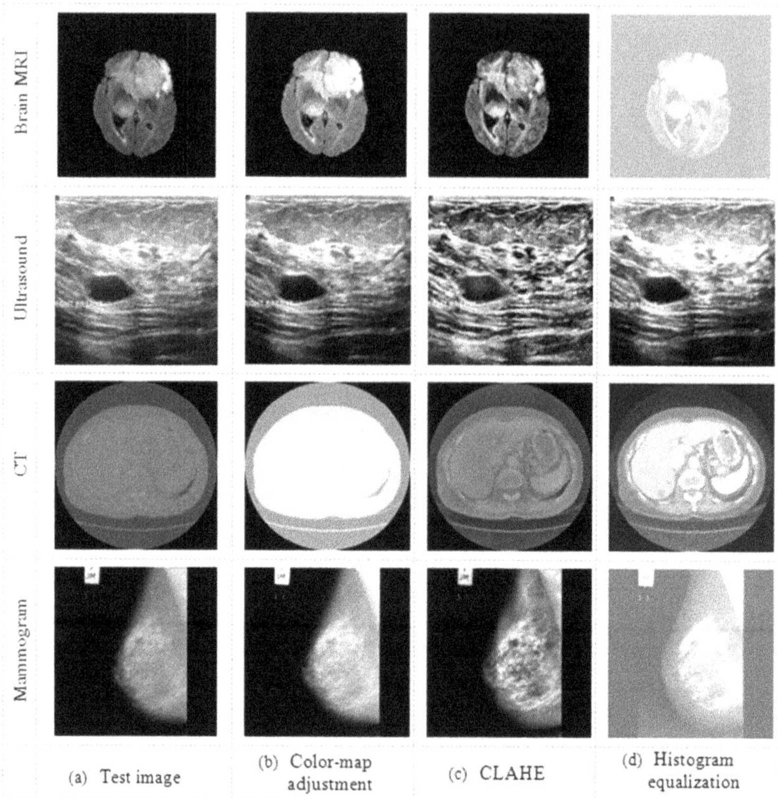

Figure 3.9. Contrast enhancements of images from various modalities: brain MRI, ultrasound, CT, and mammogram.

mammogram, is presented in figure 3.9. Figure 3.9(a) presents the chosen image for the assessment and figures 3.9(b)–(d) depict the enhanced outcomes [25, 26].

Advantages: During the computerized/personal assessment of medical images, the ROI section needs to be identified with greatest accuracy. Contrast improvement is a frequent practice and requires very little computational effort in its execution. This procedure helps to improve the pixel values of the chosen image so that the ROI section is improved considerably.

Limitations: This practice is considered during the beginning stages of image improvement; as such, most initial images will have some associated noise, which will occlude the expected outcome with contrast enhancement alone. Hence, it may not be suitable to treat noisy images, and in most cases has to be used along with a noise filter.

3.3.4 Image edge detection

Edge recognition is considered to find the outline of the ROI found in the test image. In the literature a number of edge-recognition techniques are discussed. The

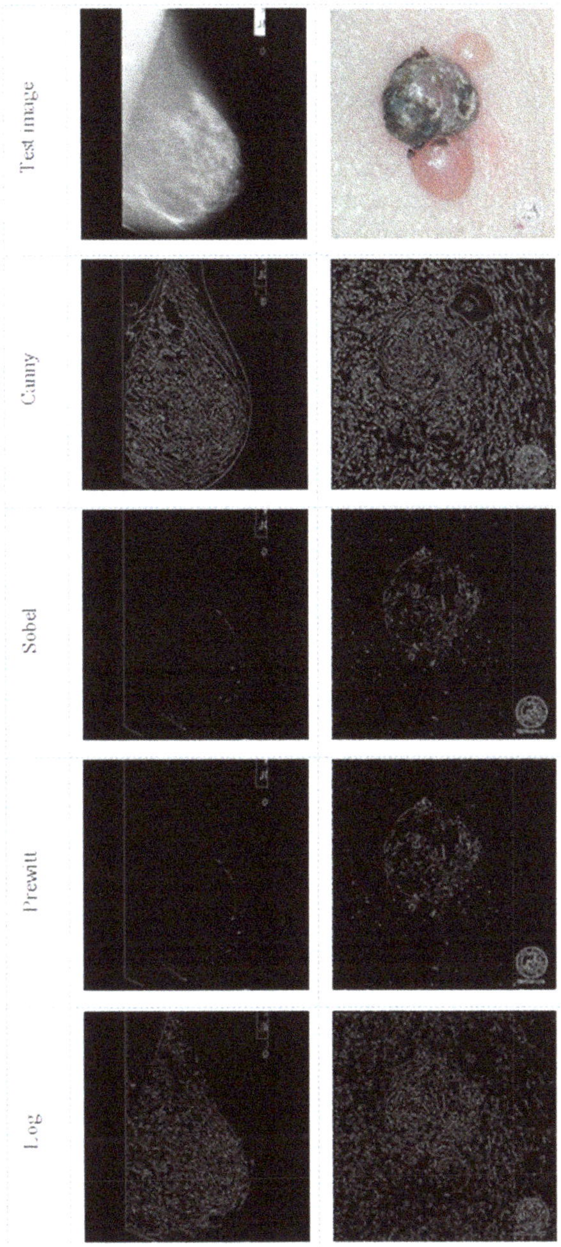

Figure 3.10. Edge detection implemented on a grayscale image.

methods, such as a Canny detector, Sobel and Prewitt operator, and Laplacian of Gaussian (LoG), are widely adopted to find grayscale and RGB edges; some sample results achieved for selected images are depicted in figure 3.10. This procedure helps to get valuable structural information from an image by decreasing other sections of the image which do not contain sufficient information [27–30]. Common conditions for edge detection include the following:

(a) Identification of border with minute error rate by precisely finding numerous edges found in the chosen test picture.
(b) The border tip of the image which is expected by the operator should precisely denote the information about the ROI.
(c) The perimeter of the image should simply be noticed once, and the existing image noise should not generate fake boundaries.

To attain the above said constraints, a Canny detector implements a calculus of variation to optimize the process. A Sobel operator is another one of the frequent methods used for edge detection adopted in the image-processing literature. Figure 3.10 confirms that the investigational outcome of a Canny detector is superior compared to other methods.

The edge-detection operation can be executed on both grayscale and RGB images, as depicted in figure 3.10, which further confirms that the results with grayscale images are better compared to RGB images.

Advantage: Execution of edge detection is essential to recognize the border and texture of the image under study; it works well on grayscale images.

Limitation: The edge-discovery procedure requires complex operations to observe the border of a given picture, and this practice may not offer an appropriate result when an RGB picture is examined.

3.3.5 Restoration

Uncertainty in medical imaging can be due to a variety of causes, and this difficulty will degrade the information existing in test pictures. Image degradation is a widespread issue and this defect can be fixed by implementing an imaging enhancement approach. During the vital picture recording procedure, reregistration of an image is not advisable; further, the picture recording process involves a considerable number of steps and preventive measures [31]. Hence, it is essential to carry out an image-restoration practice, which helps to correct/remove any uncertainty latent in initial medical images. This practice will calculate the key pixels in an image and fix any distortions in order to get an enhanced image [32–34].

Figure 3.11 depicts various images and their restored versions. Figure 3.11(a) depicts distorted images and figures 3.11(b)–(d) depict the initially corrected, enhanced, and restored images, respectively. This procedure is widely employed during the initial image registration and correction stages, and is a primary aspect of machine-learning-supported image examination.

3.3.6 Image smoothing

When medical-imaging-supported automatic disease detection is employed, the texture information in the picture plays a vital role. The obtained texture features will help to detect/classify the images with better accuracy. Before extracting the

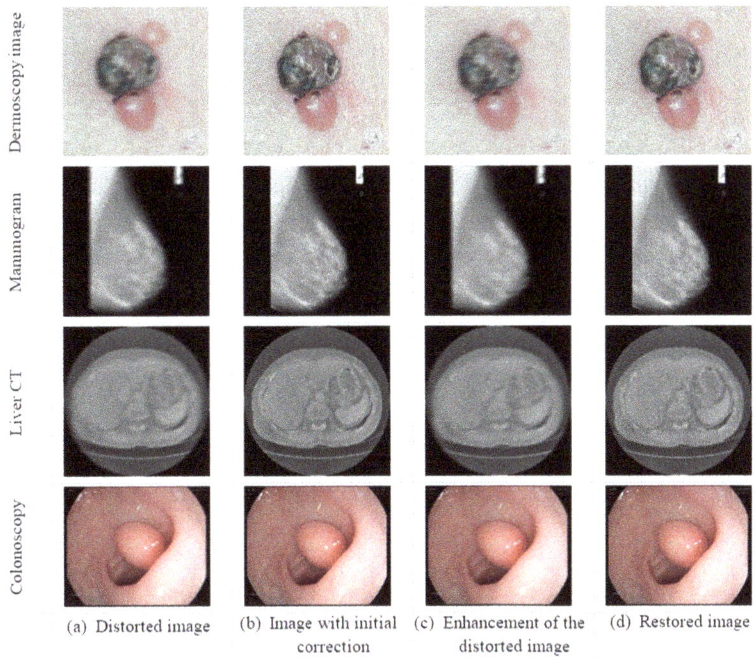

Figure 3.11. Results achieved using image-restoration technique.

exterior information from an image, it is essential to modify the raw picture with a preferred image normalization method; image surface smoothing, based on a selected filter, is broadly employed to enhance its features. Previous research has confirmed that a Gaussian filter (GF)-based texture enhancement works well to attain better perimeter features of grayscale images. Further, an earlier work confirms that a GF with a selected scale (φ) will offer better improvement of a texture pattern in the vertical and horizontal directions [35–37].

A Gaussian operator for the case of a 2D picture is presented in equation (3.1):

$$U(x, y) = \frac{1}{2\pi\varphi^2} e^{-\left(\frac{x^2+y^2}{2\varphi^2}\right)}, \tag{3.1}$$

where φ is the standard deviation and U(x, y) are the Cartesian coordinates of the picture. By changing φ, we can produce images with diverse edge enrichments.

The Laplacian in a GF is a function which helps to notice edges by detecting the zero crossings of their second derivatives, as in equation (3.2):

$$\nabla^2 U(x, y) = \frac{d^2}{dx^2} U(x, y) + \frac{d^2}{dy^2} U(x, y) = \frac{x^2 + y^2 - 2\varphi^2}{2\pi\varphi^6} e^{-\left(\frac{x^2+y^2}{2\varphi^2}\right)}. \tag{3.2}$$

Figures 3.12 and 3.13 show some selected images and their related experimental results. Figure 3.12(a) presents a horizontally smoothed lung CT slice for a chosen

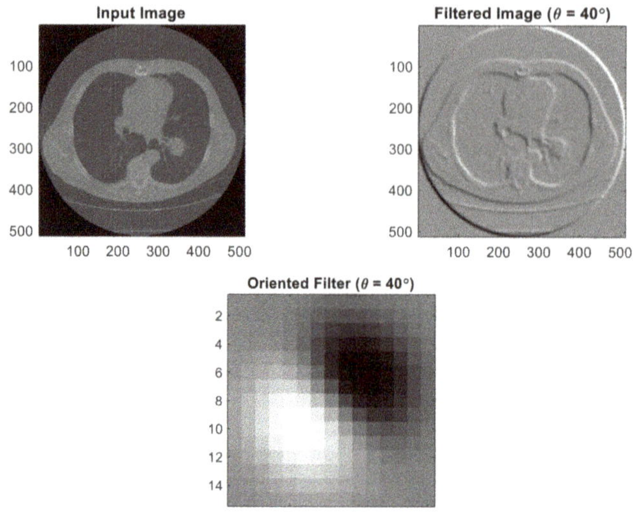

(a) Gray color map

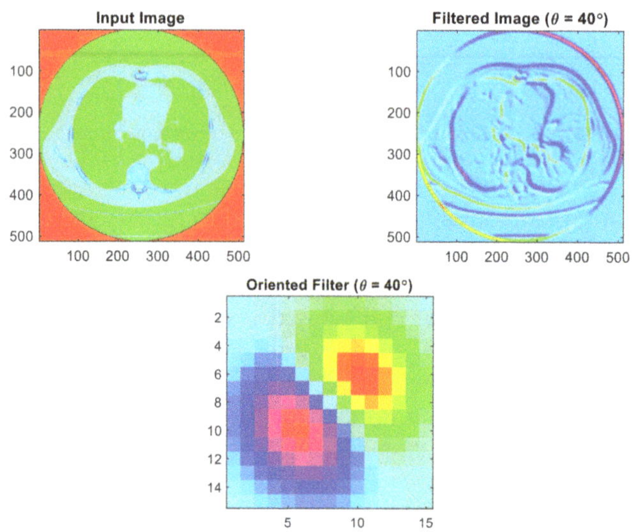

(a) HSV color map

Figure 3.12. Gaussian-filter-enhanced lung CT slice for $\varphi = 45^o$.

value of $\varphi = 45^o$, and figure 3.12(b) depicts the hue, saturation, value (HSV) color map of the enhanced image. As discussed earlier, various values of φ will help us to achieve a better result. After the probable enhancement, the surface and edge features from these images are extracted and based on these features; subsequently, the automatic disease detection schemes are trained and validated. A similar procedure is then implemented on a dermoscopy image, and the attained results are presented in figures 3.13(a) and (b), in which figure 3.13(a) presents a grayscale

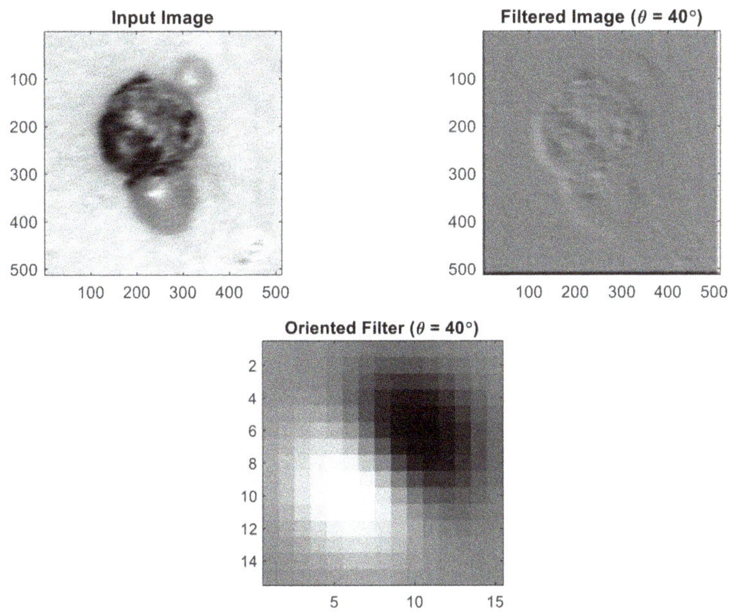

(a) Gray color map

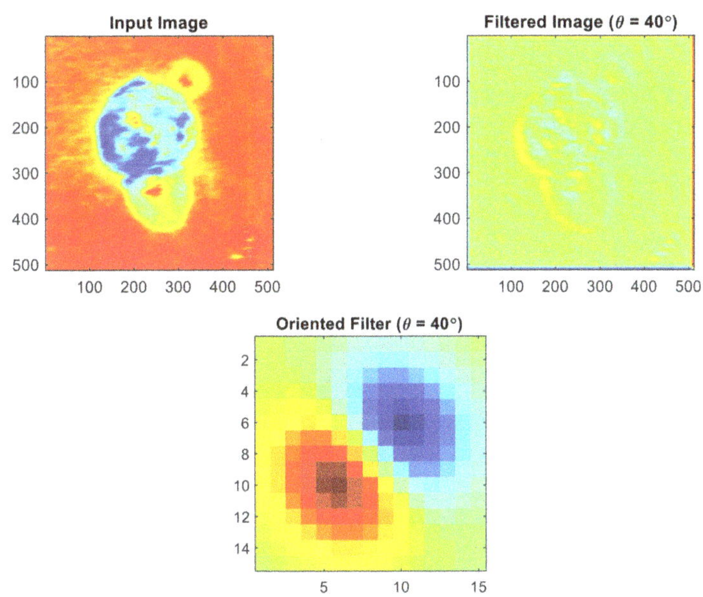

(b) Jet color map

Figure 3.13. Gaussian-filter-enhanced dermoscopy image for $\varphi = 45^o$.

version and figure 3.13(b) depicts a Jet color-map image. The images enhanced using the GF demonstrate a range of surface and border values for both the ROI and the other sections of the picture, and appraisal of these values will support an improved understanding of the imagery and its abnormalities.

Advantages: A GF-supported enhancement is considered to normalize the exteriors and boundaries of grayscale imagery of different characteristics. Further, this method can be used to generate different edge as well as texture patterns based on the chosen φ. A GF supports a range of edge and texture recognition schemes.

Limitations: The information found in the GF-enhanced examination image can be evaluated only with a chosen image assessment exercise and the information cannot be examined with a manual operator. Hence, this image evaluation can only be utilized when a computer-supported algorithm is employed.

3.3.7 Saliency detection

Saliency detection is a common image pre-processing method in which any abnormalities in the image are identified to better accuracy. The 'saliency' of an image can be considered as the ROI or the vital information which is to be evaluated with better precision. Earlier works related to saliency detection can be found in [38–40].

Figure 3.14 depicts the outcome of a chest radiographs enhanced using the saliency detection procedure. Figure 3.14(a) shows the test picture and figures 3.14(b) and (c) show a histogram and the saliency of the test image. To demonstrate the visibility of the saliency, in this work a Hot color map is considered. The detected saliency plays a vital role in obtaining the necessary image information in a range of machine-learning and deep-learning procedures.

3.3.8 Local binary pattern

A local binary pattern (LBP) is a straightforward and extremely proficient texture operator which labels the pixels of an image by thresholding the neighborhood of every pixel. The LBP modifies the considered test image and accounts its result as a binary numeral. Because of its widespread application and computational straightforwardness, a LBP consistency operator has become a common and accepted procedure in a variety of imaging examination tasks. The most significant characteristics of the LBP operator in real-world applications is its robustness to monotonic grayscale changes caused by illumination variations. In the literature, LBPs with varied weights are widely employed in machine-learning and deep-learning methods to improve disease detection accuracy [41].

In this section, a LBP with varied weights ($W = 1$–4) is demonstrated for discussion; earlier works on this process can be found in [42]. Figure 3.15 presents an example breast ultrasound image: figure 3.15(a) presents the test image and figure 3.15(b) shows the grayscale histogram. Figure 16 depicts the LBP patterns generated for the test image shown in figure 3.15(a). Figures 3.16(a)–(d) depict the various binary patterns for $W = 1$ to $W = 4$, respectively. During the image-classification task, every image provides one-dimensional features with

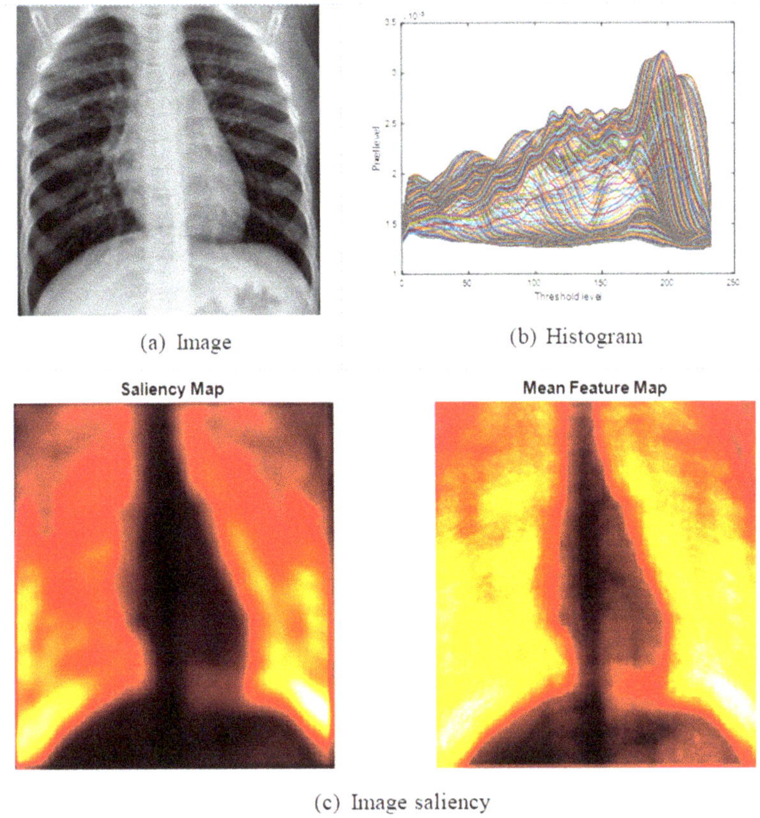

(a) Image (b) Histogram

(c) Image saliency

Figure 3.14. Chest x-ray enhanced with saliency detection.

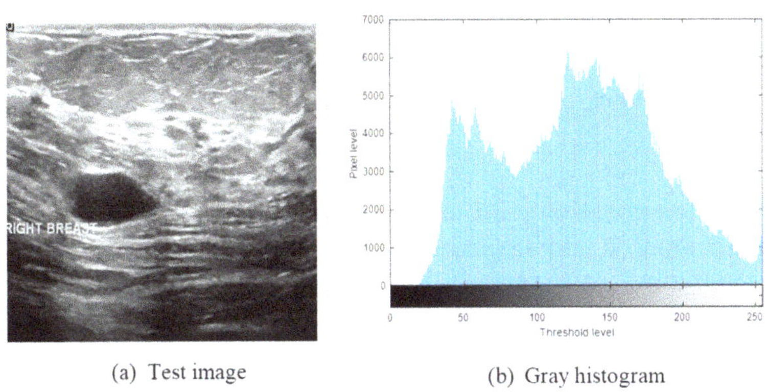

(a) Test image (b) Gray histogram

Figure 3.15. Breast ultrasound test image considered for demonstration.

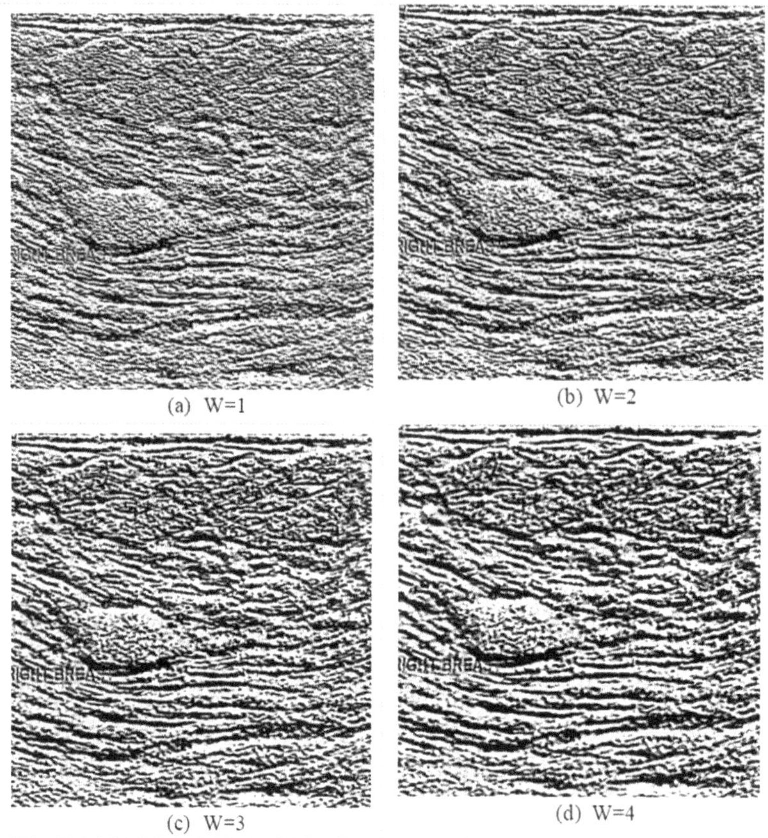

Figure 3.16. Local binary patterns for the test image for $W = 1$–4.

size 59 (i.e. 1 × 1 × 59 pixels). These features are then considered to train and validate the performance of the classifiers.

3.3.9 Image thresholding

Previously, image assessment tasks were performed by a knowledgeable operator, and the outcomes achieved by these exercises required some level of human negotiation. Further, manually enhancing an image with such procedures is complex and time consuming. Rapid advancement in science and technology has helped in furthering assistance by computer algorithms to reduce the burden on human operators; hence, a considerable number of computerized image-examination procedures are now being developed and implemented.

Recent computerized image-examination schemes support (i) semi-automated/automated procedures to enhance the picture, (ii) better operation on grayscale/RGB images, (iii) support for the implementation of different soft-computing practices, and (iv) attained outcomes that can be quickly and effectively stored and retrieved based on need. Computerized methods assist in a selection of image-evaluation procedures to enhance their performance and the image information irrespective of its modality, dimension, and pixel distribution. Further, recently a number of software solutions have been proposed to streamline computerized image-evaluation schemes without compromising their fineness, and the throughput obtained with these actions is superior compared to manually executed methods.

The recent literature confirms that computerized methods are widely employed to implement bi-level and multilevel thresholding methods. Bi-level thresholding is quite simple and needs a few steps to implement. However, multilevel thresholding is one of the most time-consuming and complex procedures and it cannot be implemented manually. Further, the complexity will rise when an RGB image is to be examined. To overcome this, thresholding methods are now combined with methods supported by heuristic algorithms. In this scheme, the heuristic algorithms are responsible for fiding the appropriate threshold for a chosen image based on the constraints to be satisfied. Thresholding combined with a chosen segmentation will help to achieve better disease detection irrespective of the modality of the medical images.

In the literature, demonstrations of image thresholding using the methods of Otsu, Kapur, Tsallis, and Shannon are very common. In this section, only Otsu's approach, supporting grayscale and RGB image thresholding, is demonstrated with a chosen medical image; similar outcomes are expected from other schemes [43–47].

3.3.9.1 Need for thresholding

Image multithresholding using a chosen methodology is widely employed to examine a class of medical images. The thresholding method applied to the medical image will help to enhance its ROI by dilating the background. In a digital picture, the allocation of the pixel plays a principal function, and alteration or grouping of these pixels are significantly favored to improve/change the information available in the figure. Thresholding with a chosen method will group similar pixels in the ROI and improve its visibility, as well as reducing the visibility of the background image.

In earlier years, bi-level thresholding was utilized to divide the raw picture into its ROI and background. In this procedure, the operator/computer algorithm is authorized to distinguish a finest threshold (FT) by means of a chosen thresholding operation.

Let the chosen picture have 256 thresholds (i.e. from 0 to 255). Among these thresholds a chosen threshold will be selected to divide the image into various pixel sections. This operation is depicted in equation (3.3):

$$0 < FT < 255. \tag{3.3}$$

The chosen threshold will function to partition the image into two segments, such as an initial segment consisting of the pixel distribution lesser than the FT and a later segment with a pixel distribution greater than the FT. This procedure partitions the picture into two pixel groups, and hence this process is called bi-level thresholding.

If the preparation is to separate the particular picture into more than two segments, then a multilevel thresholding is preferred. In a multithresholding operation, the number of FT = number of threshold levels.

If a tri-level threshold is chosen for demonstration, this operation will divide the test picture into three segments, as depicted in equation (3.4):

$$0 < FT_1 < FT_2 < 255. \tag{3.4}$$

In this case, the picture is detached into three segments, as in an initial segment (pixels between 0 and FT_1), intermediate segment (pixels between FT_1 and FT_2), and final segment (pixels between FT_2 and 255). In most medical imaging schemes, the outcome achieved with a bi-level threshold is not suitable, and hence, multithresholding is referred to pre-process grayscale/RGB images. Related works on multithresholding can be found in the literature [48, 49].

3.3.9.2 Otsu/Kapur thresholding

In medical imaging examination tasks, ROI enhancement and extraction using a chosen image-processing scheme is widely employed in a variety of machine-learning procedures. In the image extraction process, an image being subjected to a chosen thresholding procedure is necessary for the initial separation of the test picture into a ROI and background.

In a heuristic-algorithm-supported multithresholding process, a chosen heuristic algorithm is employed in selecting the appropriate threshold value based on the chosen objective function to be maximized (Otsu/Kapur). Earlier works on multithresholding confirm that this procedure works well on grayscale and RGB class images and that its complexity will increase with image dimension (since the number of pixels to be examined is larger and larger). In this work, the thresholding is implemented on an image with dimensions of 512 × 512 pixels and the results are demonstrated.

Figure 3.17 presents a thresholding process implemented for a brain MRI slice. During this operation, the chosen procedure is employed to find the finest threshold

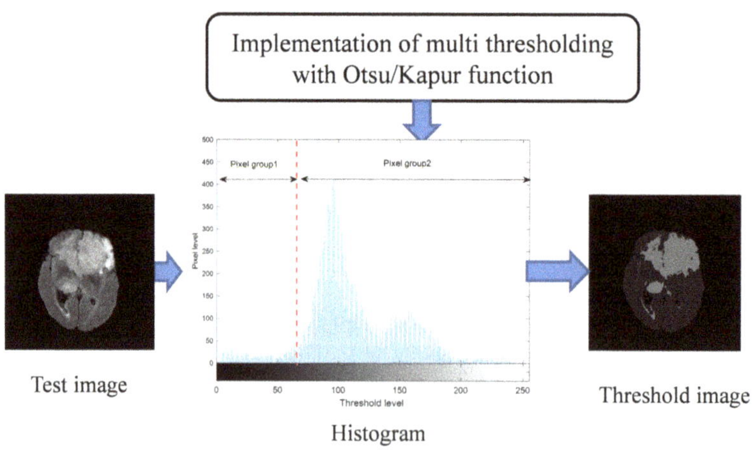

Figure 3.17. Implementation of image multithresholding.

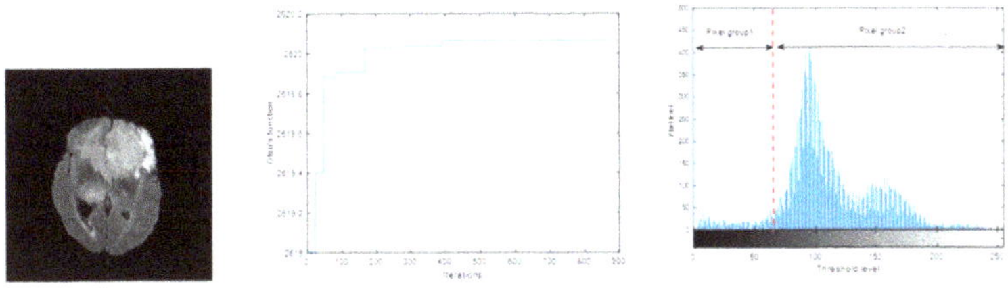

(a) Test image (b) Search convergence (c) Bi-level thresholding

Figure 3.18. Results achieved for bi-level thresholding.

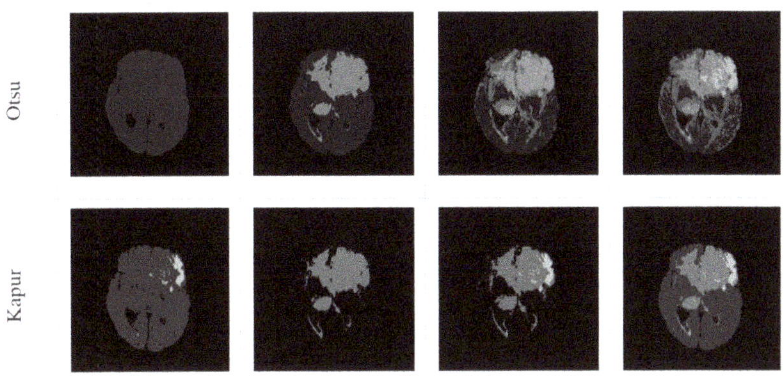

(a) FT=2 (b) FT=3 (c) FT=4 (d) FT=5

Figure 3.19. Bi-level and multilevel threshold results.

by evaluating the histogram of the image. In this work, the demonstration of the thresholding process is presented using Otsu's/Kapur's approach.

Figure 3.18 presents an example of Otsu-based bi-level thresholding implemented on a grayscale image. In this work, the selection of the finest threshold is performed with Otsu's method: the process continues till it identifies the threshold at which the image can be separated into two groups of pixels to enhance the image. Figure 3.18(a) shows the test image and figures 3.18(b) and (c) depict the convergence of Otsu's search and the identified threshold, respectively. Figure 3.18(c) shows how the bi-level threshold separates the image's pixels into two sections (pixel group 1 and 2), which helps to separate the ROI from the background.

Figure 3.19 depicts the thresholded outcome obtained with Otsu's/Kapur's methods, which confirms that the results of the bi-level threshold (figure 3.19(a)) is very poor in identifying the tumor (ROI) from the brain MRI. Hence, the thresholds (FT) are then changed into multilevels of 3, 4, and 5, and the corresponding results are demonstrated. This outcome confirms that the result of

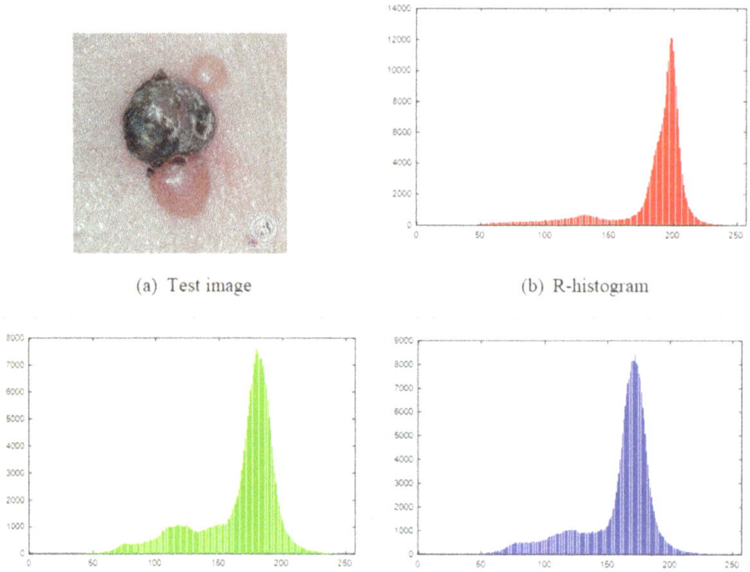

(a) Test image (b) R-histogram (c) G-histogram (d) B-histogram

Figure 3.20. RGB test image and corresponding threshold values.

threshold 2 (figure 3.19(b)) is better compared to figures 3.19(c) and (d). This demonstrates that, for medical image enhancement, tri-level thresholding is sufficient and helps to attain a better outcome compared to other methods. A similar procedure is then implemented for an RGB image (digital dermoscopy), and the achieved result is depicted in the next figure.

Figure 3.20 presents the RGB digital dermoscopy image, examined using Otsu's multithresholding method. The RGB image is more complex than the grayscale image due to its complex histogram. A RGB histogram consist of pixels belonging to red (R), green (G), and blue (B) groups. Figure 3.20(a) shows the test image and figures 3.20(b)–(d) show the thresholds obtained from the test image. Otsu's multithresholding operation is then implemented on the image and the achieved results are depicted in figure 3.21. Figures 3.21(a)–(d) demonstrate the outcome achieved for FT = 2–5, and from this it is confirmed that figures 3.21(a) and (b) provide better threshold outcomes compared to other FTs.

After executing the thresholding by means of a preferred practice, its results need to be authenticated in order to confirm the performance of the proposed method. Justification of the thresholding performance can be realized using a comparative analysis between the raw images and threshold images. During this process, frequently considered image excellence values, such as root mean squared error (RMSE), peak signal-to-noise ratio (PSNR, in dB), structural similarity index (SSIM), normalized absolute error (NAE), normalized cross-correlation (NCC), average difference (AD), and structural content (SC) are computed for every image

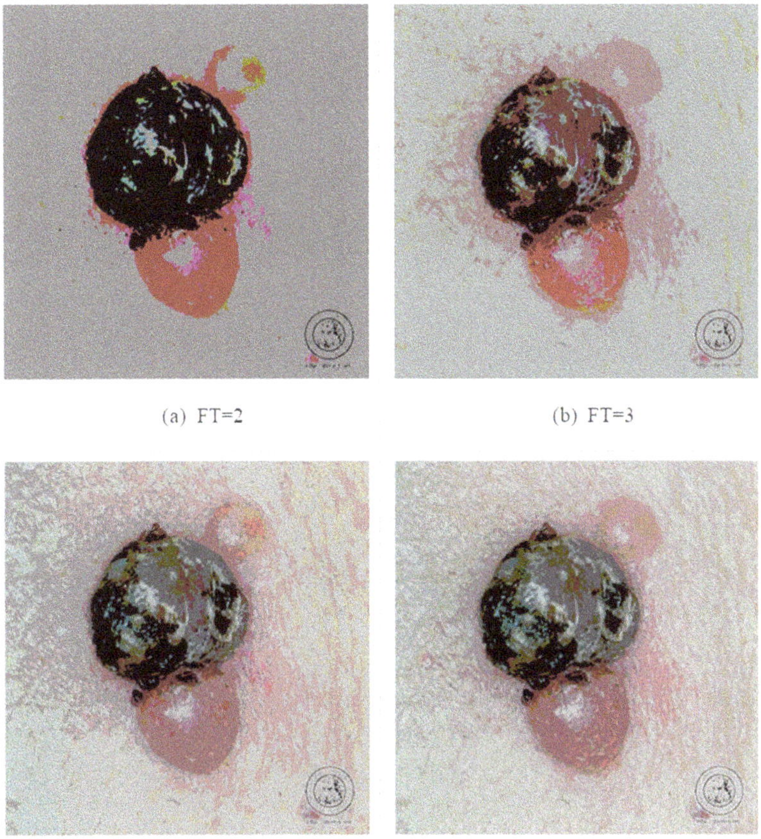

(a) FT=2 (b) FT=3

(c) FT=4 (d) FT=5

Figure 3.21. Multilevel thresholding results achieved for the RGB dermoscopy image.

and, based on these values, the performance of the implemented thresholding technique is confirmed. The procedure is depicted in figure 3.22 and the related mathematical expressions are presented in equations (3.5)–(3.11).

Mathematical expressions of the considered image quality measures are presented below [50, 51]:

$$\mathrm{PSNR}(R,\ T) = 20\log_{10}\left(\frac{255}{\sqrt{MSE(R,\ T)}}\right),\ \mathrm{dB} \tag{3.5}$$

$$\mathrm{RMSE}_{(R,\ T)} = \sqrt{\mathrm{MSE}_{(R,\ T)}} = \sqrt{\frac{1}{XY}\sum_{i=1}^{X}\sum_{j=1}^{Y}\left[R_{(i,\ j)} - T_{(i,\ j)}\right]^2}. \tag{3.6}$$

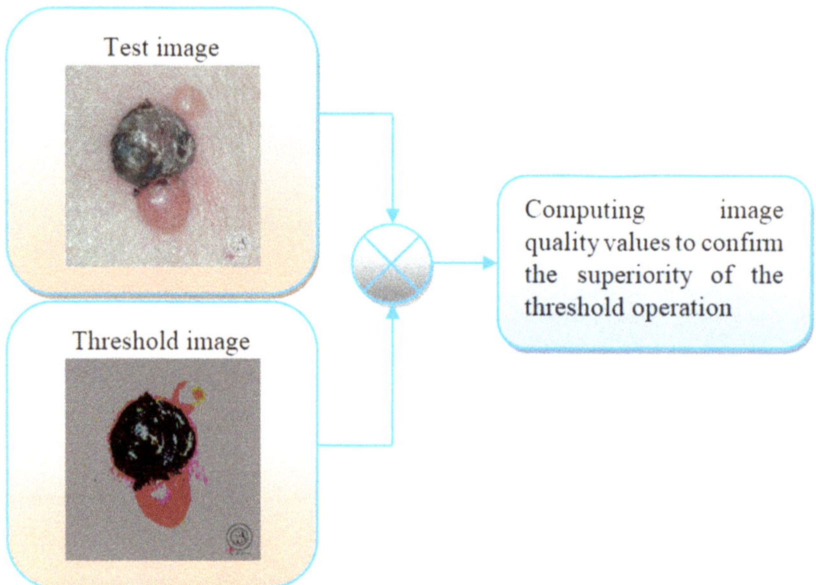

Figure 3.22. Performance confirmation between the raw and threshold image.

The mean SSIM is generally used to estimate the image superiority and interdependencies between the original and processed image:

$$\mathrm{MSSIM}_{(R,\,T)} = \frac{1}{M}\sum_{z=1}^{M}\mathrm{SSIM}(R_z,\ Tz), \tag{3.7}$$

where R_z and T_z are the image contents at the zth local window, and M is the number of local windows in the image.

$$\mathrm{NAE}(R,\ T) = \frac{\sum_{i=1}^{X}\sum_{j=1}^{Y}\left| R_{(i,\,j)} - T_{(i,\,j)} \right|}{\sum_{i=1}^{X}\sum_{j=1}^{Y}\left| R_{(i,\,j)} \right|}, \tag{3.8}$$

$$\mathrm{NCC}(R,\ T) = \frac{\sum_{i=1}^{X}\sum_{j=1}^{Y} R_{(i,\,j)} \cdot T_{(i,\,j)}}{\sum_{i=1}^{X}\sum_{j=1}^{Y} R^2_{(i,\,j)}}, \tag{3.9}$$

$$\mathrm{AD}(R,\ T) = \frac{\sum_{i=1}^{X}\sum_{j=1}^{Y} R_{(i,\,j)} - T_{(i,\,j)}}{XY}, \tag{3.10}$$

$$\mathrm{SC}(R, T) = \frac{\sum_{i=1}^{X}\sum_{j=1}^{Y} R^2_{(i,j)}}{\sum_{i=1}^{X}\sum_{j=1}^{Y} T^2_{(i,j)}}. \tag{3.11}$$

In all the expressions, $X * Y$ is the size of the considered image, R is the original test image, and S is the segmented image of a chosen threshold. Higher values of PSNR, MSSIM, NCC and lower values of RMSE, NAE, AD, SC specify a superior quality of thresholding. An improved Tsallis fitness function with minor CPU time demand during the optimization search also confirms the capability of the considered heuristic algorithm.

Advantages: Multilevel thresholding is an uncomplicated and competent image-processing technique, executable manually as well as using heuristic algorithms. Further, it supports the processing of grayscale/RGB imagery with different methods. The ROI of the trial picture can be improved with either a bi-level or a multilevel threshold selection process.

Limitations: Selection of the finest threshold and the selection of the objective function during soft-computing-based thresholding are quite difficult. Further, in most image-enhancement practices, thresholding is preferred only as a pre-processing method, and the execution time of this process is amplified with respect to the histogram's increasing complexity.

3.4 Summary

The need for the arrangement of prior image assessment and the execution of different possible image improvement procedures to adjust unprocessed trial pictures was here outlined, with suitable results given. Further, the need for image thresholding and the implementation of bi-level and multilevel thresholding were given with evidence. Implementation of thresholding procedures for grayscale/RGB imagery and their appraisal procedures were demonstrated. From the above discussion, it can be noted that image thresholding, performed by means of a well-selected scheme, can be implemented to pre-process digital test images recorded across a range of modalities. Moreover, image thresholding has emerged as a key research field due to its practical importance, and now represents one of the principal actions to be considered in medical imaging examination tasks.

References

[1] Suetens P 2017 *Fundamentals of Medical Imaging* (Cambridge: Cambridge University Press)

[2] Rajinikanth V, Raja N S M and Dey N 2020 *A Beginner's Guide to Multilevel Image Thresholding* (Boca Raton, FL: CRC Press)

[3] Estrela V V, Monteiro A C, França R P, Iano Y, Khelassi A and Navid R 2018 Health 4.0: applications, management, technologies and review: array *Med. Tech. J.* **2** 262–76

[4] Gupta L, Klinkhammer B M, Boor P, Merhof D and Gadermayr M 2019 GAN-based image enrichment in digital pathology boosts segmentation accuracy *Int. Conf. on Medical Image Computing and Computer-Assisted Intervention* pp 631–39

[5] Mohan C R and Kiran S 2018 Image enrichment using single discrete wavelet transform multi-resolution and frequency partition *Artificial Intelligence and Evolutionary Computations in Engineering Systems* (Singapore: Springer) pp 87–98

[6] Nasirahmadi A, Edwards S A, Matheson S M and Sturm B 2017 Using automated image analysis in pig behavioural research: assessment of the influence of enrichment substrate provision on lying behaviour *Appl. Animal Behav. Sci.* **196** 30–5

[7] Estrela V V, Khelassi A, Monteiro A C B, Iano Y, Razmjooy N, Martins D and Rocha D T 2019 Why software-defined radio (SDR) matters in healthcare? *Med. Tech. J.* **3** 421–29

[8] Abreu L M, Hora H R M D, Rangel J J A, Erthal M, Navid, Estrela V V and Iano Y 2020 A multi-criteria modelling for ranking CO_2 emitting G20 countries from the Kaya identity and their impacts on elderly health *Proc. Brazilian Technology Symp.* (Cham: Springer) pp 477–87

[9] Alferaidi A, Yadav K, Alharbi Y, Navid R, Viriyasitavat W, Gulati K and Dhiman G 2022 Distributed deep CNN-LSTM model for intrusion detection method in IoT-based vehicles *Math. Problems Eng.* **2022** 3424819

[10] Raja N S M, Rajinikanth V and Latha K 2014 Otsu based optimal multilevel image thresholding using firefly algorithm *Model. Sim. Eng.* **2014** 794574

[11] Dougherty 1994 *Digital Image Processing Methods* 1st edn (Boca Raton, FL: CRC Press)

[12] Satapathy S C, Raja N S M, Rajinikanth V, Ashour A S and Dey N 2018 Multi-level image thresholding using Otsu and chaotic bat algorithm *Neural Comput. Appl.* **29** 1285–307

[13] Bechara B, McMahan C A, Geha H and Noujeim M 2012 Evaluation of a cone beam CT artefact reduction algorithm *Dentomaxillofacial Radiology* **41** 422–28

[14] Rajinikanth V, Kadry S, Thanaraj K P, Kamalanand K and Seo S 2020 Firefly-algorithm supported scheme to detect COVID-19 lesion in lung CT scan images using Shannon entropy and Markov-random-field arXiv:2004.09239

[15] Rajinikanth V, Dey N, Raj A N J, Hassanien A E, Santosh K C and Raja N 2020 Harmony-search and otsu based system for coronavirus disease (COVID-19) detection using lung CT scan images arXiv:2004.03431

[16] Xu Y, Wang Y and Razmjooy N 2022 Lung cancer diagnosis in CT images based on Alexnet optimized by modified Bowerbird optimization algorithm *Biomed. Signal Process. Control* **77** 103791

[17] Wang M, Wang Q and Chanussot J 2021 Tensor low-rank constraint and $ l_0 $ total variation for hyperspectral image mixed noise removal *IEEE J. Sel. Top. Signal Process.* **15** 718–33

[18] Singh I and Verma O P 2021 Impulse noise removal in color image sequences using fuzzy logic *Multimedia Tools Appl.* **80** 18279–300

[19] Shan B P, Shiney O J, Saleem S, Rajinikanth V, Zaguia A and Singh D 2022 A post-processing algorithm for boosting contrast of MRI images *Computers Materials and Continua* **72** 2749–63

[20] He X, Wang C, Zheng R and Li X 2021 GPR image noise removal using grey wolf optimisation in the NSST domain *Remote Sensing* **13** 4416

[21] Ranjbarzadeh R, Dorosti S, Jafarzadeh Ghoushchi S, Safavi S, Razmjooy N, Tataei Sarshar N and Bendechache M 2022 Nerve optic segmentation in CT images using a deep learning model and a texture descriptor *Complex Intel. Syst.* **8** 3543–57

[22] Zuiderveld K 1994 Contrast limited adaptive histogram equalization *Graphics Gems IV* (Academic: New York) pp 474–85

[23] Jin Y, Fayad L M and Laine A F 2001 Contrast enhancement by multiscale adaptive histogram equalization *Wavelets: Applications in Signal and Image Processing IX* vol 4478 (Bellingham, WA: SPIE) pp 206–13

[24] Rajive Gandhi C and Murugesh V 2021 A contrast adaptive histogram equalization with neural learning quantization (CAHE-NLQ) for blood clot detection in brain *J. Ambient Intell. Human. Comput.* https://doi.org/10.1007/S12652-021-03132-W

[25] Dhal K G, Das A, Ray S, Gálvez J and Das S 2021 Histogram equalization variants as optimization problems: a review *Arch. Comput. Meth. Eng.* **28** 1471–96

[26] Bulut F 2021 Low dynamic range histogram equalization (LDR-HE) via quantized Haar wavelet transform *The Visual Computer* **38** 2239–55

[27] Versaci M and Morabito F C 2021 Image edge detection: a new approach based on fuzzy entropy and fuzzy divergence *Int. J. Fuzzy Syst.* **23** 918–36

[28] Chetia R, Boruah S M B and Sahu P P 2021 Quantum image edge detection using improved Sobel mask based on NEQR *Quantum Inf. Process.* **20** 21

[29] Rahmawati S, Devita R, Zain R H, Rianti E, Lubis N and Wanto A 2021 Prewitt and canny methods on inversion image edge detection: an evaluation *J. Phys.: Conf. Series* **1933** 012039

[30] Wu F, Zhu C, Xu J, Bhatt M W and Sharma A 2021 Research on image text recognition based on canny edge detection algorithm and k-means algorithm *Int. J. Syst. Assur. Eng. Manage.* **13** 72–80

[31] Alferaidi A, Yadav K, Alharbi Y, Navid R, Viriyasitavat W, Gulati K and Dhiman G 2022 Distributed deep CNN-LSTM model for intrusion detection method in IoT-based vehicles *Math. Problems Eng.* **2022** 3424819

[32] Liang J, Cao J, Sun G, Zhang K, Van Gool L and Timofte R 2021 Swinir: image restoration using swin transformer *Proc. IEEE/CVF Int. Conf. on Computer Vision* pp 1833–44

[33] Zamir S W, Arora A, Khan S, Hayat M, Khan F S, Yang M H and Shao L 2021 Multi-stage progressive image restoration *Proc. IEEE/CVF Conf. on Computer Vision and Pattern Recognition* pp 14821–31

[34] Chen L, Lu X, Zhang J, Chu X and Chen C 2021 HINet: half instance normalization network for image restoration *Proc. IEEE/CVF Conf. on Computer Vision and Pattern Recognition* pp 182–92

[35] Rajinikanth V, Sivakumar R, Hemanth D J, Kadry S, Mohanty J R, Arunmozhi S and Nhu N G 2021 Automated classification of retinal images into AMD/non-AMD class—a study using multi-threshold and gassian-filter enhanced images *Evolutionary Intelligence* **14** 1163–71

[36] Syed H H, Khan M A, Tariq U, Armghan A, Alenezi F, Khan J A and Rajinikanth V 2021 A rapid artificial intelligence-based computer-aided diagnosis system for COVID-19 classification from CT images *Behavioural Neurology* **2021** 2560388

[37] Vijayakumar K, Rajinikanth V and Kirubakaran M K 2022 Automatic detection of breast cancer in ultrasound images using mayfly algorithm optimized handcrafted features *J. X-Ray Science and Technology* **30** 751–66

[38] Rajinikanth V, Kadry S, Taniar D, Damaševičius R and Rauf H T 2021 Breast-cancer detection using thermal images with marine-predators-algorithm selected features *7th Int. Conf. on Bio Signals, Images, and Instrumentation (ICBSII)* pp 1–6
[39] Rajinikanth V, Kadry S, Damaševičius R, Taniar D and Rauf H T 2021 Machine-learning-scheme to detect choroidal-neovascularization in retinal OCT image *2021 7th Int. Conf. on Bio Signals, Images, and Instrumentation (ICBSII)* pp 1–5
[40] Zhang J, Fan D P, Dai Y, Anwar S, Saleh F, Aliakbarian S and Barnes N 2021 Uncertainty inspired RGB-D saliency detection *IEEE Trans. Pattern Anal. Mach. Intell.* **44** 5761–79
[41] Song T, Xin L, Gao C, Zhang T and Huang Y 2021 Quaternionic extended local binary pattern with adaptive structural pyramid pooling for color image representation *Pattern Recognit.* **115** 107891
[42] Gudigar A, Raghavendra U, Devasia T, Nayak K, Danish S M, Kamath G and Acharya U R 2019 Global weighted LBP based entropy features for the assessment of pulmonary hypertension *Pattern Recognit. Lett.* **125** 35–41
[43] Rajinikanth V and Couceiro M S 2015 RGB histogram based color image segmentation using firefly algorithm *Procedia Computer Science* **46** 1449–57
[44] Rajinikanth V, Dey N, Raj A N J, Hassanien A E, Santosh K C and Raja N S M 2020 Harmony-search and otsu based system for coronavirus disease (COVID-19) detection using lung CT scan images arXiv:2004.03431
[45] Dey N *et al* 2019 Social-group-optimization based tumor evaluation tool for clinical brain MRI of Flair/diffusion-weighted modality *Biocybern. Biomed. Eng* **39** 843–56
[46] Fernandes S L, Rajinikanth V and Kadry S 2019 A hybrid framework to evaluate breast abnormality using infrared thermal images *IEEE Consum. Electron. Mag* **8** 31–6
[47] Ghamisi P, Couceiro M S, Benediktsson J A and Ferreira N M F 2012 An efficient method for segmentation of images based on fractional calculus and natural selection *Expert Syst. Appl.* **39** 12407–17
[48] Manikantan K, Arun B V and Yaradonic D K S 2012 Optimal multilevel thresholds based on Tsallis entropy method using golden ratio particle swarm optimization for improved image segmentation *Procedia Engineering* **30** 364–71
[49] Rajinikanth V, Raja N S M and Latha K 2014 Optimal multilevel image thresholding: an analysis with PSO and BFO algorithms *Aust. J. Basic and Appl. Sci.* **8** 443–54
[50] Hore A and Ziou D 2010 Image quality metrics: PSNR vs. SSIM *IEEE Int. Conf. on Pattern Recognition (ICPR) (Istanbul, Turkey)* pp 2366–9
[51] Wang Z, Bovik A C, Sheikh H R and Simoncelli E P 2004 Image quality assessment: from error measurement to structural similarity *IEEE Trans. Image Process.* **13** 1–14

IOP Publishing

Frontiers of Artificial Intelligence in Medical Imaging

Navid Razmjooy and Venkatesan Rajinikanth

Chapter 4

Computer-aided-scheme for automatic classification of brain MRI slices into normal/ Alzheimer's disease

Seifedine Kadry

Recently, several methodologies have been developed to support the elderly and maintain their quality of life. However, the incidence of disease in older people gradually increases due to their reduced health conditions. When such age-related health issues are identified accurately, appropriate treatment and assistance can be provided to reduce the diseases' harshness. Alzheimer's disease (AD) is one of these age-associated illnesses which causes various problems, including dementia. This chapter aims to develop and implement a computer-aided scheme (CAS) to detect AD using T2 modality brain MRI slices. This work implements (i) a machine-learning scheme and (ii) a deep-learning scheme to detect AD. The various phases in this scheme include (i) MRI slice collection and resizing, (ii) handcrafted feature mining, (iii) deep feature mining using AlexNet, a convolutional neural network architecture, (iv) feature reduction using the firefly algorithm, and (v) binary classification. The proposed CAS is considered to classify MRI slices into normal/ AD classes using (i) handcrafted features, (ii) deep features, and (iii) hybrid features in which the series integration of handcrafted and deep features are considered. The classification task is independently executed for every feature, and the attained results are presented and discussed using the chosen binary classifiers.

4.1 Introduction

The occurrence of age-associated disease (AAD) is gradually rising in older people, and appropriate diagnosis and proper care will help reduce the impact of the disease. Even though a considerable number of AAD manifests its symptoms and can be dealt with immediately, brain-related AAD can cause severe issues [1–3]. Brain

doi:10.1088/978-0-7503-4012-0ch4

illnesses due to AAD will affect both physiological and the psychological state of the patient; hence, researchers have proposed several diagnostic tools and treatment methodologies.

AAD relating to the brain will cause mild to severe problems, such as depression, loss of communication between the brain and other body sections, memory-related issues, and psychological problems. Therefore, these diseases can severely impact older adults who are frequently about to enjoy their retirement. Alzheimer's disease (AD) is one of the AAD that affects the brain, and which is the most frequent reason for dementia in the elderly. Usually, the onset of AD is caused by the gradual death of brain cells, which causes the brain to contract. The cognitive refuse is distinguished by the regular vanishing of vital nerve cells in the cerebral cortex, particularly in the frontal/medial temporal sections of brain. AD is a considerable issue in morbidity, ranked fifth among the causes of mortality by the World Health Organization (WHO) [4]. The main characteristic feature of AD is the occurrence of amyloid plaques and neurofibrillary tangles in the brain. A recent report confirmed that roughly 5.8 million citizens in the United States over 65 years of age are living with AD. Among them, 80% of individuals are aged >75 years. Further, roughly 50 million people in the global population are living with dementia, of which 60% and 70% are likely to have AD. Because of this, many research works have been proposed and implemented to develop an appropriate computer-aided scheme (CAS) to detect AD [5–10]. The different phases of AD comprise (i) pre-dementia, (ii) a premature phase, (iii) a middle phase, and (iv) an advanced phase.

Analysis of the progress of AD involves taking account of the sickness and the occurrence of neurological/psychological symptoms. The patient's health history may be taken from relatives, and the patient's performance under various conditions can also be accounted for [10]. Clinical-level screening for AD involves a personal check using clinical protocol, and bioimaging-supported screening. Current methods use advanced biomedical imaging schemes, such as computed tomography (CT), magnetic resonance imaging (MRI), and positron emission tomography-CT (PET-CT) techniques. A CT scan is a radiological methodology that assists in recognizing dementia by scrutinizing the dimensions of different brain sections, such as the temporal lobe, hippocampus, and frontal lobe. MRI screening of the brain demonstrates the brain's arrangements, shrinkage, vascular abnormality, or any other structural change(s) which can influence cognitive dysfunction. The prime function of MRI in the diagnosis of AD is the assessment of the amount of change in feature locations, which can yield better diagnostic accuracy [11, 12]. The evaluation is frequently conducted on mesial temporal lobe atrophy (MTLA) and temporoparietal cortical atrophy (TCA). MTLA can be assessed directly or indirectly, and direct appraisal is based on assessing the volume loss of the hippocampal or para-hippocampal regions. In contrast, indirect appraisal relies on the swelling of the para-hippocampal fissure. These evaluations are frequently analyzed jointly; as a result, a high MTLA score can lead to a dementia diagnosis.

The medical importance of AD, along with other brain AAD, is that they provide a opportunity for society, in consideration of the afflicted, to develop and advance consistent and precise means of technological estimation for numerous brain conditions. Therefore, researchers have proposed implementing a variety of CASs to inspect the incidence and harshness of AD. The general framework of a CAS implemented for AD includes (i) gathering of brain images with a suggested imaging technique, (ii) image resizing and pre-processing, (iii) feature extraction with a chosen technique, (iv) feature reduction and optimal feature selection, and (v) classification and validation.

This chapter implements a CAS to categorize T2 modality brain MRI slices into normal/AD classes using binary classifiers with a fivefold cross-validation. In this work, the proposed CAS consists of (i) a machine-learning (ML) system to detect AD, (ii) a deep-learning (DL) system to detect AD, and (iii) a combined ML and DL (DL+ML) system to detect the AD.

In this work, the necessary test images are collected from well-known benchmark images, like the Alzheimer's Disease Neuroimaging Initiative (ADNI) and the Cancer Imaging Archive's (TCIA) Low-Grade-Glioma (LGG) database and Harvard's Brain Atlas Database (HBAD). Initially, the necessary test image slices are collected from T2 modality MRI, and every image is resized to pixels. In this work, 1000 images are considered for assessment (500 AD and 500 normal). All images are associated with the skull section; a classification task for this study is separately implemented with/without the skull, and the results presented.

The ML scheme is initially implemented with handcrafted features (HF). Then, a feature-mining procedure is implemented using procedures such as a discrete wavelet transform (DWT), shearlet transform (ST), complex wavelet transform (CWT), as well as local binary patterns (LBPs) and pyramid histograms of oriented gradients (PHOGs) with selected bins. In this work, the performance of the CAS is initially tested using the individual features. Then, these features are optimized with the firefly algorithm (FA), the features are serially integrated, and the classification performance is confirmed with the chosen binary classifiers. After verifying the performance of the ML scheme, an AlexNet-supported scheme is then considered to classify the MRI slices into normal/AD classes. Finally, the optimal ML and DL features are combined and the classification performance is verified. In this chapter, the performance of the developed CAS is confirmed by computing the accuracy, sensitivity, specificity, and positive predictive value (PPV) percentage.

The contributions of this chapter include the following:

(i) Assessment of MRI slices using a ML technique with chosen HF.
(ii) FA-based feature optimization to achieve better accuracy.
(iii) Assessment of MRI slices using AlexNet.
(iv) Assessment of MRI slices using ML and DL features techniques with chosen HF.

The sections of this chapter are arranged as follows: section 4.2 reviews earlier research, section 4.3 presents our methodology, and sections 4.4 and 4.5 present the experimental outcomes and conclusions.

4.2 Related work

In the medicinal field, AD analysis is necessary to protect a person's cognitive capability and community health in general. However, AD generates severe problems with individual thinking, recollection, and other everyday activities. Due to the inexorable death of nerve cells over time, an individual's essential cerebral aptitude is harshly damaged in the later stages of life. To facilitate early recognition of AD, different diagnostics practices have been developed. Although MRI is an effective means that can distinguish signs of AD in the brain, the entire scanning process consumes too much time, chiefly due to manual examination workflow bottlenecks [13–15].

Many methods have been discussed for analyzing AD with traditional, ML, and DL practices which can executed in a much more resource- and time-efficient manner than conventional schemes. The recent work of Acharya *et al* presents a detailed assessment of AD using various ML techniques with the help of benchmarks and clinically collected brain MRI slices [16].

Other recent works related to AD diagnosis are summarized in table 4.1.

Recently, the aforementioned work of Acharya *et al* proposed a ML scheme to classify clinical and benchmark brain MRI slices into normal/AD classes, which achieved considerable detection accuracy [16]. The proposed scheme is implemented using the standard image features in this work. In addition, a Student's *t*-test-based

Table 4.1. Summary of the AD detection schemes found in the literature.

Reference	Employed procedure to detect AD
Wang *et al* [6]	Recurrent neural-network-based predictive modeling technique is proposed to detect AD.
Haaksma *et al* [7]	A detailed review on AD detection is presented and the results discussed.
Malik and Robertson [8]	Evaluation methodologies available to detect AD are presented.
Braskie *et al* [12]	A thorough assessment of the methodologies and methods invented to detect AD is discussed.
Stonnington *et al* [15]	Development of a chemical score to detect AD is presented.
Beheshti *et al* [16]	Effective classification of MRI slices into normal/AD classes using ML schemes. This work employed binary classifiers and executed this task using various features to achieve a better detection accuracy.
Dimitriadis *et al* [17]	Random-forest-supported classification of AD is presented with MRI slices.
Beheshti *et al* [18]	Structural MRI-based examination of AD is presented.

feature selection is considered to find the optimal features, which helps to provide a better result. This work also initially implemented a similar procedure to detect AD using the ML scheme. Later, the proposed work is extended using the DL technique and the DL+ML feature-based approach. In this work, the feature selection is implemented using the FA, and the selected features are then considered for computing the performance of the proposed CAS. The experimental outcome of this study confirms that the proposed scheme helps to detect AD with better accuracy for brain MRI with/without the skull section. The attained results are separately presented for each approach, and the merit of the proposed scheme is discussed.

4.3 Methodology

The proposed CAS is implemented in three different procedures: (i) a ML scheme with conventional features, (ii) a DL scheme that utilizes AlexNet, and (iii) an integrated approach using deep features and handcrafted features (HF+DF). All these methods are discussed in this section and illustrated with a relevant block diagram. Similar image data sets are considered in all these works, and the attained results are discussed.

4.3.1 Proposed AD detection scheme

Automatic and accurate AD detection from the MRI slice is essential to distinguish the severity of the disease. Further, this plays a vital role in deciding the medical assistance needed for the person affected with AD.

4.3.2 Machine-learning scheme

This work initially implements a ML scheme to distinguish the MRI slices into normal/AD classes; the structure of this scheme is depicted in figure 4.1. The various stages involved in this scheme include the following:

- Image collection.
- Pre-processing of the MRI slices.
- Feature extraction using a chosen technique.
- Feature optimization using the FA.
- Performance evaluation using the binary classifier and validation.

The test images for this study were collected from the ADNI [19], TCIA [20, 21], and HBAD [2] databases. After collecting the data set, image pre-processing methods, such as resizing and skull elimination, are then implemented to treat the test images. The original MRI slices are available in 256×256×3 pixels (px) dimension; these images are resized to 227×227×3 px to satisfy the conventional dimension required for AlexNet's architecture. After resizing, the necessary features from these images are extracted using DWT, ST, CWT, LBP, and PHOG procedures. The basic features extracted are significant, and if these features are considered to verify the classifier, it may lead to an overfitting

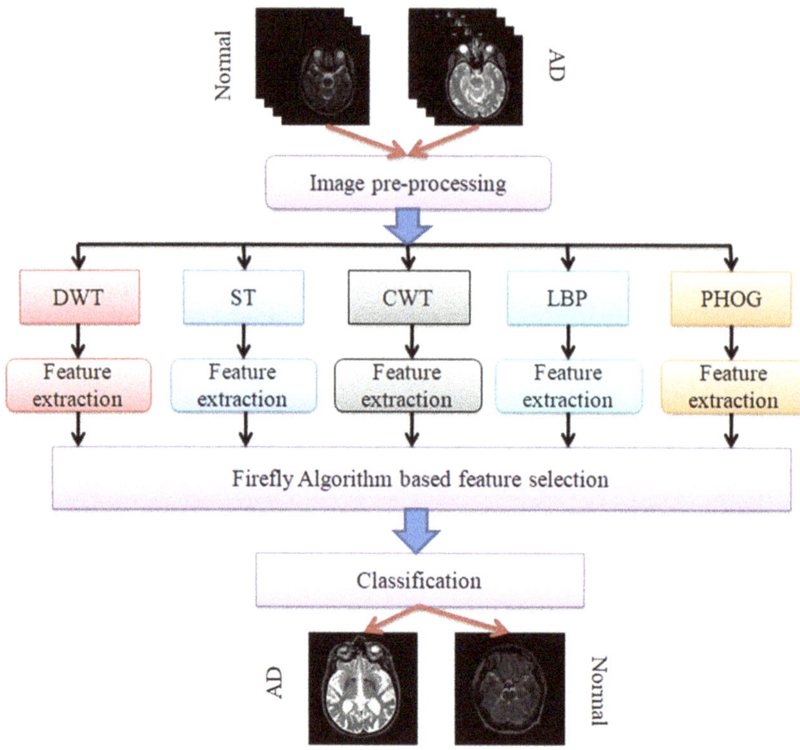

Figure 4.1. Machine-learning scheme employed to detect AD using MRI.

problem. Accordingly, a feature reduction is then employed using the FA, and the reduced features are individually considered to train, test, and validate the classifier's performance using a fivefold cross-validation process. During this task, the k-nearest neighbors (k-NN) classifier is considered, as discussed by Acharya *et al* [16]. After verifying the individual performance of the chosen features, serial concatenation is employed to get a single handcrafted feature vector (HFV), which is then considered to verify the AD detection performance of the proposed CAS with k-NN. The result of this study confirms that the considered HFV helps achieve a classification accuracy of >90% for MRI with the skull section and 91% for MRI without the skull section. The overall performance of the proposed scheme confirms that the serially concatenated HFV helps to provide a better result for the test images considered in this study.

4.3.3 Deep-learning scheme

Recently, DL schemes have been widely employed to examine a considerable number of raw and processed data sets with better accuracy. Researchers have widely employed many pre-trained and customary DL-scheme-supported medical image processing methods to evaluate benchmark and clinical data to achieve better

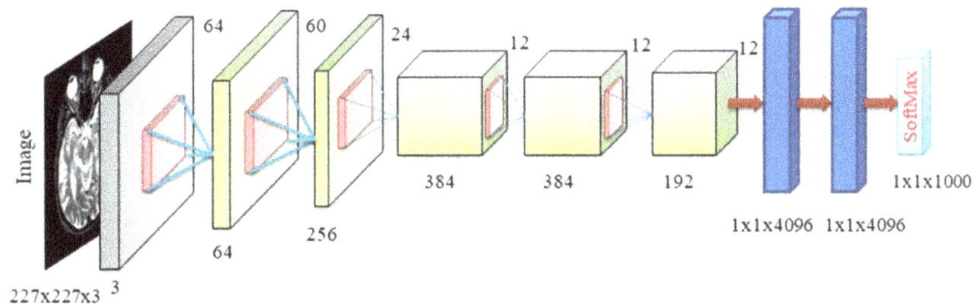

Figure 4.2. Deep-learning scheme employed to detect AD using MRI.

diagnostic accuracy [22–26]. A typical DL scheme's development and implementation requires appropriate coding skills; hence, researchers widely adopt pre-trained DL methods to help find the relevant results. Further, a pre-trained scheme will help to achieve a better result than customary models.

In this work, the considered MRI slices are evaluated using the traditional AlexNet convolutional neural network scheme, the architecture of which is depicted in figure 4.2. This presents a simple example AlexNet architecture widely employed to examine medical images. In this work, MRI slices from normal/AD classes are considered to train, test, and confirm the merit of AlexNet using the SoftMax classifier [27, 28]. The considered AlexNet is implemented using the following initial parameters: initial weights = ImageNet; batch size = 8; optimizer = Adam; pooling = average; hidden-layer activation = Relu; classifier = SoftMax; and performance metric(s) = loss value and accuracy. Initially, training images are considered so that AlexNet can learn the new data. Then, this scheme is tested and validated with the chosen images, and the classification achieved for a fivefold cross-validation is considered to confirm the merit of the proposed scheme. The experimental work detailed in this study confirms that a pre-trained AlexNet helps achieve a detection accuracy of >93% on the chosen MRI images.

4.3.4 Scheme with integrated features

Earlier research work in the literature confirms that disease detection with medical images achieves a better outcome when it is performed using deep features (DF) combined with handcrafted features (HF) [23–25]. Figure 4.3 presents the structure of such a scheme, in which the deep and handcrafted features are separately mined using test images. These features are then reduced with the FA, and a serial concatenation is implemented to get the necessary feature vector.

In this work, the deep feature is obtained from AlexNet. It helps to acquire a one-dimensional (1D) feature vector with dimensions of 1×1×1000 px, which is then reduced using the FA algorithm. The FA-based reduction helps to achieve a feature vector with dimensions of 1×1×418 px. Similar feature reduction is also applied for the integrated handcrafted feature vector; the FA-based reduction helps to achieve dimensions of 1×1×229 px. These features are then serially concatenated to get a new feature vector with a feature size of 1×1×647 px. These features are then considered

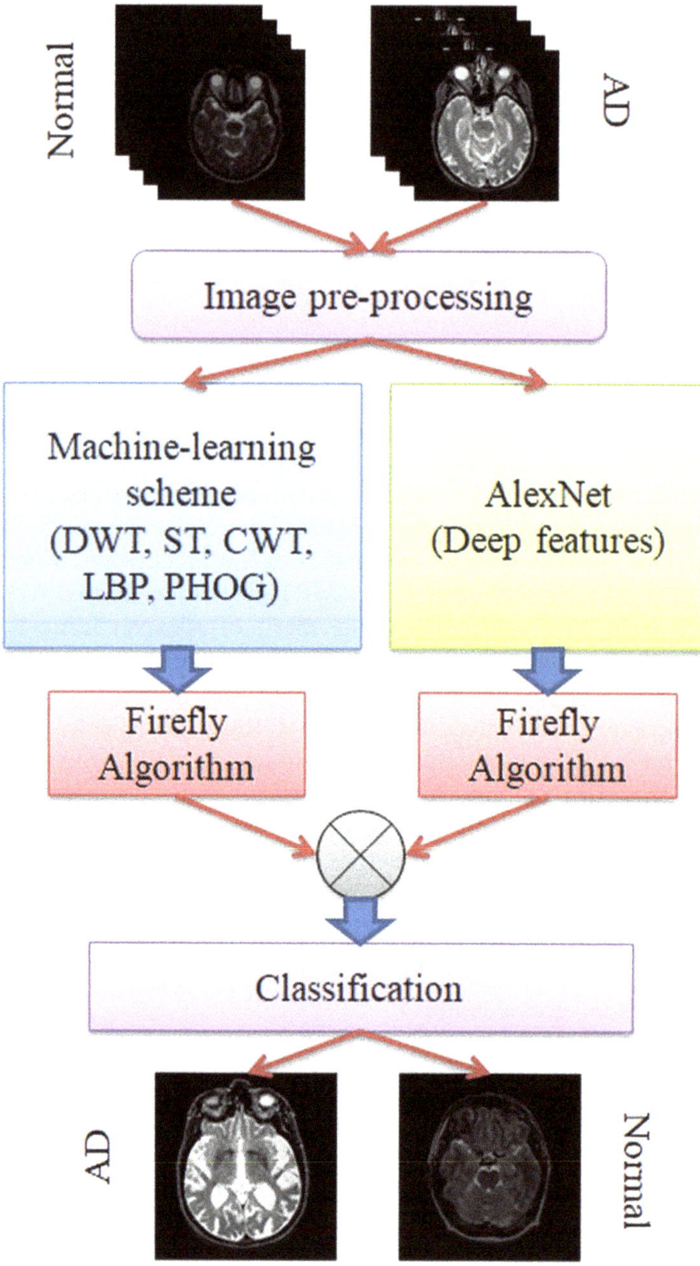

Figure 4.3. Detection of AD in MRI using the integrated features.

to classify the brain MRI slices into either normal or AD class; the classification achieved a detection accuracy of >98%. This confirms that, if a CAS is implemented with integrated deep and handcrafted features, it is possible to detect the disease with better accuracy.

4.3.5 Data collection and pre-processing

The success of the automatic disease detection process depends on the database(s) considered to train the computerized algorithm. In this work, clinical-grade MRI slices available in benchmark data sets such as ADNI, TCIA, and HBAD are considered. The collected MRI slices are then resized to $227 \times 227 \times 3$ px and the existing skull section is then removed using a threshold filter. The threshold filter helps to separate the MRI slice into the brain segment and the skull using a chosen threshold value; information about this procedure can be found in [29, 30].

In this work 1000 MRI slices (500 normal and 500 AD) are considered for assessment. During the classification task 80% of the images are considered to train the CAS and 20% of the images are given to test the performance of the system. The performance evaluation of the developed CAS is done using the MRI slices with/without the skull. The proposed CAS is separately executed with (i) handcrafted features (HF), (ii) deep features (DF), and (iii) integrated deep and handcrafted features (HF + DF), and the resulting performance is separately evaluated to confirm the merit and complexity of the developed CAS.

Figure 4.4 depicts sample test images collected from ADNI, TCIA, and HBAD for both the normal and AD classes. The skull-stripping process from these images is achieved with a threshold filter, and this process is depicted in figure 4.5.

Skull stripping during MRI slice assessment is commonly performed to increase detection accuracy. Earlier works that implement a skull-stripping step when assessing brain MRI slices can be found in [31]. In this work, the skull stripping is employed using the thresholding filter [29, 30]. During this operation, a chosen threshold value is assigned to group the image pixels into two groups: the brain region and the non-brain region (i.e. skull and other artifacts). This process is graphically depicted in figure 4.5. As is shown, the test image is separated into skull and brain sections using the employed filter. The threshold value for this work is assigned manually using a trial and error method, and the assigned value is considered for all the images to extract the skull.

Let us consider that the image has a threshold value (Th) ranging from 0 to 256; then, the selected Th must be between 0 and 256, as in $0 < \text{Th} < 256$, which separates the skull. Figure 4.6 depicts the various images and their related gray-level histograms. From this it can be observed that the proposed technique separates the image (histogram) based on a chosen threshold value. In this work, the proposed CAS is initially implemented on MRI scans with the skull and a similar procedure is then validated on MRI scans without the skull, and the attained results are then presented.

4.3.6 Feature extraction and selection

The performance of the automatic disease detection depends on the features considered to identify the images with improved accuracy. In the proposed CAS, features such as (i) handcrafted features, (ii) deep features, and (iii) integrated features are considered.

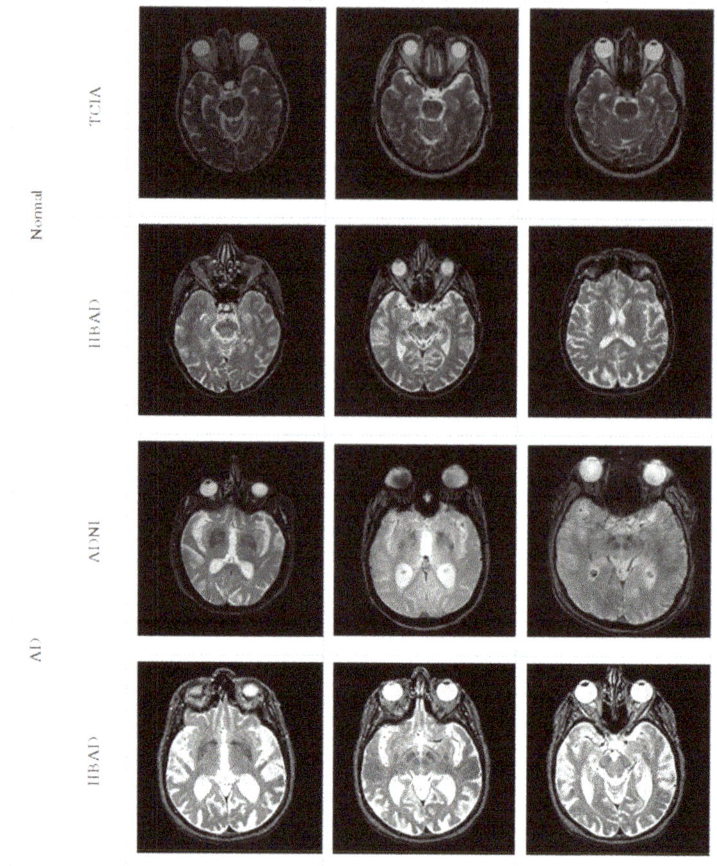

Figure 4.4. Sample test images considered in this study.

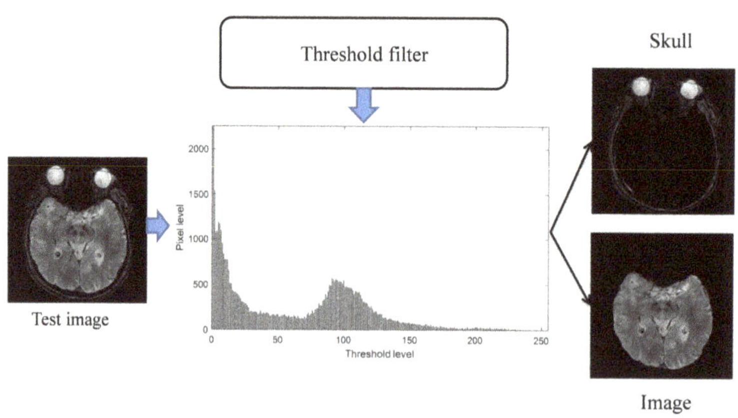

Figure 4.5. Implementation of threshold filter to separate skull and brain sections.

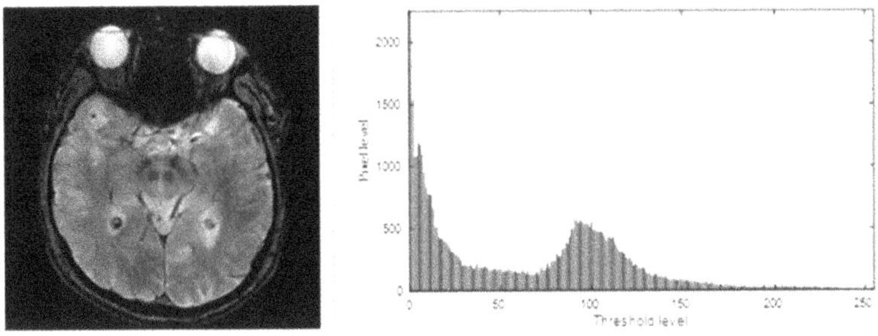

(a) Test image along its gray-hisogram

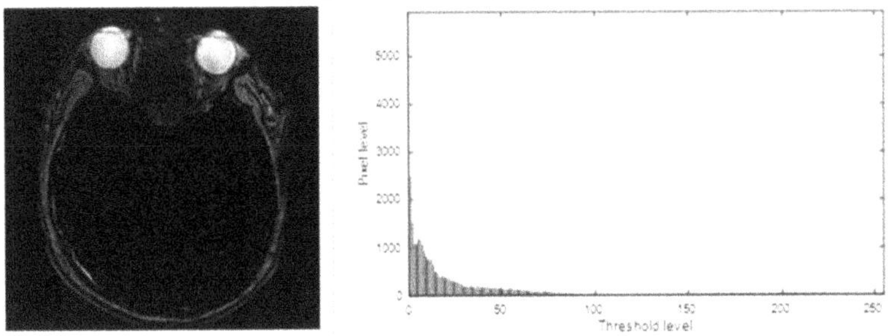

(b) Skull section along its gray-hisogram

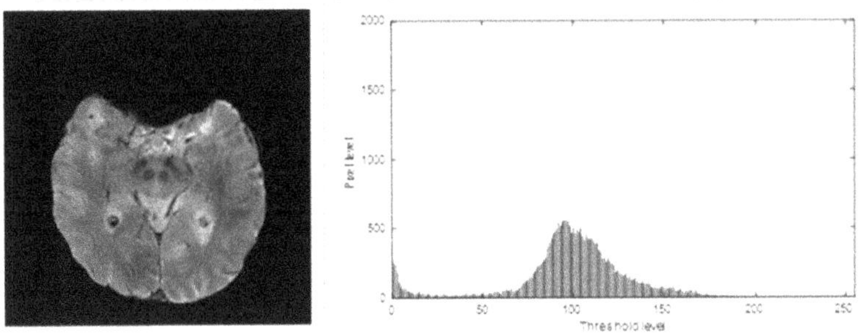

(c) MRI without section along its gray-hisogram

Figure 4.6. Various class images and their gray-level histograms.

4.3.6.1 Handcrafted features

This work builds on the methodology that Acharya *et al* (2019) implemented to detect AD using MRI slices [16]. The necessary image features are initially extracted from the MRI slice using the aforementioned procedures, e.g. DWTs, STs, CWTs, LBPs, and PHOGs.

The mined features are then reduced using the FA; this procedure is depicted graphically in figure 7. FA is a nature-inspired heuristic algorithm proposed by Yang in 2008 [32–34]. Due to its advantages and optimization exactitude,

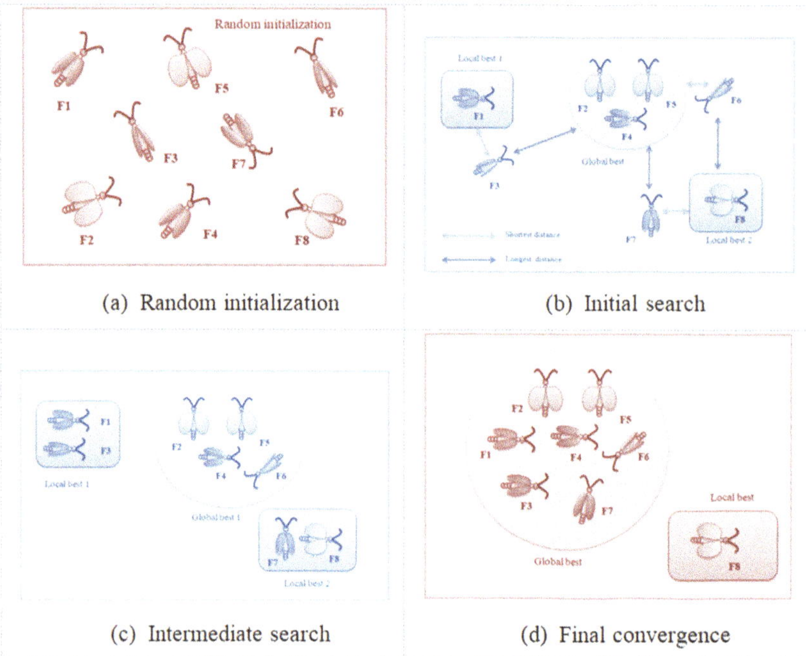

(a) Random initialization (b) Initial search

(c) Intermediate search (d) Final convergence

Figure 4.7. Working principle of firefly algorithm.

researchers have extensively adopted it to discover solutions for various optimization problems. The FA was developed by mimicking the community behaviors of fireflies. The early versions of the FA adopted a Lévy flight (LF) scheme to execute convergence. In order to enhance the performance of this conventional FA, a substantial number of improvements have been made by replacing the LF with other operators [35]. A Brownian walk (BW) is one of the known methodologies adopted by researchers to improve the FA's convergence towards the best optimal solution. Earlier works on this can be found in [36, 37]. Compared to FA with LF, the merit of this scheme is that it provides a steady and optimal answer for the chosen optimization problem. Therefore, a FA with BW is selected to find the optimal features in this work.

Figure 4.7 shows step-by-step images examining the association of fireflies from a random location towards an optimal location. Figure 4.7(a) shows the scattered fireflies in the search area, and figure 4.7(b) demonstrates the initial movement among the fireflies towards the optimal location by computing the Cartesian distance (CD) between the flies. Finally, figures 4.7(c) and (d) present the flies' intermediate and final converged positions towards the optimized result. The complete working methodology can be found in [36, 37].

The mathematical expression of the FA is depicted below.

Let us consider, in a search space, that there exist two groups of fireflies, labeled i and j. Due to a process of attraction, as observed in nature, firefly group i will move closer to firefly group j. This procedure can be denoted as follows:

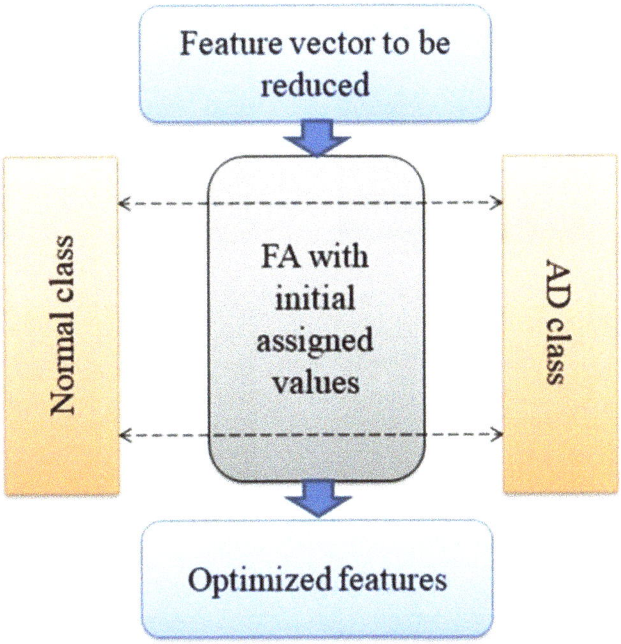

Figure 4.8. Firefly-algorithm-supported feature selection process.

$$X_i^{t+1} = X_i^t + \beta_0 e^{-\gamma d_{ij}^t}\left(X_j^t - X_i^t\right) + BW, \tag{4.1}$$

where X_i^t is the initial position of firefly i, X_j^t is the initial position of firefly j, BW stands for Brownian walk, β_0 is the attractiveness coefficient, γ is the light absorption coefficient, and d_{ij}^t is the CD between flies. In this work, the FA is initialized with the following parameters: No. of flies = 50; search dimension = feature to be selected; iteration value = 3000; const function = maximized CD; terminating criteria = maximal iteration.

A graphical representation of the feature reduction is clearly presented in figure 4.8, in which the FA is responsible for selecting the optimal features based on the CD.

During this task, the firefly algorithm aims to find the CD between the features of the normal and AD class images; the feature which has the maximal CD is considered, and the features which show a minimal CD are discarded. This is the concept behind FA-supported feature reduction; similar procedures can be found in the literature. In this work, the FA is utilized to find optimal values in handcrafted and deep features.

DWT feature extraction is widely adopted in image examination tasks. It separates an image into four subgroups, such as approximate, a vertical, horizontal and diagonal coefficients. The DWT features from these processed images are mined, as discussed by Acharya *et al* [16]. Figure 4.9 depicts the DWT -treated

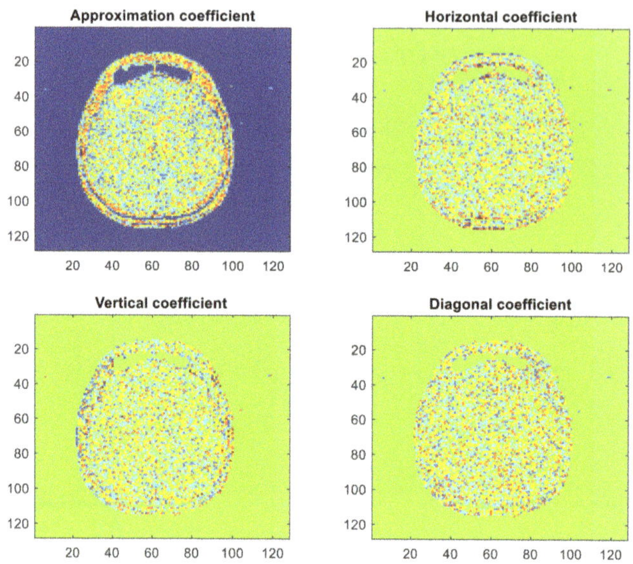

(a) Normal class MRI

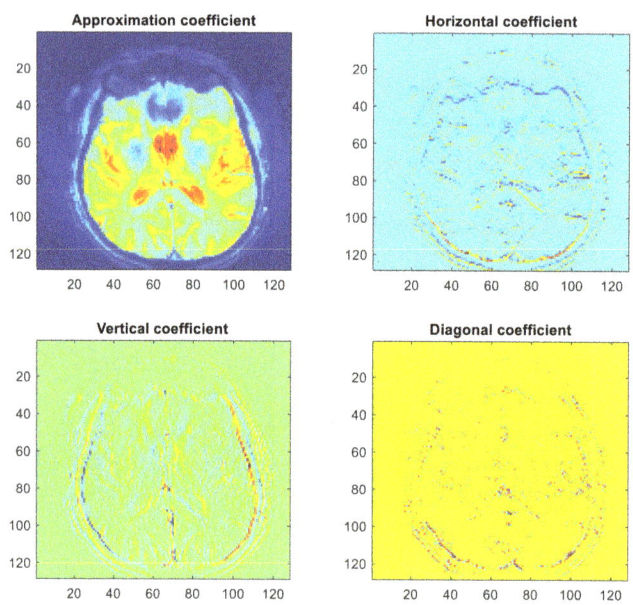

(b) AD class MRI

Figure 4.9. MRI slices processed with DWT scheme.

image section for normal (figure 4.9(a)) and AD class brain MRI scans (figure 4.9(b)). After extracting the features, FA-based feature reduction is employed to select the best features. In this case, the procedure helped to achieve 40 features, as in equation (4.2):

Table 4.2. Feature table using shearlet transform.

	Normal		AD			
Features (entropy)	Mean	SD	Mean	SD	*p*-value	*t*-value
$KapurEntropy_{Vertical}$	0.5335	0.1866	0.7715	0.1253	0.0001	5.7252
$YagerEntropy_{Vertical}$	0.6477	0.1474	0.5024	0.2005	0.0001	5.6615
VadjaEntropyss	0.6118	0.1758	0.2263	0.1274	0.0001	5.3753
$KapurEntropy_{Vertical}$	0.7479	0.1116	0.5112	0.1653	0.0002	5.3695
Max $Entropy_{Vertical}$	0.5593	0.1096	0.2145	0.1085	0.0007	5.3318
Max Entropys	0.6478	0.1363	0.2643	0.2075	0.0001	5.3085
$Energy_{Horizontal}$	0.6024	0.1166	0.5163	0.1163	0.0008	5.2864
$FuzzyEntropy_{Vertical}$	0.4166	0.1232	0.7885	0.1753	0.0004	5.2661
$FuzzyEntropy_{Vertical}$	0.4755	0.1007	0.7622	0.1085	0.0001	5.2265
$FuzzyEntropy_{Horizontal}$	0.4007	0.1464	0.5008	0.2046	0.0001	5.2221
$KapurEntropy_{Vertical}$	0.3164	0.1337	0.7113	0.1334	0.0001	5.2207
$FuzzyEntropy_{Vertical}$	0.2899	0.1075	0.7274	0.2001	0.0001	5.2202
Max $Entropy_{Horizontal}$	0.6477	0.1442	0.2173	0.1657	0.0005	5.2107
$VadjaEntropy_{Horizontal}$	0.4702	0.1788	0.3396	0.1703	0.0002	5.2054
$VadjaEntropy_{Vertical}$	0.3376	0.1812	0.4163	0.1454	0.0002	5.1884

$$DWT_{(1 \times 1 \times 400)} = DWT_{(1,1)}, DWT_{(1,2)}, \ldots, DWT_{(1,40)}. \tag{4.2}$$

The ST features (entropies) extracted for this data set have dimensions of $1 \times 1 \times 280$ px. FA-assisted feature reduction is then implemented to reduce these features by discarding the values whose p-value is <0.005. In this work, only 15 types of features are collected; these features are calculated as in equation (4.3):

$$ST_{(1 \times 1 \times 415)} = STT_{(1,1)}, ST_{(1,2)}, \ldots, s_{(1,15)}. \tag{4.3}$$

The statistically collected ST features are shown in table 4.2, and the ranges of these features are presented in figure 4.10 using box plots. These values confirm that the proposed scheme will well evaluate the considered MRI data set.

Along with the DWT and ST, other features, like a CWT [38], LBP [39, 40] and PHOG [41, 42], are also mined from these images. The complete information about the extracted CWT features can be found in [38] and the number of features extracted and selected with the FA is denoted in equation (4.4):

$$CWT_{(1 \times 1 \times 28)} = CWT_{(1,1)}, CWT_{(1,2)}, \ldots, CWT_{(1,28)}. \tag{4.4}$$

LBPs are widely employed by researchers to achieve better detection accuracy during ML- and DL-based automatic image examination. In this work, the weighted LBP presented by Gudigar *et al* is considered [40]. Every image is processed using a chosen binary weight (W) with a value between 1 to 4, and the achieved images are

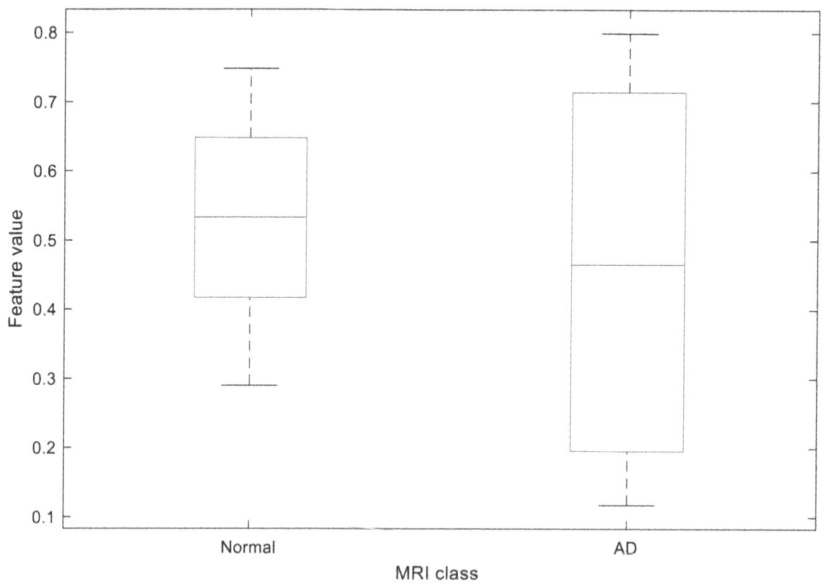

Figure 4.10. Values of ST features depicted as box plots.

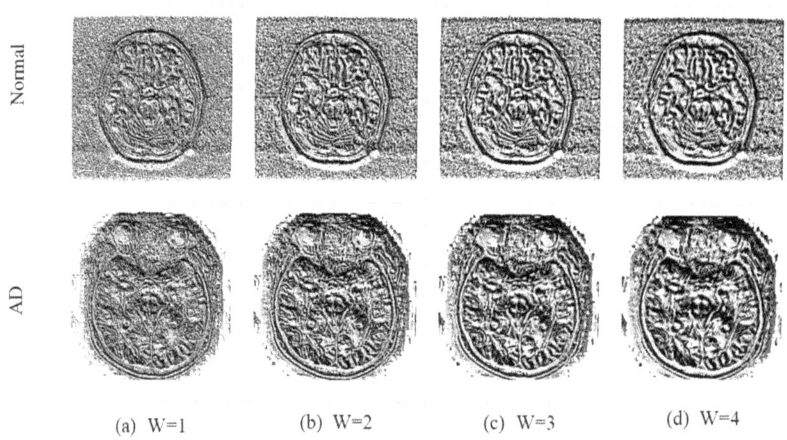

Figure 4.11. MRI image pre-processed using LBP with different weights.

then considered for assessment. The outcome of this procedure is depicted in figure 4.11. Every image is capable of providing $1 \times 1 \times 59$ features; these values are presented in equations (4.5)–(4.8), and the total LBP features considered in this work is depicted in equation (4.9):

$$LBP_1(1 \times 1 \times 59) = LBP_1(1,1), LBP_1(1,2), \ldots, LBP_1(1,59), \tag{4.5}$$

$$LBP_2(1 \times 1 \times 59) = LBP_2(1,1), LBP_2(1,2), \ldots, LBP_2(1,59), \tag{4.6}$$

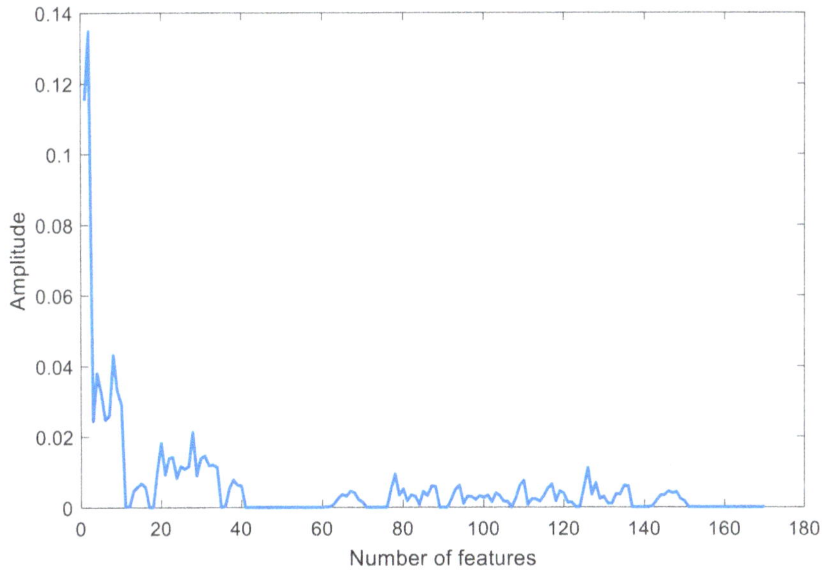

Figure 4.12. PHOG feature achieved for bin = 3.

$$\text{LBP}_3(1 \times 1 \times 59) = \text{LBP}_3(1,1),\ \text{LBP}_3(1,2),\ \ldots,\ \text{LBP}_3(1,59), \tag{4.7}$$

$$\text{LBP}_4(1 \times 1 \times 59) = \text{LBP}_4(1,1),\ \text{LBP}_4(1,2),\ \ldots,\ \text{LBP}_4(1,59), \tag{4.8}$$

$$\text{LBP}_{(1 \times 1 \times 236)} = \text{LBP}_1 + \text{LBP}_2 + \text{LBP}_3 + \text{LBP}_4. \tag{4.9}$$

PHOGs are another important image processing procedure, which help to detect an image's class with better accuracy. Earlier works on PHOGs can be found in [41, 42]; in this work, a PHOG extracted for bin = 3 is considered, and its outcome is shown in figure 4.12. The PHOG helps to acquire a feature vector with a dimension as depicted in equation (4.10):

$$\text{PHOG}_{(1 \times 1 \times 168)} = \text{PHOG}_{(1,1)},\ \text{PHOG}_{(1,2)},\ \ldots,\ \text{PHOG}_{(1,168)}. \tag{4.10}$$

After extracting the necessary handcrafted features, the classification performance if then executed using the k-NN classifier, as presented in Acharya *et al* [16]. Like former classifiers, the k-NN needs similar training and testing using image features. The arithmetical presentation of k-NN is as follows.

Let there exist two feature vectors of D dimensions, $M = (M_1, M_2, \ldots M_n)^T$ and $N = (N_1, N_2, \ldots N_n)^T$. Then, the Euclidean distance can be shown as

$$\text{Euclidean distance}\left(\overrightarrow{M}, \overrightarrow{N}\right) = \sqrt{(M_1 - N_1)^2 + (M_2 - N_2)^2 +, \ldots, (M_D - N_1)^2}. \tag{4.11}$$

The collected and reduced feature set using a Student's t-test is then considered to train and validate the detection performance of the k-NN classifier. To demonstrate the performance of the k-NN on individual features, the feature subsets of the DWT,

ST, and CWT are considered and the achieved results are discussed for various features ranging from feature dimension 2 to its maximal value; the achieved results are presented in figure 4.13. This work initially computes measures, such as true-positive (TP) rate, true-negative (TN) rate, false-positive (FP) rate, and false-

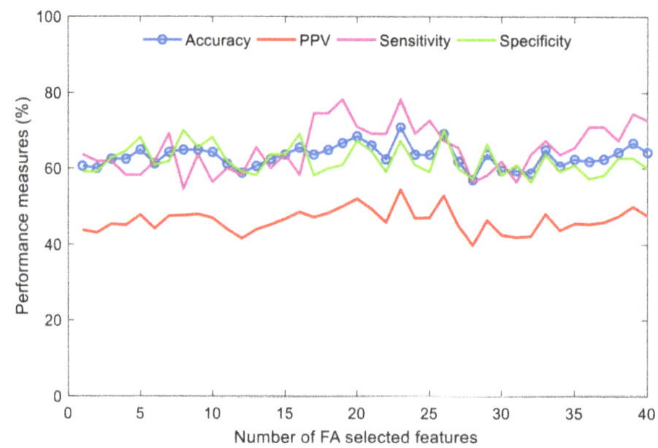

(a) DWT features

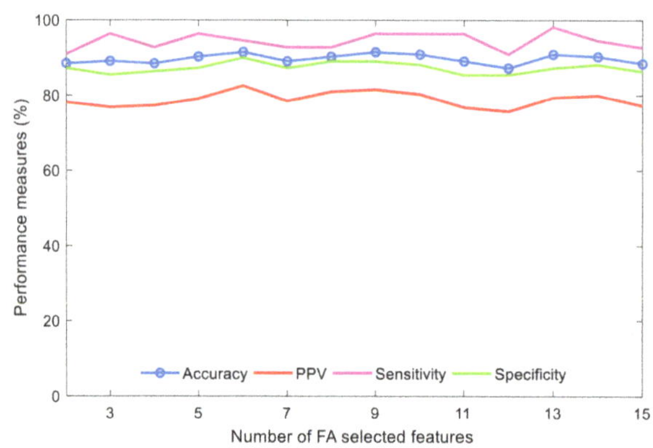

(b) ST features

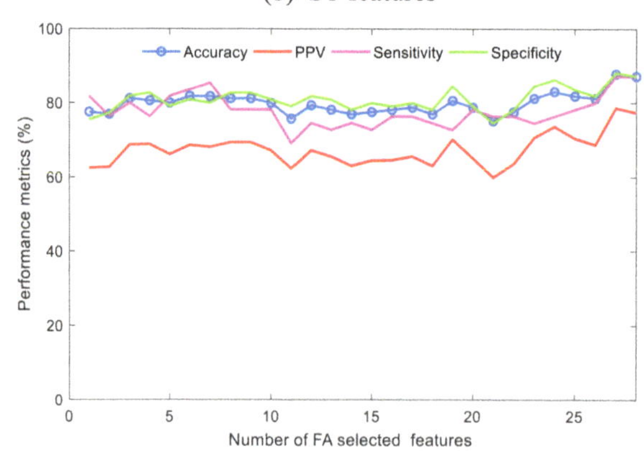

(c) CWT features

Figure 4.13. Individual performance evaluation of DWT, ST, and CWT features.

negative (FN) rate, and from these values, the metrics, such as accuracy, positive predictive value (PPV), sensitivity, and specificity are derived.

Figure 4.13(a) presents the classification results achieved with the DWT for a feature vector with dimensions 2–40; the maximum accuracy achieved with this feature subset is <75%. Figure 4.13(b) presents the classification results obtained with the ST for feature values of 2–15, which helps to achieve a classification accuracy of >88%. Figure 4.13(c) presents the AD detection using CWT features with values 2–28, and this procedure also helped to achieve a detection accuracy of >88%. Hence, in this work a combined feature vector is considered in order to achieve better detection accuracy during the examination of normal/AD class MRI slices.

4.3.6.2 Deep features

Deep-feature-supported disease detection is widely employed due to its enhanced detection accuracy. Presently, pre-trained DL systems are widely employed in analyzing medical-grade images, and in this work the AlexNet architecture is considered to classify the MRI slices into normal/AD classes. This work initially extracts $1 \times 1 \times 4096$ features and, after a possible dropout, the SoftMax function receives a feature vector of $1 \times 1 \times 1000$. This feature is then utilized to detect AD from the MRI. Conventional deep feature dimensions are large, and hence a feature reduction is then employed using the FA, which helps to generate a reduced feature vector of $1 \times 1 \times 418$.

Equations (4.11) and (4.12) present the actual and reduced DF:

$$DF_{(1 \times 1 \times 1000)} = DF_{(1,1)}, DF_{(1,2)}, \ldots, DF_{(1,1000)}, \tag{4.12}$$

$$DF_{(1 \times 1 \times 418)} = DF_{(1,1)}, DF_{(1,2)}, \ldots, DF_{(1,418)}. \tag{4.13}$$

4.3.6.3 Integrated deep and handcrafted features

Earlier research works have confirmed that an integrated DF and HF implementation helps to achieve a better outcome during the medical image examination process. In this work, the FA-optimized HF and DF are combined to achieve a new feature vector (HF + DF), as shown in equations (4.14) and (4.15):

$$HF_{(1 \times 1 \times 229)} = HF_{(1,1)}, HF_{(1,2)}, \ldots, HF_{(1,229)s}, \tag{4.14}$$

$$DF + HF_{(1 \times 1 \times 647)} = DF_{(1 \times 1 \times 418)} + HF_{(1 \times 1 \times 229)}. \tag{4.15}$$

The above discussed features are then considered to test the performance of the developed CAS using various binary classifiers with fivefold cross-validation.

4.3.7 Validation

The implentation of the CAS was validated by calculating the necessary performance metrics, such as accuracy, PPV, sensitivity, and specificity [43]. In order to develop the assessment ability, a fivefold cross-validation was employed. The obtained values are computed using equations (4.16)–(4.19):

$$\text{Accuracy} = (T_P + T_N)/(T_P + T_N + F_P + F_N), \tag{4.16}$$

$$\text{Precision} = \text{PPV} = T_P/(T_P + F_P), \tag{4.17}$$

$$\text{Sensitvity} = \text{Recall} = T_P/(T_P + F_N), \tag{4.18}$$

$$\text{Specificity} = T_N/(T_N + F_P). \tag{4.19}$$

4.4 Results and discussions

This section presents the experimental results and discussion. The proposed method is verified using MRI slices, the classification of which is achieved using the above detailed ML and DL methods. The investigation is repeated separately for the images with/without the skull section and the results are presented.

HF-based classification of MRI into normal/AD is initially executed using the FA-selected and serially concatenated DWT, ST, CWT, LBP, and PHOG features. This provides a 1D feature vector of dimension 1×1×229 (as in equation (4.14)), which is then executed using the chosen binary classifiers; the achieved results for the images (with/without skull) are presented in tables 4.3 and 4.4. The experimental results of table 4.3 confirm that the classification accuracy (84.5%) using a support

Table 4.3. HF-based experimental outcome for MRI scans with the skull.

Classifier	TP	FN	TN	FP	Accuracy	PPV	Sensitivity	Specificity
k-NN	85	15	83	17	84.0000	83.3333	85.0000	83.0000
DT	84	16	81	19	82.5000	81.5534	84.0000	81.0000
RF	83	17	83	17	83.0000	83.0000	83.0000	83.0000
NB	82	18	86	14	84.0000	85.4167	82.0000	86.0000
SVM-L	86	14	83	17	84.5000	83.4951	86.0000	83.0000
SVM-RBF	85	15	84	16	84.5000	84.1584	85.0000	84.0000

Table 4.4. HF-based experimental outcome for MRI scans without the skull.

Classifier	TP	FN	TN	FP	Accuracy	PPV	Sensitivity	Specificity
k-NN	84	16	88	12	86.0000	87.5000	84.0000	88.0000
DT	85	15	87	13	86.0000	86.7347	85.0000	87.0000
RF	87	13	87	13	87.0000	87.0000	87.0000	87.0000
NB	86	14	86	14	86.0000	86.0000	86.0000	86.0000
SVM-L	88	12	86	14	87.0000	86.2745	88.0000	86.0000
SVM-RBF	87	13	86	14	86.5000	86.1386	87.0000	86.0000

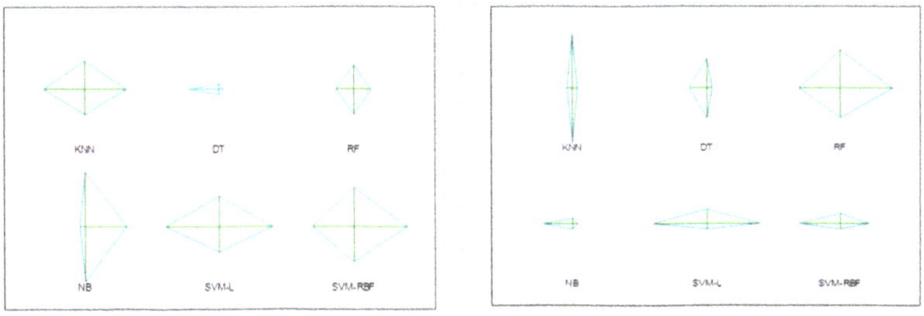

(a) With skull (b) Without skull

Figure 4.14. Glyph plot to demonstrate the overall merit of the classification tasks.

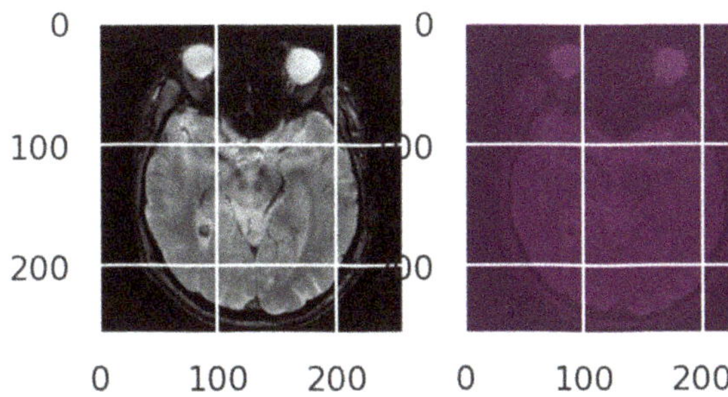

Figure 4.15. Saliency map for a chosen test image.

vector machine (SVM) is better than compared to other schemes. The results of table 4.4 further verify that the accuracy (87%) of the support vector machines with linear kernel (SVM-L) and support vector machines with radial basis function (SVM-RBF) is better. This confirms that the MRI scans without the skull offer better results compared to MRI scans with the skull. The overall performance is represented graphically using a glyph plot (figure 4.14). Figures 4.14(a) and (b) present the outcomes for brain MRI slices with/without the skull.

After verifying the AD detection performance with the HF, the pre-trained AlexNet is then utilized to classify the test images into normal/AD classes using the binary classifiers. During this task, a 1D feature vector of dimensions 1×1×1000 is considered, and during the experiment fivefold cross-validation is adopted to achieve a consistent result. During this process, along with the results, other outcomes from the various layers of the AlexNet are extracted and presented.

Figure 4.15 presents an enhanced sample test images at the initial layer of the AlexNet and then after training; the images extracted from the various convolutional layers are shown in figure 4.16. Figures 4.16(a)–(d) show the extracted images from convolutional layers 1–4, which demonstrate the learning of the AlexNet for a given image. The training and testing is executed for 100 epochs, and the achieved results are separately stored for the model accuracy and loss functions, as depicted in figures 4.17(a) and (b). This result is achieved with the SoftMax classifier, and a similar procedure is then repeated using other the classifiers considered in this study.

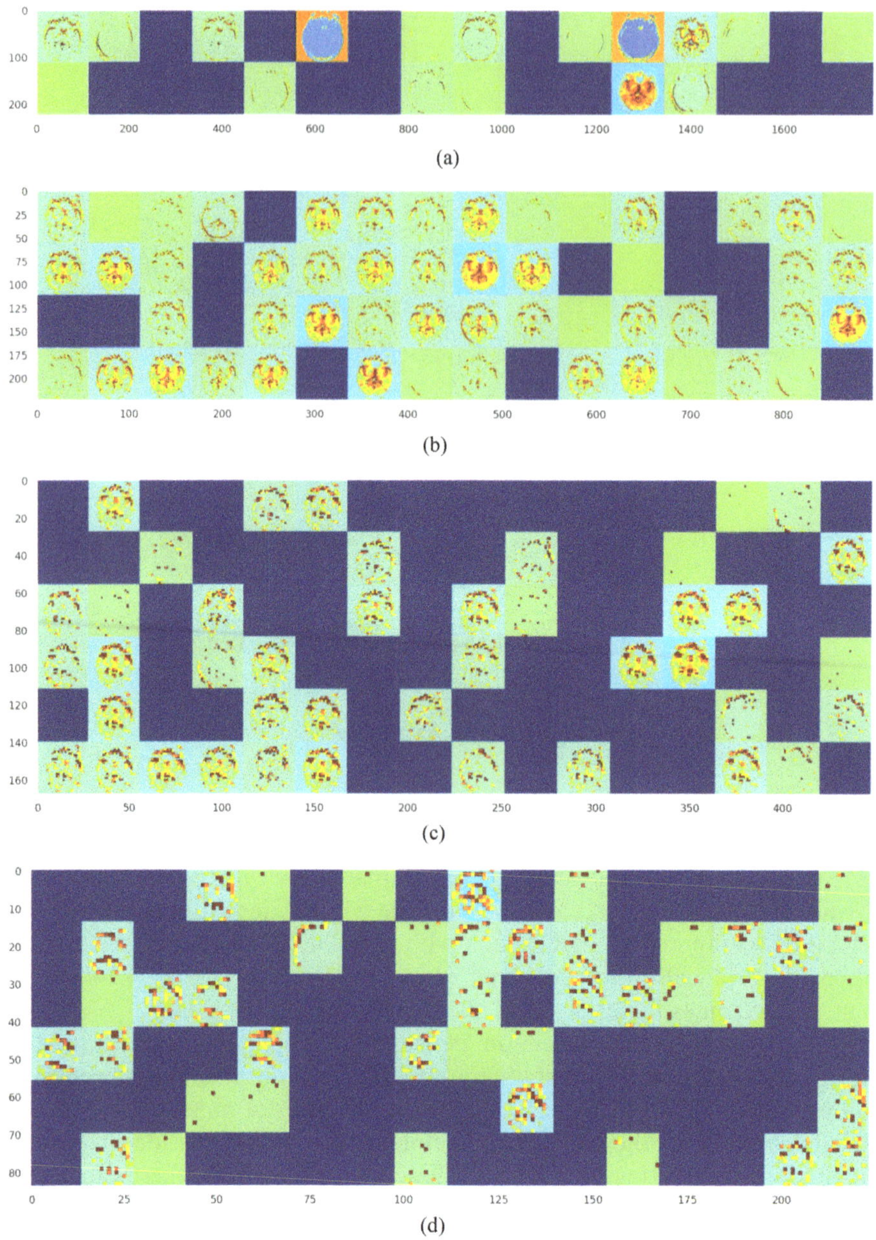

Figure 4.16. Various convolutional layer results by AlexNet.

The obtained confusion matrix (CM) and the receiver operating characteristic curve are depicted in figures 4.18 and 4.19, respectively. The parameters of the CM help to compute the other essential performance metrics such accuracy, PPV, sensitivity, and specificity and, based on these values, the merit of the proposed scheme is verified.

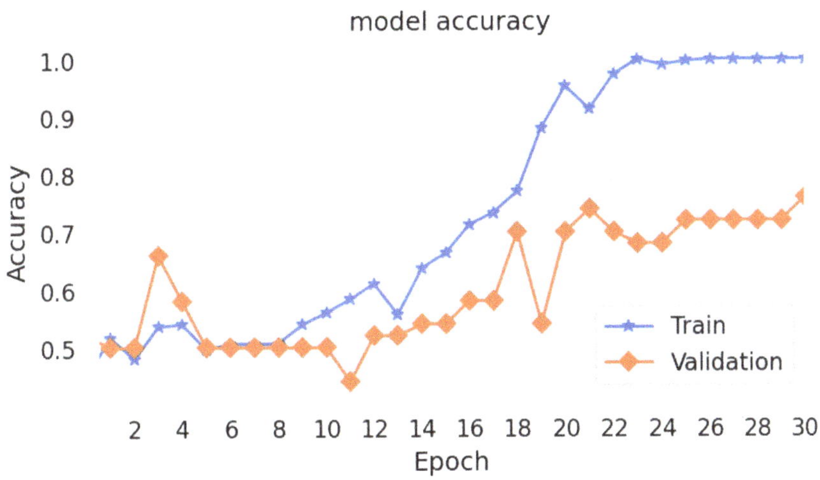

(a)

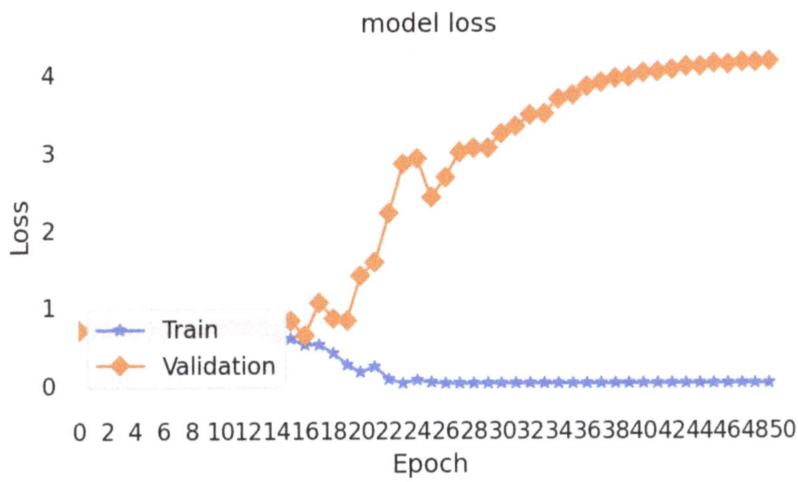

(b)

Figure 4.17. Search convergences for AlexNet with SoftMax classifier.

The results achieved with this configuration of AlexNet and binary classifiers for MRI scans with/without skull are then examined individually; the achieved outcomes are shown in tables 4.5 and 4.6, respectively. The values given in table 4.5 confirm a classification accuracy of 91% with SVM-L, and table 4.6 verifies that the accuracy of SVM-L is better (92%) than compared to other classifiers. The overall merit of this experiment is then verified with a glyph plot (figure 4.20), which confirms that the results achieved with the MRI scans without skull are superior to the MRI scans with skull. To improve the detection accuracy further, this task is then repeated with the integrated HF+DF using the feature vector depicted in equation (4.15) and the results are presented.

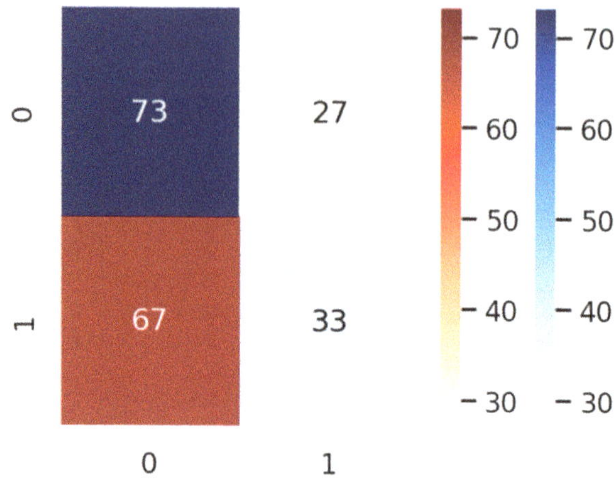

Figure 4.18. Confusion matrix.

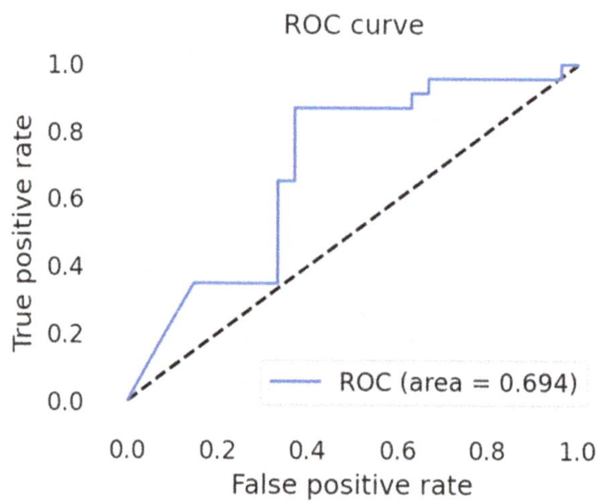

Figure 4.19. Receiver operating characteristic (ROC) curve.

Table 4.5. DF-based experimental outcome for the MRI scans with skull.

Classifier	TP	FN	TN	FP	Accuracy	PPV	Sensitivity	Specificity
SoftMax	88	12	89	11	88.5000	88.8889	88.0000	89.0000
k-NN	90	10	91	9	90.5000	90.9091	90.0000	91.0000
DT	89	11	89	11	89.0000	89.0000	89.0000	89.0000
RF	90	10	88	12	89.0000	88.2353	90.0000	88.0000
NB	91	9	89	11	90.0000	89.2157	91.0000	89.0000
SVM-L	91	9	91	9	91.0000	91.0000	91.0000	91.0000
SVM-RBF	90	10	91	9	90.5000	90.9091	90.0000	91.0000

Table 4.6. DF-based experimental outcome for the MRI scans without skull.

Classifier	TP	FN	TN	FP	Accuracy	PPV	Sensitivity	Specificity
SoftMax	90	10	91	9	90.5000	90.9091	90.0000	91.0000
k-NN	92	8	91	9	91.5000	91.0891	92.0000	91.0000
DT	91	9	91	9	91.0000	91.0000	91.0000	91.0000
RF	90	10	92	8	91.0000	91.8367	90.0000	92.0000
NB	91	9	92	8	91.5000	91.9192	91.0000	92.0000
SVM-L	91	9	93	7	92.0000	92.8571	91.0000	93.0000
SVM-RBF	89	11	91	9	90.0000	90.8163	89.0000	91.0000

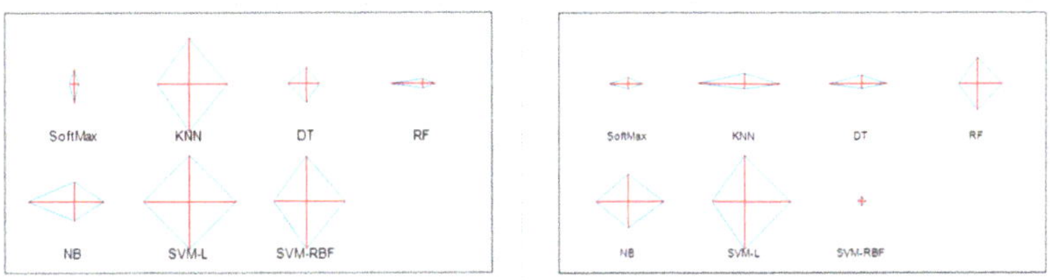

(a) With skull (b) Without skull

Figure 4.20. Glyph plot to demonstrate the overall merit of AlexNet.

The performance of the AlexNet is then verified using new normal/AD class MRI images, and the results are presented in figure 4.21. These results confirm that the DF-based AD detection helps achieve a better detection accuracy (>90%) for the MRI slices with/without the skull. A similar procedure is repeated with the HF+DF; the results are presented in tables 4.7 and 4.8, and a graphical comparison is presented in figure 4.22. These results confirm that the proposed scheme helps achieve an accuracy of 95.5% for MRI scans with skull and 97.5% for MRI scans without skull. This confirms that the proposed scheme helps to detect AD to better accuracy, and that in the future this scheme can be considered to classify clinical-grade MRI images into normal/AD classes.

This chapter has thus presented a detailed study on the detection of normal/AD class MRI slices using DF, FA-selected HF and FA-selected HF+DF, and demonstrated better outcomes with MRI slices without the skull section. This work considered only the AlexNet scheme and achieved a detection accuracy of 97.5%. In future, other DL architectures should be considered to improve the accuracy to as close to 100% as possible. Further, the FA-based feature selection can be replaced with other recent heuristic algorithms in the literature.

4.5 Conclusion

In this research, examination of T2-weighted axial-plane brain MRI was considered, and a newly devised task was executed for MRI scans with/without the skull section. The purpose of this research is to develop a proficient CAS to detect AD from a

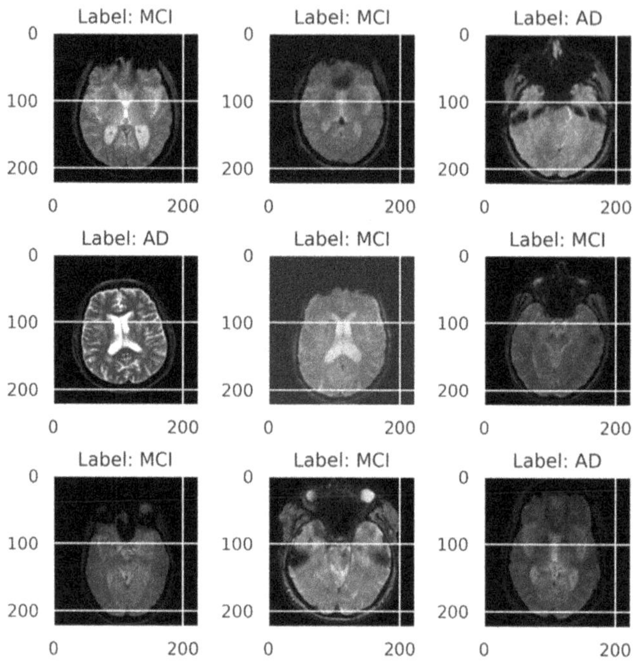

Figure 4.21. Classification outcome during the validation process.

Table 4.7. HF+DF-based experimental outcome for the MRI scans with skull.

Classifier	TP	FN	TN	FP	Accuracy	PPV	Sensitivity	Specificity
k-NN	95	5	96	4	0.9550	0.9596	0.9500	0.9600
DT	93	7	92	8	0.9250	0.9208	0.9300	0.9200
RF	95	5	91	9	0.9300	0.9135	0.9500	0.9100
NB	90	10	93	7	0.9150	0.9278	0.9000	0.9300
SVM-L	93	7	94	6	0.9350	0.9394	0.9300	0.9400
SVM-RBF	95	5	95	5	0.9500	0.9500	0.9500	0.9500

Table 4.8. HF+DF-based experimental outcome for the MRI scans without the skull.

Classifier	TP	FN	TN	FP	Accuracy	PPV	Sensitivity	Specificity
k-NN	98	2	97	3	0.9750	0.9703	0.9800	0.9700
DT	94	6	94	6	0.9400	0.9400	0.9400	0.9400
RF	95	5	95	5	0.9500	0.9500	0.9500	0.9500
NB	96	4	98	2	0.9700	0.9796	0.9600	0.9800
SVM-L	97	3	97	3	0.9700	0.9700	0.9700	0.9700
SVM-RBF	94	6	97	3	0.9550	.9691	0.9400	0.9700

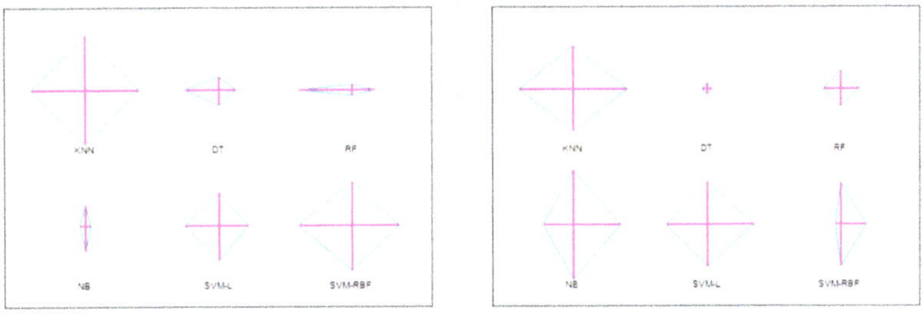

(a) With skull (b) Without skull

Figure 4.22. Glyph plot to demonstrate the overall merit of HF+DF classification.

chosen test image. The experimental investigation was performed with (i) HF, (ii) DF, and (iii) HF+DF. In this work, FA-based feature selection is employed to reduce the HF and DF to avoid any overfitting issues during classification. The results of this study confirm that the detection implemented with HF+DF along with the *k*-NN classifier helped to achieve an accuracy of 97.5%. The outcomes of this work attest to the clinical significance of the proposed technique, and in future it can be considered to examine clinical MRI.

It is important to be able to assess the severity of brain abnormalities caused by AD without resorting to slower manual techniques, which may even be more cost prohibitive when providing supportive care. A detailed evaluation of existing feature extraction procedures is also presented in this chapter, using feature selection implemented based on Student's *t*-test. The outcome of this work confirms that the ST+*k*-NN technique offers better results than the alternatives. Further, the number of features required for the ST+*k*-NN is very few (four) compared to other techniques. The proposed procedure offered better results on brain MRI scans obtained from both a medical clinic and from benchmark AD data sets. In the future, the performance of this system may be improved by replacing the *k*-NN classifier with other existing classifiers.

Conflict of interest

The authors declare that they have no conflict of interest.

References

[1] Fang P, Ge R, She Y, Zhao J, Yan J, Yu X and Zhang Z 2022 Adipose tissue spexin in physical exercise and age-associated diseases *Ageing Res. Rev.* **73** 101509

[2] Rajinikanth V, Kadry S, Taniar D, Kamalanand K, Elaziz M A and Thanaraj K P 2022 Detecting epilepsy in EEG signals using synchro-extracting-transform (SET) supported classification technique *J. Ambient Intell. Human. Comput.* https://doi.org/10.1007/s12652-021-03676-x

[3] Rajinikanth V, Sivakumar R, Hemanth D J, Kadry S, Mohanty J R, Arunmozhi S and Nhu N G 2021 Automated classification of retinal images into AMD/non-AMD class—a study

using multi-threshold and Gaussian-filter enhanced images *Evolutionary Intelligence* **14** 1163–71

[4] WHO 2020 The top 10 causes of death https://who.int/news-room/fact-sheets/detail/the-top-10-causes-of-death

[5] Head E, Powell D, Gold B T and Schmitt F A 2014 Alzheimer's disease in down syndrome *Eur. J. Neurodegener Dis.* **1** 353–64

[6] Wang T, Qiu R G and Yu M 2018 Predictive modeling of the progression of Alzheimer's disease with recurrent neural networks *Sci. Rep.* **8** 9161

[7] Haaksma M L *et al* 2017 Comorbidity and progression of late onset Alzheimer's disease: a systematic review *PLoS One* **12** e0177044

[8] Malik G A and Robertson N P 2017 Treatments in Alzheimer's disease *J. Neurol.* **264** 416–18

[9] Editorial 2011 The three stages of Alzheimer's disease *Lancet* **377** P1465

[10] Neugroschl J and Wang S 2011 Alzheimer's disease: diagnosis and treatment across the spectrum of disease severity *Mt. Sinai. J. Med.* **78** 596–612

[11] Merlo Pich E *et al* 2014 Imaging as a biomarker in drug discovery for Alzheimer's disease: is MRI a suitable technology? *Alzheimer's Research and Therapy* **6** 51

[12] Braskie M N, Toga A W and Thompson P M 2013 Recent advances in imaging Alzheimer's disease *J. Alzheimers Dis.* **33** S313–327

[13] Norfray J F and Provenzale J M 2004 Alzheimer's disease: neuropathologic findings and recent advances in imaging *AJR Am. J. Roentgenol* **182** 3–13

[14] Whalley L J 2012 Spatial distribution and secular trends in the epidemiology of Alzheimer's disease *Neuroimaging Clin. N. Am.* **22** 1–10

[15] Stonnington C M *et al* 2010 Predicting clinical scores from magnetic resonance scans in Alzheimer's disease *NeuroImage* **5** 1405–413

[16] Acharya U R, Fernandes S L, WeiKoh J E, Ciaccio E J, Fabell M K M, Tanik U J and Yeong C H 2019 Automated detection of Alzheimer's disease using brain MRI images–a study with various feature extraction techniques *J. Med. Syst.* **43** 302

[17] Dimitriadis S I, Liparas D and Tsolaki M N 2018 Random forest feature selection, fusion and ensemble strategy: combining multiple morphological MRI measures to discriminate among healhy elderly, MCI, cMCI and Alzheimer's disease patients: from the Alzheimer's disease neuroimaging initiative (ADNI) database *J. Neurosci. Methods* **302** 14–23

[18] Beheshti I, Demirel H and Matsuda H 2017 Classification of Alzheimer's disease and prediction of mild cognitive impairment-to-Alzheimer's conversion from structural magnetic resource imaging using feature ranking and a genetic algorithm *Comput. Biol. Med.* **83** 109–19

[19] Petersen R C, Aisen P S, Beckett L A, Donohue M C, Gamst A C, Harvey D J and Weiner M W 2010 Alzheimer's disease neuroimaging initiative (ADNI): clinical characterization *Neurology* **74** 201–9

[20] Pedano N, Flanders A E, Scarpace L, Mikkelsen T, Eschbacher J M, Hermes B and Ostrom Q 2016 The Cancer Imaging Archive: Radiology data from the cancer genome atlas low grade glioma [TCGA-LGG] collection https://doi.org/10.7937/K9/TCIA.2016.L4LTD3TK

[21] Clark K *et al* 2013 The cancer imaging archive (TCIA): maintaining and operating a public information repository *J. Digital Imaging* **26** 1045–57

[22] Syed H H, Khan M A, Tariq U, Armghan A, Alenezi F, Khan J A and Rajinikanth V 2021 A rapid artificial intelligence-based computer-aided diagnosis system for COVID-19 classification from CT images *Behav. Neurol.* **2021**

[23] Khan M A, Rajinikanth V, Satapathy S C, Taniar D, Mohanty J R, Tariq U and Damaševičius R 2021 VGG19 network assisted joint segmentation and classification of lung nodules in CT images *Diagnostics* **11** 2208
[24] Kadry S, Rajinikanth V, González Crespo R and Verdú E 2021 Automated detection of age-related macular degeneration using a pre-trained deep-learning scheme *J. Supercomput.* **78** 7321–40
[25] Kadry S, Taniar D, Damaševičius R and Rajinikanth V 2021 Automated detection of schizophrenia from brain MRI slices using optimized deep-features *7th Int. Conf. on Bio Signals, Images, and Instrumentation (ICBSII)* pp 1–5
[26] Iandola F N, Han S, Moskewicz M W, Ashraf K, Dally W J and Keutzer K 2016 SqueezeNet: AlexNet-level accuracy with 50x fewer parameters and <0.5MB model size arXiv:1602.07360
[27] Bhandary A, Prabhu G A, Rajinikanth V, Thanaraj K P, Satapathy S C, Robbins D E and Raja N S M 2020 Deep-learning framework to detect lung abnormality—a study with chest x-ray and lung CT scan images *Pattern Recognit. Lett.* **129** 271–8
[28] Dey N, Zhang Y D, Rajinikanth V, Pugalenthi R and Raja N S M 2021 Customized VGG19 architecture for pneumonia detection in chest x-rays *Pattern Recognit. Lett.* **143** 67–74
[29] Kadry S, Rajinikanth V, Rho S, Raja N S M, Rao V S and Thanaraj K P 2020 Development of a machine-learning system to classify lung CT scan images into normal/COVID-19 class arXiv:2004.13122
[30] Rajinikanth V, Raja N S M and Kamalanand K 2017 Firefly algorithm assisted segmentation of tumor from brain MRI using Tsallis function and Markov random field *J. Control Engineering and Applied Informatics* **19** 97–106
[31] Yang X S 2010 Firefly algorithm, stochastic test functions and design optimisation arXiv:1003.1409
[32] Yang X S 2013 Chaos-enhanced firefly algorithm with automatic parameter tuning *Recent Algorithms and Applications in Swarm Intelligence Research* (Hershey, PA: IGI Global) pp 125–36
[33] Yang X S 2013 Multiobjective firefly algorithm for continuous optimization *Eng. Comput.* **29** 175–84
[34] Li J, Wei X, Li B and Zeng Z 2022 A survey on firefly algorithms *Neurocomputing* **500** 662–78
[35] Raja N S M, Manic K S and Rajinikanth V 2013 Firefly algorithm with various randomization parameters: an analysis *Int. Conf. on Swarm, Evolutionary, and Memetic Computing* pp 110–21
[36] Sri Madhava Raja N, Rajinikanth V and Latha K 2014 Otsu based optimal multilevel image thresholding using firefly algorithm *Model. Simul. Eng.* **2014** 794574
[37] Begum M, Ferdush J and Uddin M S 2021 A hybrid robust watermarking system based on discrete cosine transform, discrete wavelet transform, and singular value decomposition *J. King Saud University-Computer and Information Sciences* **34** 5856–67
[38] Francis A and Pandian I A 2021 Early detection of Alzheimer's disease using local binary pattern and convolutional neural network *Multimedia Tools Appl.* **80** 29585–600
[39] Gudigar A, Raghavendra U, Devasia T, Nayak K, Danish S M, Kamath G and Acharya U R 2019 Global weighted LBP based entropy features for the assessment of pulmonary hypertension *Pattern Recognit. Lett.* **125** 35–41

[40] Shang J, Guan H P, Liu Y, Bi H, Yang L and Wang M 2021 A novel method for vehicle headlights detection using salient region segmentation and PHOG feature *Multimedia Tools Appl.* **80** 22821–41

[41] Nasir I M, Bibi A, Shah J H, Khan M A, Sharif M, Iqbal K and Kadry S 2021 Deep learning-based classification of fruit diseases: An application for precision agriculture *Comp. Mater. Continua* **66** 1949–62

[42] Vijayakumar K, Rajinikanth V and Kirubakaran M K 2022 Automatic detection of breast cancer in ultrasound images using Mayfly algorithm optimized handcrafted features *J. X-Ray Sci. Technol.* **30** 751–66

[43] Daniel J, Rose J T, Vinnarasi F and Rajinikanth V 2022 VGG-UNet/VGG-SegNet supported automatic segmentation of endoplasmic reticulum network in fluorescence microscopy images *Scanning* **2022** 7733860

Chapter 5

Design of a system for melanoma diagnosis using image processing and hybrid optimization techniques

Venkatesan Rajinikanth, Navid Razmjooy and Noradin Ghadimi

Melanoma is the most dangerous type of skin cancer, which can occur on any part of the skin or around moles. Melanoma can also form in the eyes and, more rarely, elsewhere in the body, such as the nose or throat. This type of cancer develops as a result of the uncontrolled proliferation of melanocytes (skin pigment cells) and, as a result, is usually seen as black or brown, although it may have other colors such as red or white. To early diagnose melanoma and prevent its progression and serious consequences, it is necessary to examine all moles and dark spots on the body, first by the person and, if necessary, by a dermatologist. One proper technique for increasing the accuracy of this diagnosis is to use image processing and machine vision. An artificial neural network is a kind of black box technique that is commonly used in contemporary cancer diagnosis. The goal of neural network training is to find the size of weights and biases in a way that minimizes training data error. Therefore, neural network training can be considered as an optimization problem whose purpose is to optimize weighting coefficients and biases to achieve the minimum training error. Conventional methods use neural network propagation algorithms and other gradient methods to train neural networks. These methods show their weakness and inefficiency in cases where the form of the function is nonlinear and complex. In this chapter, a new hybrid meta-heuristic algorithm, called a developed electromagnetic field optimization algorithm, has been utilized for neural network training. The use of this algorithm in neural network training and its comparison with an error post-propagation training algorithm show that in complex problems with nonlinear processes the use of the new algorithm is more efficient. Finally, the results of the implementation of the proposed algorithm on two issues and its comparison with a post-publication training method are given.

doi:10.1088/978-0-7503-4012-0ch5

5.1 Introduction

5.1.1 Conception

The skin is the body's first point of contact with the outside world and the environment. This organ is not completely straight and has lines, grooves, depressions and, in some areas, extensions such as hair. The skin in an adult with an average body size comprises an area more than 2 square meters in size, and is the heaviest part of the body after the skeletal muscles. The thickness of the skin is not the same in all parts of the body: in places such as the palms of the hands and feet, the skin is very thick and in areas such as the face, it is very thin and delicate. There are two types of skin in the human body, one hairless and the other hairy.

The first type of skin is found on the palms of the hands and feet and lacks hair follicles and sebaceous glands. Its epidermis is very thick and there are many sensory organs in its dermis. In the second type of skin, there are both hair follicles and sebaceous glands. The scalp and face are of this type. Large follicles and thick hair are abundant on the scalp, while facial skin has a large number of sebaceous glands and very fine, fluffy hairs. A cross-section of the skin represents the four main and distinct layers in its structure, which are, from the surface to the deepest layer, respectively: the epidermis, dermis and hypodermis, and melanocytes. Figure 5.1 shows the structure of the skin.

In the following, the main parts of the skin are explained briefly. The *epidermis* is the most superficial layer of the skin, which itself is composed of different parts. These layers from, surface to depth, are the stratum corneum and the live epidermis. The stratum corneum is the outermost layer of the skin. This layer is the main barrier and protection against external factors, and the task of the live epidermis is to produce this layer and maintain its natural and desirable state. The stratum corneum is made up of dead, water-resistant cells that are joined together by

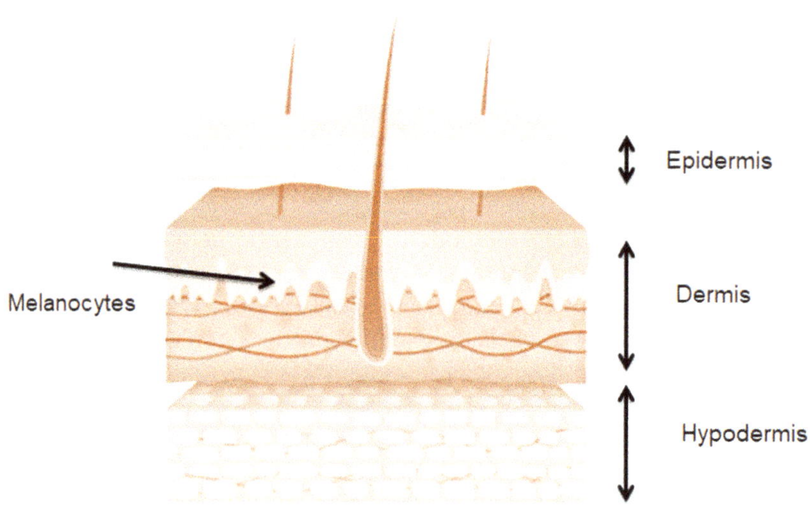

Figure 5.1. The structure of the skin.

complex fatty compounds. These fatty compounds play a key role in preventing water loss through the skin. The thickness of this layer varies in different areas of the body. The epidermis is very thin in the eyelid area and the thickest in the palm and foot area. This layer is constantly forming and the upper layers are continually gradually peeling off and being replaced by new layers from the bottom. It takes about two weeks to replace the cell layers in this area. Under normal circumstances, no microbes, whether bacteria or viruses, can pass through the stratum corneum and enter the body.

The second layer in the epidermis is live epidermis. The living epidermis refers to the cells beneath the cells of the stratum corneum that are distinct from the cells of the stratum corneum from above and the dermis from below. These cells are round and cubic in the deepest part and, gradually, when they reach the surface of the skin, they expand and dry and lose their water on the surface of the skin and form a horny (corneum) layer. The living epidermis is divided into the following sections:

- The germ layer, or basal layer, is a cell layer of cubic or cylindrical cells for which no specific characteristic can be considered.
- A prickly layer made up of cells with a sharp, thorn-like surface.
- A granular layer that contains specific grains of keratohyalin that, after staining under a microscope, are seen as granules.
- A clear layer that contains clear, transparent cells.

In addition to the cells described, there are other types of cells in the epidermis that are very important. These cells are called melanocytes, whose role is to produce the pigment melanin. On average, each melanocyte cell is associated with 36 normal cells in the epidermal layer and distributes pigment between them. Interestingly, the number of these pigment-producing cells is the same in all humans, whether black or white, but what causes the difference in human color is the distribution and size of the pigment accumulations.

The *dermis* is considered as a framework and substrate that supports and supports the epidermis. This layer also nourishes the epidermis with its many blood vessels. Unlike the epidermis, this layer is full of blood vessels, nerves, and skin appendages such as sweat glands, hair follicles, and sebaceous glands. Unlike the epidermis layer, which has a cellular structure, this layer consists of a connective tissue, most of which is made up of protein fibers such as collagen and elastin. Collagen protein is responsible for the strength and power of the skin, as well as the consistency of the skin. In people with this protein disorder, the skin shrinks and loses its freshness and beauty.

Another protein in the dermis is elastin, which is responsible for the elasticity and flexibility of the skin. This means that if you pull the skin, the elastin is responsible for returning it to normal. In the elderly, this protein loses its original properties and the skin does not have the flexibility of the past. Collagen and elastin cannot be absorbed from the skin surface and therefore topical application of these two proteins cannot affect skin wrinkles.

The *hypodermis* is located below the dermis as a layer of fat. The cells of this layer are responsible for the synthesis and storage of fat and as a source of human energy storage. Furthermore, the hypodermis has a protective role against low ambient temperatures and acts as a shock absorber to mitigate physical shocks to the skin. This layer naturally makes the skin beautiful. However, if it accumulates too much and does not distribute fat evenly, it can cause a bulging and unpleasant appearance on the skin.

The other layer is composed of *melanocytes*. This layer produces pigment in the cells in the skin, hair, and eyes that determine the color of these organs. The main determinant of color is not the number of melanocytes but their activity. Melanin production occurs in a part of the cell called the amino acid tyrosine melanosome. Skin, hair, and dark pigmented skin contain melanosomes with higher levels of melanin.

Skin cancer is the most common malignant cancer of the body. It is estimated that more than one million people worldwide faces skin cancer each year. There are different types of skin cancer, the main difference being based on the type of cell that develops the cancer. The three main types are basal cell carcinoma, squamous cell carcinoma, and malignant melanoma.

Malignant melanoma, which is the deadliest type of skin cancer, originates from skin pigment cells (melanocytes). In this disease, cancer cells continue to pigment, so that in this type of cancer different shades of light brown, brown, or black can be seen. Of course, melanoma can sometimes be white or red. Malignant melanoma has a high tendency to spread to other parts of the body, so its diagnosis and treatment in the early stages is very important.

Melanoma may occur suddenly and without warning signs, or it may start on or around a mole. Therefore, it is necessary to know the location of the moles on the body as well as their shape so that one can notice any change in the shape and size of the moles quickly. Melanoma is considered as the 19th most commonly occurring cancer among the other cancers in society, such that about 300 000 new cases were found in 2018. As a typical example of its occurrence rate, 4740 males and 2490 females died due to melanoma during 2019 [1]. Figure 5.2 shows the top 20 countries with the highest melanoma rates in 2018 [2].

Prolonged exposure to the Sun, especially in cases where sunburn has occurred, is the most important factor in the development of melanoma and should be prevented. Avoiding the Sun is especially important in people with fair skin. Heredity also plays a role in melanoma. So, if a member of the family has at some point developed melanoma, the chances of developing malignant melanoma cancer increase. People who have abnormal moles (dysplastic type) and those who have a large number of moles on their body are at higher risk for melanoma.

The presence of dark skin color (brown or black) does not guarantee the absence of melanoma. Melanoma may also be found in dark-skinned people. It is especially seen on the palms of the hands and feet, under the nails, or inside the mouth.

Regular checkups are the best way to get acquainted with moles and blemishes on the skin. This is done by the patient themself and with the help of a family member or friend so that inaccessible points are not overlooked. Areas such as the mouth, back, scalp, buttocks, etc, should also be examined.

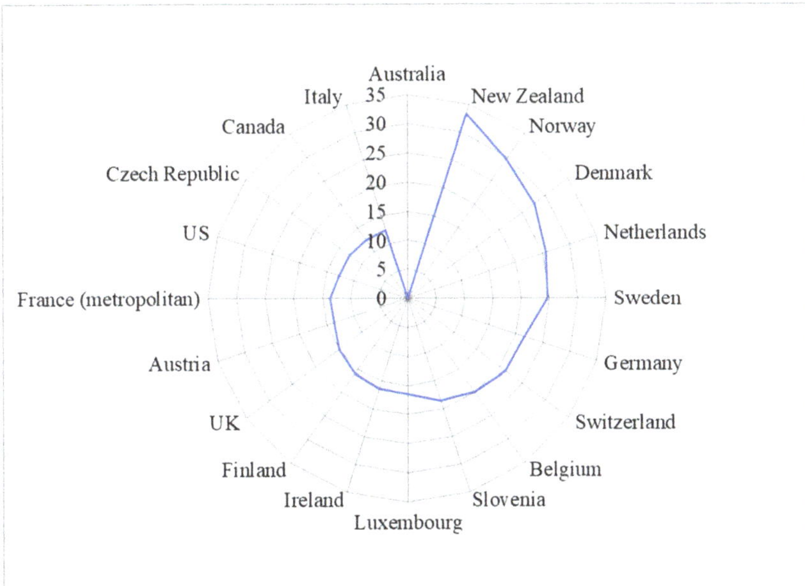

Figure 5.2. Radar plot for the age-standardized rate of melanoma in 2018 [2].

When examining moles one should pay special attention to their size, shape, edges, and color. Early detection of melanoma potentially equals a 100% improvement. But, in the late stages, treatment cannot stop the cancer from developing uncontrollably.

The following criteria help distinguish melanoma from a common mole:

- Asymmetry: ordinary moles are often circular and symmetrical, but malignant melanoma lesions are usually asymmetric, so that if we want to draw a hypothetical line from the center of the lesion, it cannot divide the lesion into equal and symmetrical parts.
- Irregular edges: the edges of benign lesions are usually uniform, but the edges of malignant melanoma lesions are often irregular and serrated.
- Color: benign lesions are usually uniformly light brown, dark brown, or black, but in malignant melanoma lesions there is often a range of different colors (light brown, dark brown, black, and even blue and red).
- Diameter: ordinary spots are often less than 6 mm in diameter (roughly equivalent to the size of a pencil eraser), although melanoma is larger in size and is usually more than 6 mm in diameter. Figure 5.7 shows some examples of melanoma.

Malignant skin cancer initially presents with pre-cancerous lesions. Pre-cancerous lesions are skin lesions that are not cancerous but become cancerous over time. If anyone knows the warning signs of skin cancer, they should do something quickly because it can be treated if skin cancer is diagnosed early.

Diagnosis of melanoma is in many cases difficult, and sometimes impossible because of its clinical resemblance to benign pigmented lesions. In other words, definitive diagnosis of pigmented lesions based on their clinical appearance is of little sensitivity and specificity. Therefore, one approach can be the removal of all pigmented lesions of the oral mucosa, especially single permanent lesions.

However, since many patients have multiple and benign pigmented lesions, such procedure(s) will be difficult and costly in many cases, where in most cases the lesions being removed are completely benign and do not rightfully require surgery. Due to these cases, there is a serious need for a noninvasive method with high sensitivity and specificity in the diagnosis of pigmented lesions; dermoscopy (microscopic or dermatoscopic epiluminescence) as an *in vivo* method has in various studies shown that in the diagnosis of melanocytic pigmented lesions, being able to tell non-melanocytic and benign from malignant is very helpful.

Normally, light emitted to the surface of the skin or mucosa is absorbed, broken, or reflected depending on the reflection coefficient of the prickly layer, so the underlying structures are not always clearly visible; however, if immersion liquids are used on the surface of the skin or mucosa, the amount of reflection is reduced from the surface and many of the subsurface structures below can be seen. Squeezing a glass slide on the surface of the skin or mucosa to even out the surface as well as using light magnification can help with better diagnosis.

The patterns visible after irradiation take different forms, and each of them plays a role in determining the type of pigment and whether the lesion is benign or malignant, which has been discussed in detail. This step is called pattern analysis. For example, the presence of multiple patterns, and asymmetry in different patterns and colors suggests more melanoma, but homogeneity, symmetry, and dominance of one color will be more indicative of benign lesions.

Therefore, due to the higher sensitivity and specificity of dermoscopy compared to clinical evaluation of the appearance of a lesion in differentiating benign from malignant pigmented lesions, as well as its being noninvasive and easy to work with, it is strongly recommended along with all usual diagnostic steps. By using dermoscopy, it is no longer necessary to remove all the individual pigmented lesions of the oral mucosa unless examination of the lesion by dermoscopy or its clinical presentation is suspected of malignancy.

Dermoscopic images have great potential for early detection of malignant melanoma, but their interpretation is time consuming even for experienced dermatologists. Therefore, special attention has been paid to the development of computer-based diagnostic systems, which can be of great help to dermatologists' analysis. To reduce the diagnostic error caused by human perceptual and visual factors, the development of computer image analysis is of great importance. Automatic border detection is often the first step in automatic analysis of dermoscopic images. Usually, the standard method in automatic dermoscopic image analysis consists of three steps:

(1) Image segmentation.
(2) Feature extraction.
(3) Classification and cancer diagnosis.

The segmentation stage is one of the most important parts, due to its great knock-on effect on the accuracy of the next stages. However, segmentation is difficult due to its different types in terms of shape, size, and color among different types of cancerous tissues. In addition, some cancers have a blurred border and, in some cases, there is a very soft area between the skin and the cancer. Other problems include the prevalence of black hair which covers cancerous spots, and the presence of reflections in images.

To overcome this problem, several different algorithms have been proposed. These methods are generally classified into threshold-based methods, edge-based methods, and zoning-based methods. An example of thresholding methods can be found in [9]: in this method, a combined method including global thresholding techniques, adaptive thresholding, and clustering was used.

5.2 Literature review

With the advancement of science in recent years, digital dermatoscope devices with the ability to capture and store skin images have replaced conventional dermatoscopes. Therefore, it is possible to provide commercial software packages to help diagnose some skin lesions, populate databases, and create a medical resume for each patient. Studies show that the most effective step in processing dermatoscopic images of melanocyte lesions is lesion demarcation. In fact, the extent of the lesion, the shape of the border, and the amount of intensity distance in the area between the lesion and the background are considered as key parameters in the diagnosis of cancer. Though visual diagnosis of the exact borders of lesions, especially in the early stages of the disease, is very difficult and in some cases impossible, on the other hand timely initiation of the treatment process has a direct effect on reducing mortality due to skin cancer. Thus, helping to determine the cancer area has been a hot focus of recent research.

This method of skin imaging makes the subcutaneous structures of the skin more visible compared to traditional clinical methods. This method, in turn, reduces the coverage error and increases the resolution in cases such as ambiguous complications. Dermoscopy is a noninvasive diagnostic method for observation *in vivo* to examine injured skin pigments.

As aforementioned, dermoscopic images have great potential for the early detection of malignant melanoma, but their interpretation is time consuming even for experienced dermatologists. Therefore, special attention has been paid to the development of computer-based diagnostic systems that can assist dermatologists' analysis. To reduce the diagnostic error caused by human perceptual and visual factors, the development of computer image analysis is of crucial importance. For example, Bansal *et al* [3] proposed a technique for automatic skin cancer diagnosis using deep-learning-based image feature extraction. They used a convolutional neural network (CNN) based on transfer learning for feature extraction of images during a pipeline process which comprised k-nearest neighbor (k-NN), AdaBoost, and random forest (RF) methods to determine melanoma based on the features extracted from the CNN. Their final results showed desirable performance for the introduced method.

In 2006 [4], Xiaojing Yuan *et al* proposed a decision support system for fast diagnosis of skin cancer in cross-polarization imaging. They used a support vector machine (SVM) for the classification. Texture features were used for the diagnosis of the cancer and benign groups, and the total accuracy was achieved 86.9%.

In 2008, Celebi *et al* presented a clustering-based method based on statistical region merging for skin cancer diagnosis in dermoscopy images. They used their method on 90 dermoscopy images. The method was compared with four state-of-the-art diagnosis methods including a dermatologist-like tumor extraction algorithm, Fuzzy C-Means (FCM), mean-shift clustering, and a modified *J*-measure-based segmentation method. Simulation results showed that employing the suggested method improved the accuracy and speed in comparison to the aforementioned methods.

In 2013, Razmjooy *et al* proposed another technique, assuming the ABCD rule. They first employed an artifact removal system to eliminate extraneous hairs from the image. Then, an image segmentation was performed to the images to highlight the doubtful region. After, new features, termed AIBQ, were used to extract the main feature. Finally, the images were grouped into two groups of benign and malignant based on a SVM. Final results indicated that they obtained around a 95% accuracy ratio for melanoma diagnosis [5].

In 2013, Sheykhahmad *et al* proposed a diagnosis system for borderline detection of skin cancer in dermoscopy images. The main purpose was to offer a well-organized technique utilizing histograms for the diagnosis of cancerous regions in input images. Simulation results of the proposed method on a standard data set showed a feasible technique for the diagnosis of lesion areas [6].

In 2018, Razmjooy *et al* presented an optimization approach for melanoma detection from dermoscopy images using soft computing. The method was first pre-processed to remove noise and artifacts. Segmentation was then performed for lesion detection. Their segmentation method was a technique based on an optimized version of a neural network. Optimization was performed based on the World Cup optimization algorithm to select the optimal weights and biases of the network. Finally, mathematical morphology was performed for post-processing of the images to remove extra zones. The final results indicated the good performance of the presented technique with regard to other comparable methods [7].

In 2019, Jadhav *et al* proposed a method for skin cancer border diagnosis using a CNN and SVM classifier. The main purpose was to use deep learning for the border detection. Simulation results were validated on 15×15 and 50×50 pixel image sizes. Their results showed that using a 15×15 pixel size for the input data provides the best efficiency. The algorithm obtained around a 95.85% accurate performance with an *F*-value of 94.14% [8].

In 2016, Pennisi *et al* [9] presented a melanoma image diagnosis approach from dermoscopy images. The method was based on Delaunay triangulation. They performed their work on a publicly available dermoscopic images benchmark, and the results indicated a 93.5% sensitivity for the proposed method.

In 2018, Heller *et al* [10] introduced another method for detection of melanoma. The method was based on a mathematical morphology feature. Simulation results showed that the proposed method possessed good efficiency for this purpose.

Somfai *et al* [11] proposed another method based on machine vision for skin cancer diagnosis. They proposed a new detection system using a deep-learning technique to deliver a precise methodology with a low false negative ratio. This technique was utilized using a U-net CNN for automatic melanoma segmentation. It was then used to extract features, and the tailored neural networks were used for features processing. The results showed advancements in all aspects over baseline.

Vocaturo *et al* [12] introduced a method based on epiluminescence microscopy (ELM) for the diagnosis of melanoma. They utilized the ELM methodology to identify the main features of the skin cancer images, which can be utilized as a beneficial tool for the other researchers.

Sreelatha *et al* [13] introduced a method for skin cancer detection using dermoscopy images, based on gradient and feature adaptive contour (GFAC). They utilized noise removal pre-processing to increase the speed and accuracy. The presented GFAC model provided a noise-free solution. The method was then performed on the PH^2 data set and compared with other state-of-the-art methods from the literature.

Dey *et al* [14] presented another optimal melanoma diagnosis system based on machine vision. They utilized the bat algorithm to optimize their technique and to obtain higher-effectiveness images. After applying pre-processing on the input images, a distance regularized level set (DRLS) segmentation was used for the main processing. The performance of the method was verified based on evaluation of defined image performance metrics. The results indicated that the method mollify the final target compared with some other state-of-the-art methods.

Tschandl *et al* [15] proposed a classification-based methodology based on a CNN by training 7895 dermoscopy images. The suggested CNN method was applied to a set of 2072 test cases, and the results were compared with some other methods.

Fan *et al* [16] employed spectral and spatial features to simplify skin cancer diagnosis from other materials. They first employed a spectral pre-processing method on microscopic hyperspectral images. Afterward, three supervised classification methods were utilized based on a CNN, SVM, and maximum likelihood classification (MLC) to apply the final diagnosis. The final results evaluated the classifiers' accuracy to select the best classification method.

Hekler *et al* [17] presented an automatic method for the diagnosis of skin cancer using artificial intelligence. They used dermoscopy images for the validation of their method to divide the images into five groups. They used a deep-learning method to train a single CNN. They then applied their method to a collection from 13 German university hospitals. Simulation results indicated better results from the proposed method.

Tan *et al* [18] introduced an optimized technique for skin cancer diagnosis using an improved version of the particle swarm optimization (PSO) algorithm. The proposed modified PSO algorithm was then employed to optimize the features present in dermoscopy images. This technique was then applied to various benchmarks to indicate the PSO's dominance in terms of performance against some well-known techniques.

5.3 Materials and methods

Soft computing refers to a set of new computing methods in computer science, artificial intelligence, machine learning, and many other fields. In all these fields, it is necessary to study, model, and analyze very complex phenomena that precise scientific methods in the past have not succeeded in solving easily, analytically, and completely. In this chapter, the idea is to introduce the concepts of artificial neural networks (ANNs) and meta-heuristic algorithms as two popular tools of soft computing for the diagnosis of skin cancer.

5.3.1 Artificial neural networks

5.3.2 Concept

An ANN is an method for information processing that is inspired by the biological neural system and processes information in a way similar to the brain. A key element of this idea is the new structure of the information processing system. This system is made up of a large number of highly interconnected processing elements, called neurons, that work together to solve a problem. ANNs, like humans, learn by example, and a neural network is set up to perform specific tasks, such as identifying patterns and categorizing information, during a learning process. In biological systems, learning involves the adjustment of synaptic connections between nerves. This method is also used in neural networks.

ANNs transfer experimental data, knowledge, or laws behind the data to the network structure, which is called learning. In essence, the ability to learn is the most important feature of an intelligent system. A learning system is more flexible and easier to program, so it can better respond to new problems and equations.

A neural network is a data-processing system that, like the human brain, delegates data processing to many small interconnected processors that act as parallel networks to solve a problem. In these networks, with the help of programming knowledge, a data structure is designed that can act like a neuron. This data structure is referred to as a node. In this structure, a network is trained by creating links between these nodes and applying a training algorithm to them. In this memory or neural network nodes have two active states (on or off) and inactive (0), and each edge (synapse or connection between nodes) has a weight. Positive-weight edges stimulate or activate the next inactive node, and negative-weight edges inactivate or inhibit the next connected node (if active).

5.3.3 Mathematical modeling of an ANN

When modeling nerves, their complexity is ignored and only the basic concepts are considered, because otherwise the modeling approach will be very difficult. At a simple glance, a model of a nerve should include inputs that act as synapses. These inputs are multiplied by weights to determine signal strength. Finally, a mathematical operator decides whether the neuron is activated or not and, if the solution is proper, determines the output. Therefore, the ANN processes information using a

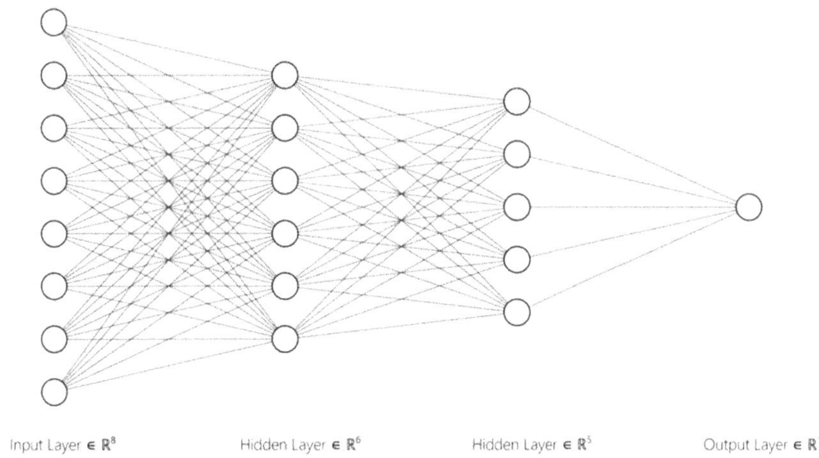

Figure 5.3. A model of an ANN.

simplified model of a real nerve. Based on these explanations, a simple model can be proposed to describe a neuron (a node in an ANN). This model is shown in figure 5.3.

Apart from the simplifications applied, the main difference between this model and a real neural networks is that in the real networks the inputs are time signals, while in this model real numbers are the inputs.

Learning in natural systems takes place adaptively. This means that as a result of learning, changes occur in the synapses. The same is true of ANNs. In these networks, learning is done by several examples. This means that often (but not always) a set of correct inputs and outputs is given to the neural network, and the neural network uses these examples to change the weight of its communications in such a way that it produces the correct solutions if new inputs are given. In fact, neural network knowledge is stored in the weight of its communications.

One of the most widely used types of networks is a multilayer perceptron (MLP) network. This type of network is one of the most important structures of ANNs. Typically, these networks consist of a set of sensory units (basic neurons) that make up the input layer, one or more hidden layers, and an output layer. The input signal is transmitted layer by layer throughout the network and through a forward path.

In the present study, a three-layer MLP network has been used. A sigmoid activation function (hyperbolic tangent) is used between the input layer and the hidden layer, and a linear activation function is used between the hidden layer and the output layer.

Among the different methods of post-error propagation training, a Levenberg–Marquardt algorithm has been selected for use in the present study due to its faster convergence in training medium-sized networks. The backpropagation algorithm changes the network weights and bias values in such a way that the performance function decreases more quickly. The backpropagation algorithm can be shown as follows:

$$x_{k+1} = x_k - \alpha_k g_k, \tag{5.1}$$

where x_k describes the weight and bias in the kth iteration, α_k represents the training rate in the kth iteration, and g_k defines the gradient in the kth iteration. The Levenberg–Marquardt algorithm has been developed to achieve faster network training and uses the following relationship:

$$x_{k+1} = x_k - [J^T J + \mu I]^{-1} J^T e, \tag{5.2}$$

where x_k describes the vectors and bias in the kth iteration, J is the Jacobin matrix containing the first derivatives of the lattice error with respect to the weights and biases, e is the lattice vector of the vectors, I is the matrix of the unit, and μ is a scalar quantity. μ decreases after each successful step and also increases if a single step increases the performance function. In this way, the performance function will be reduced in each iteration of the algorithm. In this study, an initial value of 0.001 for μ has been used.

In general, neural networks have a very good capability for use in predictive problems. Although the use of backpropagation algorithms has become very prevalent in recent years for neural network training, the use of this method in some cases can lead to problems. These barriers include slow convergence in education and early convergence in the local minimum. Recently, the application of evolutionary search algorithms to train neural networks instead of conventional training methods has been considered by researchers.

In this chapter, the structural parameters of the neural network are considered as decision variables of an optimization problem, and the performance function of the neural network is optimized by a hybrid meta-heuristic algorithm. The neural networks tested in this study were used to classify data. The practical results of various experiments on various experimental data (in the dimensions of feature space, number of samples, and class interference) clearly demonstrate the efficiency of the proposed method.

5.4 Meta-heuristics

In engineering and computer science, optimization is a technique that aims to find the best solutions from a set of possible solutions. Many different methods have been introduced for solving optimization problems, but a problem that remains in solving optimization problems is that different resources are needed to solve the problems. Among the resources required to solve a problem are the number of processors (in parallel processing), time (time required to solve the problem), and space (memory required). Part of computational theory examines the resources needed to solve a problem, known as 'complexity theory.' This theory is a branch of mathematical and computer science that examines the difficulty of solving problems by computer.

According to complexity theory, problems are divided into complexity classes so that the problems of a class are similar in terms of the time or space required. Polynomial (P) problems are classes of problems for which there are fast algorithms, i.e. polynomials, to find the solution, and non-deterministic polynomial problems (NPs) are classes of problems for which, although it may take a long time to find the solution, it is possible to find the correct solution. Taken together, the two classes, P and NP, are the most important classes; most optimization problems fall into the NP class.

Given the resources needed to solve optimization problems and different classes of problems, the point to be noted here is that the use of basic optimization methods, including linear programming, integer programming, dynamic programming, and nonlinear programming, has some associated issues. Given that most problems are in the NP class, the most important problem is that it is time consuming to solve large problems with them; so that even with today's advanced computing technologies, solving a large-scale problem with the mentioned techniques can take several years. The emergence of this problem put an end to the illusions that were created at the beginning of the formation of research knowledge in operations, assuming that optimal solutions could be found for all world problems using this knowledge. The emergence of this problem has forced researchers to adjust their expectations of this new knowledge in order to find the best possible solution, and to suffice with good enough solutions that can be applied, even for large-scale problems, in a reasonable time. The general definition of optimization is as follows:

$$\begin{aligned} &\underset{x \in \Re^n}{\text{minimize}} f_i(x), \quad (i = 1, 2, \ldots, M), \\ &s.t. \ h_j(x) = 0, \quad (j = 1, 2, \ldots, J) \\ &g_k(x) \leqslant 0, \quad (k = 1, 2, \ldots, K), \end{aligned} \tag{5.3}$$

where $f_i(x)$, $h_j(x)$ and $g_k(x)$ represent some functions of a vector. Each element x_i of x is called a decision variable, which can be real, discrete, or a combination of the two. There are a few points about this definition that should here be considered:

- The functions $f_i(x)$, where $i = 1, 2, \ldots, M$, are called the objective function or the cost function.
- If $M = 1$, the objective function will be called a single objective function; if $M > 1$, the objective function will be called a multi-objective function.
- The space divided by the decision variables is called the R^n search space.
- The space formed by the values of the objective function is called the solution space or the search space.
- Equations $h_j(x)$ and inequalities $g_k(x)$ are called problem constraints.

Note that all inequalities can be rewritten as $\geqslant 0$. The objective function of the problem can also be rewritten as a maximization problem.

Optimization problems in the real world are similar to the example of finding treasure. Given the importance of such problems, many researchers have tried to find different ways of solving them. The classification of optimization algorithms can be done in various ways. The easiest way is to consider the nature of the algorithms. Therefore, they can be classified into two categories: definite and probable. Definite

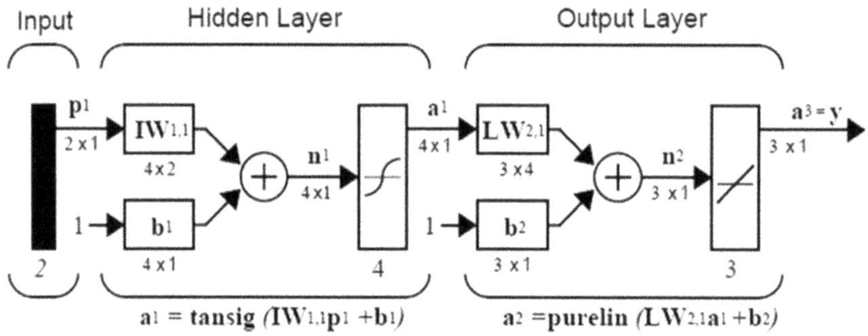

Figure 5.4. Schematic representation of a multilayer perceptron network.

algorithms are algorithms in which each time the algorithm is executed with the same inputs the same solution is achieved as before.

A hill-climbing algorithm is an example of a definite algorithm that achieves the same path in each execution using the same starting point. Probabilistic algorithms operate randomly and produce different solutions in each execution.

Genetic algorithms are a good example of probabilistic algorithms. A genetic algorithm uses different random numbers in each run. The end results are not greatly different from each other, but each candidate's paths are not repeated.

There is a third category, which is a combination of these two categories. For example, a hill-climbing algorithm with a random start would fall into this third category. The basic idea is to use a definite algorithm but commence with different starting points. The advantage of this method is that it prevents falling at the local optimal point.

Meta-heuristic algorithms are used to find an approximate optimal solution to difficult optimization problems for which there is no definitive solution available in a reasonable time frame. A meta-heuristic algorithm is defined as a problem-independent algorithm that can find approximate solutions to difficult problems. Meta-heuristic algorithms are inspired by nature and try to solve problems by imitating various sciences such as biology and physics; a genetic algorithm, explained previously, is an example of these algorithms.

There are different methods for classifying and describing meta-heuristic algorithms. Depending on the features selected to differentiate between them, several classifications are possible. In this chapter, we use an electromagnetic field optimization (EFO) algorithm to optimize the ANN.

5.5 Electromagnetic field optimization algorithm

An electric magnet is a type of magnet in which an electric current produces a magnetic field. Unlike a permanent magnet, an electric magnet has a single polarity (positive or negative) that is determined by the direction of the electric current and can be changed by changing the direction of the electric current. In addition, there are two different forces among electric magnets: absorption and repulsion. Electric magnets with similar polarity repel each other, and those with opposite polarity attract each other. The force of gravity is stronger among electric magnets (5%–10%) than the repulsive force. Our algorithm uses these concepts and replaces the ratio between absorption and repulsion forces with the golden ratio. This helps the particles to sufficiently explore the search space of the problem and find an almost optimal solution [19].

An electromagnetic optimization algorithm is a population-based algorithm in which each response vector is represented by a set of magnets (electromagnetic particles). The number of electric magnets in an electromagnetic particle is determined by the number of variables in the optimization problem. Thus, each electric magnet of an electromagnetic particle corresponds to a variable of the optimization problem. In addition, all electromagnetic magnets have the same polarity as an electromagnetic particle. However, any electromagnetic magnet can exert a force of attraction or repulsion on magnets that are related to the same variable of the optimization problem.

The EFO algorithm consists of four steps: initial population generation, a local search, calculation of the total force vector for each member moving in the direction of the incoming force vector, and using the local search in the neighborhoods to find the local optimal. The steps of implementing this algorithm are described below.

First, a population of electromagnetic particles is randomly generated and the suitability of each particle with proper performance is evaluated. The particles are then arranged according to their fitness value. Then, the classified particles are divided into three groups, and a portion of the electromagnetic population is assigned to each group. The first group is called the positive field and consists of the most suitable electromagnetic particles with positive polarity; the second group is called the negative field and consists of electromagnetic particles with the least proportion and negative polarity. The remaining electromagnetic particles form a group called the neutral field which has a negative polarity of about zero.

Finally, in each iteration of the algorithm a new electromagnetic particle with a fitness function is formed and evaluated. If the generated electromagnetic particle is more suitable than the worst electromagnetic particle in the population, the generated particle is placed in a classified population according to its proportion, obtained based on its position in the polar population. In addition, the worst particle will be destroyed. This process continues until the maximum number of iterations is reached or the expected near-optimal solution is found. The EFO algorithm determines the position of each generated electromagnetic part of an electromagnetic particle as follows.

From the electromagnetic particles of each electromagnetic field (positive, negative, and neutral), three random electromagnetic fields are selected (one electromagnetic magnet from each field). Then, the electric magnet generated from the neutral field receives the position and polarity (small negative pole) of the selected electromagnet and is influenced by the intensity of the random force of the magnets selected from the positive field (gravity) and the negative field (repulsion). In other words, the electric magnet generated distances itself from bad responses and approaches good responses. Figure 5.5 shows the direction of forces between electric magnets of different fields.

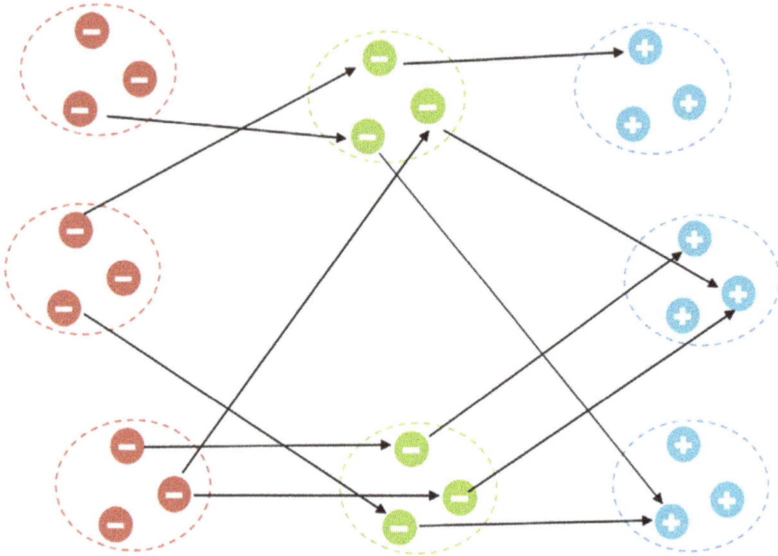

Figure 5.5. The direction of forces between electric magnets of different fields. The positive, neutral, and negative backgrounds are blue, green, and red, respectively.

As shown in figure 5.5, the positive, neutral, and negative backgrounds are blue, green, and red, respectively. Each electric magnet of a neutral field electromagnetic particle is affected by two random magnetic fields of negative field (repulsion) and positive field (gravity).

The coexistence of two opposing forces among magnets and the fact that the new solution is created by distancing from bad solutions and approaching good ones leads to an effective search and fast convergence. However, in order to maintain diversity and avoid local minima, randomness is an essential part of an EFO algorithm.

Therefore, for some (but not all) electromagnetic particles, only one magnet is produced with one magnet. The reason for random actions on some electromagnetic particles is that the presence of random variables in all solutions prevents a good solution from being found. However, random use of some solutions causes population diversity and avoids local minima.

In the algorithm, a randomly selected electromagnet from a neutral field is subjected to electromagnetic magnets selected from a positive field (gravity) and a negative field (repulsion) to determine the position of the generated magnet. The steps for solving the mathematical model of the algorithm are as follows. Initially, after generating the initial population, the new position is calculated as follows:

$$\mathrm{EMP}_j^{\mathrm{New}} = \mathrm{EMP}_j^{K_j} + \left((\phi \times r) \times \left(\mathrm{EMP}_j^{P_j} - \mathrm{EMP}_j^{K_j}\right)\right) - \left(r \times \left(\mathrm{EMP}_j^{N_j} - \mathrm{EMP}_j^{K_j}\right)\right)l, \tag{5.4}$$

where EMP is an electromagnetic particle, r describes a random value in a range between 0 and 1 (generated once for each electromagnetic particle), j is a variable index (the magnet index is generated), K is a random index of the neutral field (produced for each electric magnet of the generated particle), P defines the random index of the positive field (produced for each particle electric magnet produced), and N is the random index of the negative field (produced for each particle electric magnet produced).

To generate a new electromagnetic particle, the above equation is calculated for all magnets (variables) of electromagnetic particles produced (solution). This means that several particles work together to produce a new electromagnetic particle. The minimum number of participating particles to form a new particle is 3, when for all generated electric magnets the particle selects a random function of magnets from the same particles and the maximum number of participating particles by multiplying the number of problem variables by 3. For example, when the number of problem variables is 5, the minimum number of common particles to form a new particle is 3 and the maximum is 15. Meanwhile, in other optimization algorithms, this number is significantly lower than in the EFO. For example, in a genetic algorithm (GA), only two solutions (parents) form a new solution, and in a PSO algorithm, three different positions (current position, best personal position, and best global position) determine the new position of the particles.

Equation (5.4) consists of two parts: the first part calculates the distance between randomly selected electromagnets from the positive field and the neutral field using equation (5.5), and the second part calculates the distance between randomly selected electric magnets from the negative field and is a neutral field using equation (5.6). In order for the neutral electromagnetic magnet to move towards the positive magnet and assume a distance from the negative magnet, we use equation (5.5) to add the neutral magnetic position to a random part of the calculated distance. As mentioned earlier, the force of a positive field force is greater than the force of a negative field force. Therefore, in equation (5.7) we multiply the calculated distance between positive and neutral magnets by ϕ (approximately 1.61), which proved to have the best performance based on experiments. Therefore, by combining equations (5.5)–(5.7), equation (5.4) is obtained:

$$D_j^{P_jK_j} = \mathrm{EMP}_j^{P_j} - \mathrm{EMP}_j^{K_j}, \tag{5.5}$$

$$D_j^{N_jK_j} = \mathrm{EMP}_j^{N_j} - \mathrm{EMP}_j^{K_j}, \tag{5.6}$$

$$\mathrm{EMP}_j^{\mathrm{New}} = \mathrm{EMP}_j^{K_j} + \left((\phi \times r) \times D_j^{P_jK_j}\right) - \left(r \times D_j^{N_jK_j}\right). \tag{5.7}$$

5.6 Developed electromagnetic field optimization algorithm

It can be inferred from the literature that the EFO algorithm provides satisfying results for optimization problems. However, in some cases it has a notable shortcoming [20–22]: the EFO sometimes becomes stuck on the local optimum value and gives a premature convergence that leads to incorrect solutions.

In this research, two modifications have been used to resolve or mitigate against this shortcoming as much as possible.

The random nature of the population initialization in the EFO provides high population diversity; however, by performing the updating formulation, the difference between the electromagnets is reduced gradually, and consequently the population diversity is decreased. This can lead to a local optimum value for the problem. Therefore, a mutation mechanism has been introduced to correct this issue in the original EFO algorithm. In this method, the advantages of the basic EFO and an evolutionary algorithm are combined to maintain the search efficiency. The expression of diversity of an EFO is given below:

$$\delta^t = \frac{1}{m \times \sigma} \times \sum_{i=1}^{m} \sqrt{\sum_{j=1}^{m} \sqrt{\left(\mathrm{EMP}_j^{K_j} - \overline{\mathrm{EMP}_j^{K_j}}\right)^2}}, \tag{5.8}$$

where $\overline{\mathrm{EMP}_j^{K_j}}$ describes the mean value of the $\mathrm{EMP}_j^{K_j}$ and σ signifies the length of the longest diagonal line in the solution space.

Further, in the basic EFO algorithm, the K parameter is considered as a random value in a range between 0 and 1. In this study, we use an anti-cosine mechanism as the learning factor function. This function is formulated below:

$$K = K_{\min} + (K_{\max} - K_{\min}) \times \left(1 - \arccos\left(\frac{\left(-2 \times \frac{t}{T} + 1\right)}{\pi}\right)\right), \tag{5.9}$$

where $K_{\min}$ and $K_{\max}$ are the minimum and the maximum values of K, where the initial value is $[K_{\min}, K_{\max}] = [0.05, 1]$, t describes the present number of iterations, and T stands for the maximum quantity of iterations.

To validate the effectiveness of the proposed method, it is applied to some standard benchmark functions and its results are compared with various other metaheuristics, including the World Cup optimization algorithm (WCO) [23], elephant herding behavior optimization (EHO) algorithm [24], emperor penguin optimizer (EPO) [25], and the original EFO algorithm. The formulations of the studied benchmark functions are given in the following:

$$\mathrm{Sphere} = \sum_{i=1}^{D} x_i^2 \ \text{Constraint: } [-512, 512], \tag{5.10}$$

$$\mathrm{Rastrigin} = 10D + \sum_{i=1}^{D} (x_i^2 - 10\cos(2\pi x_i)) \ \text{Constraint: } [-512, 512], \tag{5.11}$$

$$\mathrm{Rosenbrock} = \sum_{i=1}^{D-1} \left(100(x_i^2 - x_{i+1}) + (x_i - 1)^2\right) \ \text{Constraint: } [-2.045, 2.045], \tag{5.12}$$

Table 5.1. The validation results of the developed EFO (DEFO) algorithm in comparison with other algorithms.

Function		DEFO	EFO [19]	EHO [24]	WCO [23]	EPO [25]
Ackley	MV	0.00	1.69×10^{-20}	4.96×10^{-4}	4.39×10^{3}	4.36×10^{-16}
	Std	0.00	0.00	2.08×10^{-4}	6.51×10^{-3}	3.33×10^{-3}
Rastrigin	MV	0.00	10.19	8.37	5.12	1.05
	Std	0.00	2.30	2.26	4.73	3.93
Rosenbrock	MV	3.26	3.18	8.50	7.85	6.17
	Std	2.19	1.99	10.29	4.03	5.90
Sphere	MV	0.00	7.29×10^{-17}	7.22×10^{-7}	5.68×10^{-9}	7.03×10^{-12}
	Std	0.00	6.24×10^{-21}	2.36×10^{-7}	1.04×10^{-9}	4.39×10^{-16}

$$\text{Ackley} = -20\exp\left(-0.2\sqrt{\frac{1}{D}\sum_{i=1}^{D} x_i^2}\right) - \exp\left(\frac{1}{D}\sum_{i=1}^{D}\cos(2\pi x_i)\right) + 20 + e \quad \text{Constraint: } [-10, 10], \tag{5.13}$$

where the results of the analysis based on the mean value (MV) and the standard deviation value (Std) are given in table 5.1.

As can be inferred from table 5.1, it is clear that the proposed developed EFO (DEFO) provides the minimum values for MD among the other algorithms. This indicates that the suggested method has the best accuracy among comparable methods. Further, it can be observed from the results that the standard deviation results of the proposed algorithm provide better results than the algorithms (even the basic EFO), which shows its excellence in terms of the precision.

5.7 Simulation results

Diagnosis of skin cancer based on machine vision is a step-by-step procedure that begins with receiving suspicious skin images. There are few publicly available skin image data sets that can be used for this purpose. Suspicious skin images collected may contain various artifacts. As such, before further processing it is better to apply pre-processing to the images to remove air bubbles, hair, and excess parts of the image. The next step is to separate or segment the target area from the pre-processed image. Before beginning image classification, it is necessary to separate and define the rich feature set from the image background, which can be extracted from the segmented image. The complete diagnosis process can be seen in figure 5.6.

5.7.1 Image acquisition

This section details the skin cancer image databases that are available publicly. The present research mainly uses two types of images in skin cancer diagnosis:

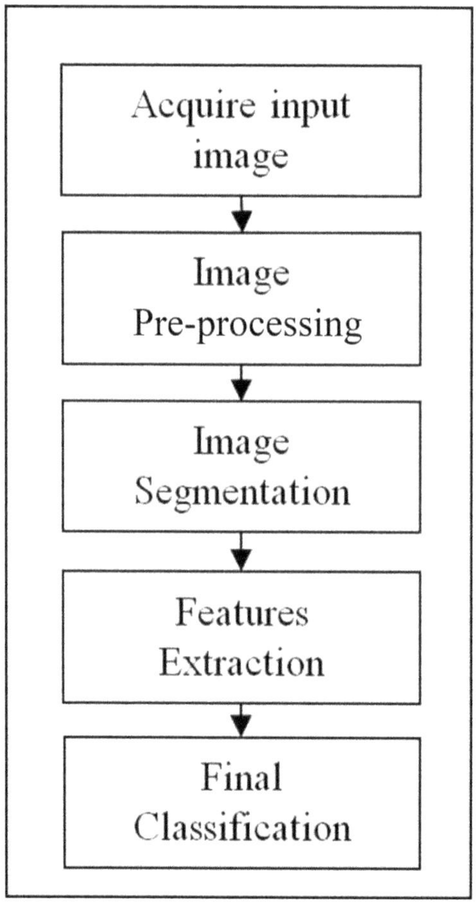

Figure 5.6. General method of skin cancer diagnosis.

dermoscopic images and digital images. Dermoscopic images are recorded by a special system in a medical center that is focused on the desired areas with high magnification (for example, 20×). Alternatively, digital images are recorded by any digital image recording system with little focus on the target area. Dermoscopic images are better for diagnosis but require a dermatologist to diagnose skin cancer. There is a huge demand for digital imaging technology for skin cancer. This study uses two data sets. All skin images have diagnostic tags for their images. For each skin image, only one disease label is assigned. These diagnostic tags are used to train skin disease classifiers. The data sets used in this study are collected from two digital databases: Dermquest [26] and DermIS [27]. General information about these two databases is explained below:

(1) DermIS Digital Database: the DermIS Digital Database is a visual atlas of different types of skin cancers used for medical imaging applications. DermIS is the largest online database on the Internet.

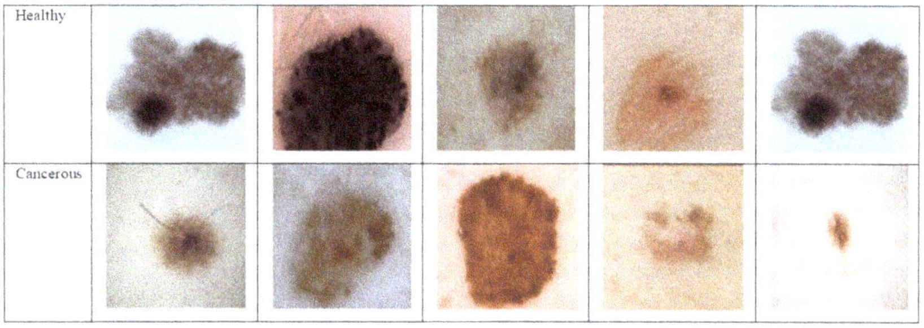

Figure 5.7. Some examples of images extracted from the Dermquest and DermIS databases.

(2) Dermquest Database: this database is an online medical atlas for health professionals and dermatologists. Images in this database have been reviewed and approved by internationally recognized editorial boards. The database contains a wide range of clinical images, including more than 22 000 clinical images.

Figure 5.7 shows some examples of Dermquest and DermIS database images.

5.7.2 Pre-processing stage

As mentioned before, the first step in processing medical images for any purpose is to perform some pre-processing to improve the quality of the original images and simplify the next steps. Skin images usually include some artifacts such as light reflection, the presence of hair, lines on the skin, air bubbles, and shadows that affect the image segmentation stage.

- *Median filtering*

A simple way to improve image quality by removing artifacts is to use a median filter. In fact, this filter can be used to remove image noise and, as a result, it softens high-frequency artifacts such as noise, extra lines, and hair without losing information about the rest, thus creating precise segmentation. A median filter is a nonlinear process that, unlike linear filters, smoothens the edges of images by holding the original image without blur. This filter may be used to smooth out skin lesions in addition to removing artifacts, preserving the edges of the lesion. To create an operational filter, the average filter mask size should be commensurate with the original image. This study uses a 9×9 convolution mask on images. While other masks do not produce a smooth image with a good level of noise reduction, they replace the median filter of 1 pixel with the center of the whole pixels adjacent to w, i.e.

$$y[m, n] = \text{median}\ (x[i, j], (i, j) \in w), \tag{5.14}$$

where w defines the area specified by the user and its center corresponds to the location $[m, n]$ in the image.

By considering a two-dimensional disk window for the center filter, the center pixel will be replaced by the average of all the pixel values inside the window. The main operation in this filter is sorting. Several sorting algorithms have been introduced for this purpose with complexity ($n\log_2 n$). However, in this study, with a limited number of pixels, a simple sorting method with complexity is used (n^2). The pseudo-code of this method is given below:

Algorithm 1

```
for (i = 0; i<n-1; i++)
  for (j = i+1; j<n; j++)
  if ( bin[i] < \;bin[j]) {
  w = bin[i]; bin[i] = bin[j]; bin[j] = w;
  }
```

Figure 5.8 shows two examples of median filtering for skin cancer images.

- Contrast enhancement

Contrast enhancement is a digital image processing method that is used to increase the contrast of medical images in multiplicity. As such, contrast enhancement is one of the main digital image processing techniques used to improve image quality. Contrast enhancement is based on the histogram of an image. A histogram is a representation of an image's frequency distribution. This form is the basis of many spatial domain processing techniques. Histogram manipulation can be used to

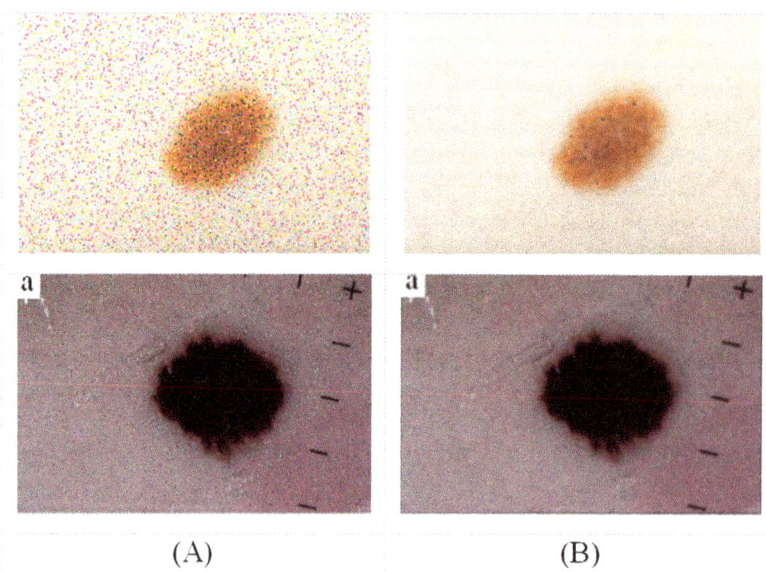

Figure 5.8. An example of median filtering for skin cancer images: (a) noisy image, and (b) filtered image.

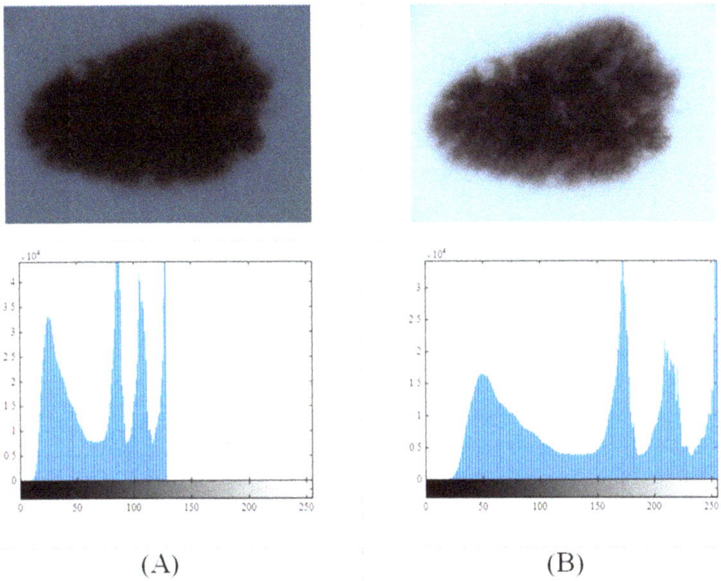

Figure 5.9. An example of a contrast-enhanced image: (a) the input image and its histogram, and (b) the image after improving the contrast and its histogram.

improve images. Contrast is defined as the difference in intensity between two objects in an image; if the contrast is too low, it is impossible to distinguish between two objects and they will be seen as a single object. Histogram matching and contrast enhancement are popular contrast enhancement methods that are widely used in medical image processing due to their high efficiency and simplicity. Figure 5.9 shows an example of a contrast enhancement method.

As can be inferred from figure 5.8, the image quality has been adequately improved.

5.7.3 Processing stage

• *Optimal thresholding based on Kapur's method and developed EFO algorithm*

Kapur's entropy thresholding method is one of the available thresholding methods that is used in two-level thresholding and has frequently been applied by researchers in the field of multi-level thresholding (MT). Kapur's entropy method is an effective image division method based on the threshold distribution and the histogram probability of an image. When the optimal threshold is assigned correctly, the entropy is at a maximum. Entropy is used to measure compaction and resolution between categories. The purpose of this method is to find the optimal threshold and produce the maximum entropy. This method extracts the brightness level from a grayscale or red-green-blue image. Assume the gray levels in an image with N pixels, where L are the gray levels in a range $[0, 1, \ldots, L-1]$. In this case, if $h(i)$ is the number of occurrences of gray area i in the image, then the average occurrence of the gray area i is defined as follows:

$$p_i = h(i)/N. \tag{5.15}$$

When providing an M-class segmentation for an image, the $M - 1$ threshold is required. The image is divided into M classes of $C_1 \tilde{} C_M$ according to the obtained thresholds. The range of gray levels for each class, according to the optimal achieved thresholds $\{t_1^*, t_2^*, \dots, t_{M-1}^*\}$, is defined as follows:

$$C_i: [t_{i-1}^*, \dots, t_i^* - 1] i = 1, \dots, M, \tag{5.16}$$

where $t_0 = 0$, $t_M - 1 = L - 1$.

For each C_k interval as defined above, the value W_k is defined as the probability of distributing the gray surfaces of the C_k interval member as follows:

$$w_k = \sum_{j=t_{k-1}}^{t_k - 1} P_j. \tag{5.17}$$

Kapur's method obtains thresholds based on maximizing Kapur entropy and on the information obtained from the histogram of the gray surfaces, which is defined as follows in the case of a two-level segmentation:

$$\text{Maximize}\{f_1(t)\} = H(0, t) + H(t, L), \tag{5.18}$$

where

$$H(0, t) = -\sum_{i=0}^{t-1} \frac{P_i}{w_0} ln \frac{P_i}{w_0}, \; w_0 = \sum_{i=0}^{t-1} P_i,, \tag{5.19}$$

$$H(t, L) = -\sum_{i=t}^{L-1} \frac{P_i}{w_1} ln \frac{P_i}{w_1}, \; w_1 = \sum_{i=t}^{L-1} P_i. \tag{5.20}$$

The value of the optimal threshold is the value of the gray surface t that maximizes the function f_1. Figure 5.10 shows an example of applying Kapur's method to an image.

In the present study, the developed EFO (DEFO) algorithm is used to find the optimal value of this threshold. Here, the electromagnetic candidates select k elements as the problem variables for optimization. These variables represent a different threshold that is used to segment the image. Therefore, the total population is determined as follows:

$$HM = [x_1^c, x_2^c, \dots, x_{HMS}^c]^T, x_i^c = [th_1^c, th_2^c, \dots, th_k^c], \; c = 1, 2, 3, \tag{5.21}$$

where T describes the transposition matrix operator, HM represents the magnitude of the electromagnetic candidates, x_i signifies the ith element of HM, and c represents the dimension of the image (here R, G, and B). In other words, if c equals 1, it indicates that our input is gray.

- *Morphological operations*

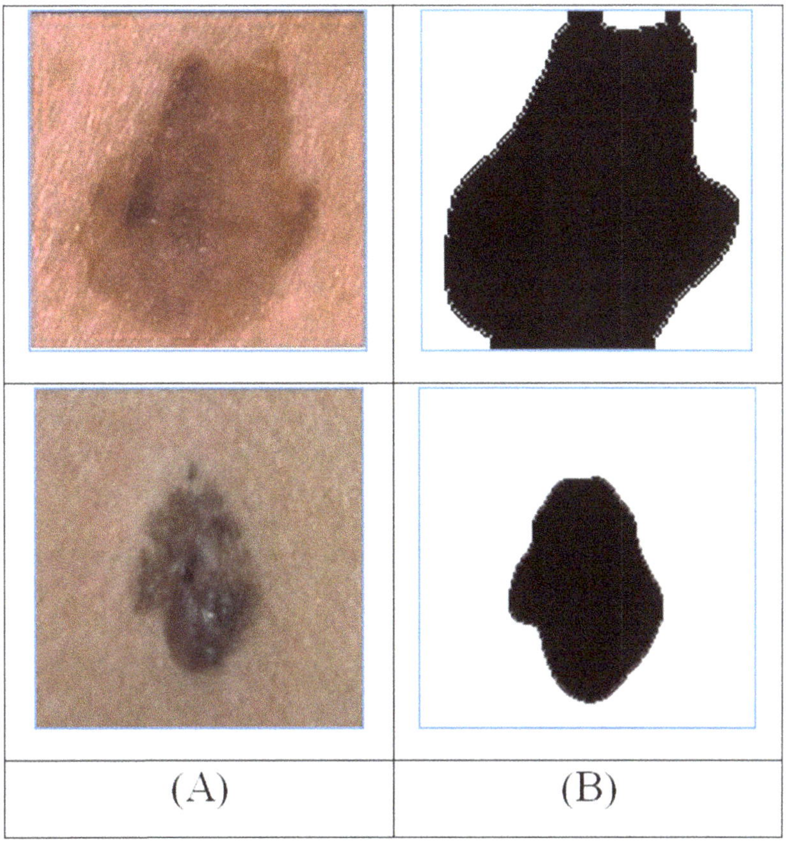

Figure 5.10. An example of applying Kapur's method to an image: (a) input image, (b) image after Kapur thresholding.

A set of nonlinear operations related to the shape or morphology of an image is known as a morphological operation (mathematical morphology) in image processing. Morphological operations rely only on the relative order of pixel values and not on their numerical values, and are therefore particularly suitable for processing binary images. These techniques can also be extended to images on a gray scale in such a way that their light transmission function is unknown and therefore their absolute pixel values are not of interest or partial.

A small shape or pattern called a 'structuring element,' a matrix that identifies the pixel in the image being processed and the location used to process each pixel, is used to explore an image in these morphological techniques, located in all possible places in the input image and compared with the neighborhood of the corresponding pixels.

The main point of using mathematical morphology is to choose a threshold level to convert an image into a binary image. In addition, the morphological operations of the gray surface soften the image and, in addition, so does the filtering itself, which greatly eliminates the need to filter the image.

This action eliminates dark and light noise or artifacts in the image, for particles that are regular in shape and lighter than the background. There are four basic operations of mathematical morphology: erosion, dilation, opening, and closing. Mathematical morphology uses a structural element to gather information about the image when a probe is constantly moving in the image. The particular morphological operations applied in our project include opening and closing in order of priority, which are summarized below.

In the next step, an opening operation is performed on the formed image. The opening operation is morphological with increasing size, and is generally used to remove small bright details without manipulating other gray surfaces. The formula for this operation is given below:

$$A \circ B = (A \ominus B) \oplus B, \tag{5.21}$$

where A and B are the range and structural element, and $\oplus$ and $\ominus$ are dilation and erosion operations, respectively.

The dilation action expands the binary image, and in addition to dilating the image it eliminates the holes in it and repairs the damaged edges. The formula for this operation is as follows:

$$A \oplus B = (z \in E \mid (B^s)_z \bigcap A \neq \Phi), \tag{5.22}$$

where z is as follows:

$$B^s = (x \in E \mid -x \in B). \tag{5.23}$$

In the above statement, B has a center whose location is at the center of E.

The erosion morphological operation is another one of the most basic operators in image processing. The erosion operator analyzes the white areas of the binary image and shrinks the white image and removes the extra parts. This operation is similar to the contraction of white areas. The formula for this operation is as follows:

$$A \ominus B = (z \in E \mid B_z \subseteq A), \tag{5.24}$$

where

$$B_z = (b + z \mid b \in B) \quad . \tag{5.25}$$

The second morphology operator used in this work is the closing morphology operator. In this work, the purpose of the operation is to connect the narrow parts together:

$$A \bullet B = (A \oplus B) \ominus B. \tag{5.26}$$

The structural element in this work is a single cube with a size of 9×9, i.e.

$$\begin{bmatrix} 1 & \cdots & 1 \\ \vdots & \ddots & \vdots \\ 1 & \cdots & 1 \end{bmatrix}_{9\times 9} . \tag{5.27}$$

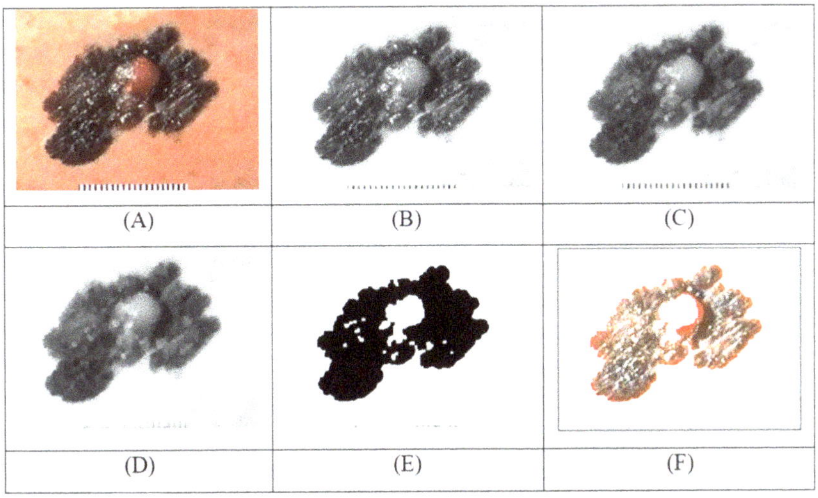

Figure 5.11. An example of the general process of applying optimal segmentation: (a) the input image, (b) the gray image, (c) the image after morphological opening, (d) image (c) after morphological closing, (e) the image after the proposed optimal thresholding, and (f) the segmented part.

Note that the morphological operations in this study were performed before thresholding. Figure 5.11 shows an example of the general process of applying optimal segmentation based on the proposed DEFO algorithm.

As can be seen, by applying different operations, the image segmentation quality has been greatly increased. Figure 5.12 shows the final results for some other examples.

• *Feature extraction.*

Extraction is a process of dimensional reduction in which an initial set of raw data is reduced to more controllable groups for processing. This large data set is characterized by a large number of variables that require a lot of computational resources for processing. Attribute extraction is the name of the method that selects or combines variables into attributes, thereby effectively reducing the amount of data to be processed, while still accurately describing the original data set.

The feature extraction process is useful when there is a need to reduce the number of resources required for processing without losing important or relevant information. Feature extraction can also reduce the amount of redundant data for a given analysis. In addition, reducing the data and the device trying to create variable combinations (features) facilitates the learning speed and generalization steps in a machine-learning process. Feature extraction can be done manually or automatically.

Manual feature extraction requires identifying and describing features related to a particular problem and implementing a method for extracting these features. In many situations, having a good understanding of the context or domain can help make informed decisions about which feature might be useful. Through decades of research, engineers and scientists have developed feature extraction methods for

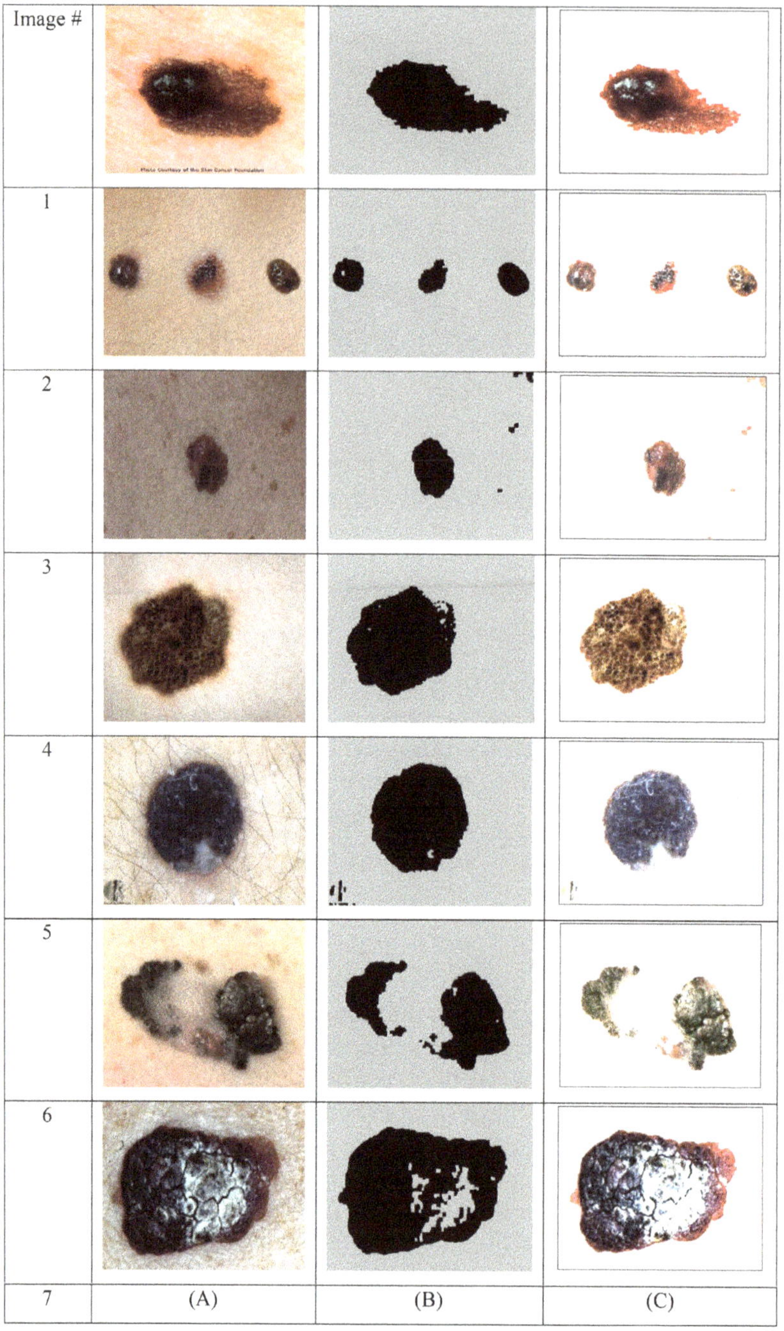

Figure 5.12. The final results for some different examples: (a) input image, (b) thresholding (a), and (c) image after segmentation.

images, signals, and text. An example of a simple feature is the average of a window in a signal.

Automatic feature extraction automatically extracts features from signals or images using specialized algorithms or deep networks without the need for human intervention. This method can be very useful when there is an aim to move quickly from raw data to the development of machine-learning algorithms. Wavelet scattering is an example of automatic feature extraction. As deep-learning techniques have progressed, feature extraction has been largely replaced by the first layers of deep grids, although more so for image data. For signal and time series programs, feature extraction is the first challenge that requires considerable skill before building effective predictive models.

Nowadays, feature extraction has become a significant part of signal and image processing for various applications, including the identification and classification of disease. This process forms the next step in diagnosing cancer after image segmentation.

The main data extracted from the segmented image are very important, although it might not provide any immediately useful information about the image. The use of feature extraction techniques at this time is thus very useful for exploiting the useful features extracted from the raw data. In this study, we used the following geometric properties, tissue properties, and statistical properties:

- *Geometric features*. Strength, area, size, equivalent diameter, centrifuge, convex area, environment, and irregularity index.
- *Tissue properties*. Correlation, entropy, contrast, homogeneity, and energy.
- *Statistical characteristics*. Mean, variance, standard deviation, fixed moments.

The feature formulas considered are shown below:

$$\text{Area} = \sum_{i=1}^{M}\sum_{j=1}^{N} p(i, j), \tag{5.28}$$

$$\text{Correlation} = \sum_{i=1}^{M}\sum_{j=1}^{N} \frac{p(i, j) - \mu_r \mu_c}{\sigma_r \sigma_c}, \tag{5.29}$$

$$\text{Rectangularity} = \frac{\text{Area}}{a \times b}, \tag{5.30}$$

$$\text{Homogeneity} = \sum_{i=1}^{M}\sum_{j=1}^{N} \frac{p(i, j)}{1 + |\, i - j \,|}, \tag{5.31}$$

$$\text{Perimeter} = \sum_{i=1}^{M}\sum_{j=1}^{N} b_p(i, j), \tag{5.32}$$

$$\text{Entropy} = \sum_{i=1}^{M}\sum_{j=1}^{N} p(i, j) \log \text{p}(i, j), \tag{5.33}$$

$$\text{Elongation} = \frac{2\sqrt{\text{Area}}}{a\sqrt{\pi}}, \tag{5.34}$$

$$\text{Mean} = \frac{1}{MN}\sum_{i=1}^{M}\sum_{j=1}^{N} p(i, j), \tag{5.35}$$

$$\text{Solidity} = \frac{\text{Area}}{\text{Convex Area}}, \tag{5.36}$$

$$\text{Variance} = \frac{1}{MN}\sum_{i=1}^{M}\sum_{j=1}^{N} (p(i, j) - \mu), \tag{5.37}$$

$$\text{Irregularity index} = 4\pi \times \frac{\text{Area}}{\text{Perimeter}^2}, \tag{5.38}$$

$$\text{Standard deviation} = \text{variance}\ \frac{1}{2}, \tag{5.39}$$

$$\text{Eccentricity} = 2a^{-1}(a^2 - b^2)^{0.5}, \tag{5.40}$$

$$\text{Form factor} = \frac{\text{Area}}{a^2}, \tag{5.41}$$

$$\text{Energy} = \sum_{i=1}^{M}\sum_{j=1}^{N} p^2(i, j) \tag{5.42}$$

$$\text{Contrast} = \sum_{i=1}^{M}\sum_{j=1}^{N} p^2(i, j). \tag{5.43}$$

The invariant moments are denoted by the following:

$\varphi_1 = \eta_{20} + \eta_{02}$

$\varphi_2 = (\eta_{20} - \eta_{02})^2 + 4\eta_{11}^2$

$\varphi_3 = (\eta_{30} - 3\eta_{12})^2 + (3\eta_{21} - \mu_{03})^2$

$$\varphi_3 = (\eta_{30} + 3\eta_{12})^2 + \left(3\eta_{21} + \mu_{03}\right)^2, \tag{5.44}$$

where b_p describes the length of the outer side of the border pixel, $p(i, j)$ is the value of the pixel intensity in (i, j), MN defines the image size, a and b represent the major and minor axes, respectively, and μ and σ are the mean and the standard deviation, respectively.

For example, some extracted features from figure 5.12 are reported in tables 5.2 and 5.3.

Table 5.2. Some extracted features from figure 5.11.

Image #	Contrast	Energy	Entropy	Mean	Variance	Correlation	Homogeneity
1	0.0031	0.8911	0.2308	2.372	0.662	0.951	−0.916
2	0.0049	0.749	0.424	2.357	0.711	0.9617	−0.900
3	0.0024	0.8903	0.2274	2.68	0.374	0.9637	−0.884
4	0.0086	0.6421	0.5764	2.472	0.21	0.957	−0.891
5	0.0031	0.9595	0.101	2.517	0.091	0.9247	−0.911
6	0.0015	0.984	0.0444	2.532	0.075	0.9515	−0.895
7	0.0035	0.9226	0.1792	2.308	0.43	0.9413	−0.915

Table 5. 3. Some extracted features from figure 5.11.

Image #	ϕ_4	ϕ_3	ϕ_2	ϕ_1
1	0	0	0.454	0.709
2	0	0	0.454	0.709
3	0	0	0.459	0.698
4	0	0	0.439	0.739
5	0	0	0.498	0.547
6	0	0	0.468	0.628
7	0	0	0.439	0.663

After extracting the image properties, this information must be injected into a classifier to make the final classification. In the following section, the use of classification is described.

5.7.4 Classification

Image classification is a complex process that can be influenced by many factors. Classification involves a range of theoretical decision-making approaches to identifying images (or parts of them). All classification algorithms are based on the assumption that the image represents one or more attributes, and each of these attributes belongs to one of several distinct and unique classes. Classification algorithms typically use two processing steps: training and testing. In the initial training phase, the characteristic features of the typical image are separated and, based on this, a unique description of each classification group, for example the training class, is created. In the next step (experiment), these feature space partitions are used to classify the image's properties. Classes may be specified by an analyst (such as supervised classification) or automatically clustered (i.e. in unattended classification) in a set of prototype classes, where the analyzer specifies only the desired number of categories.

• *Supervised classification.*
Supervised classification is based on the idea that the user can select sample pixels in the image that represent specific classes and then direct the image processing software to use them as references for classifying other image pixels. Experimental data are selected based on user knowledge. The user also sets boundaries to group other pixels. These ranges are often determined by the spectral characteristics of the trained area. The user also determines the number of classes in which the image is classified. Once a statistical description has been obtained for each data class, the image is categorized by examining the reflection for each pixel and deciding which class is more similar. Supervised classification uses classification algorithms and regression techniques to develop prediction models. These algorithms include, for instance, linear regression, logistic regression, neural networks, decision trees, SVMs, random forests, Bayesian methods, and nearest neighbors.

• *Unsupervised classification.*
Unsupervised classification is where the results (grouping of pixels with common features) are based on software analysis of an image without the aid of a user specifying sample classes. The computer uses techniques to determine how the pixels relate to each other and subsequently groups them into classes. The user can specify which algorithm the software uses and the desired number of output classes, but otherwise does not help the classification process. However, when grouping pixels with computer-generated common features relates to real properties, the user should be aware of the area being classified. Some of the most common algorithms used in unsupervised learning include cluster analysis, anomaly detection, neural networks, and latent variable model learning approaches. Figure 5.13 shows an overview of the types of classification.

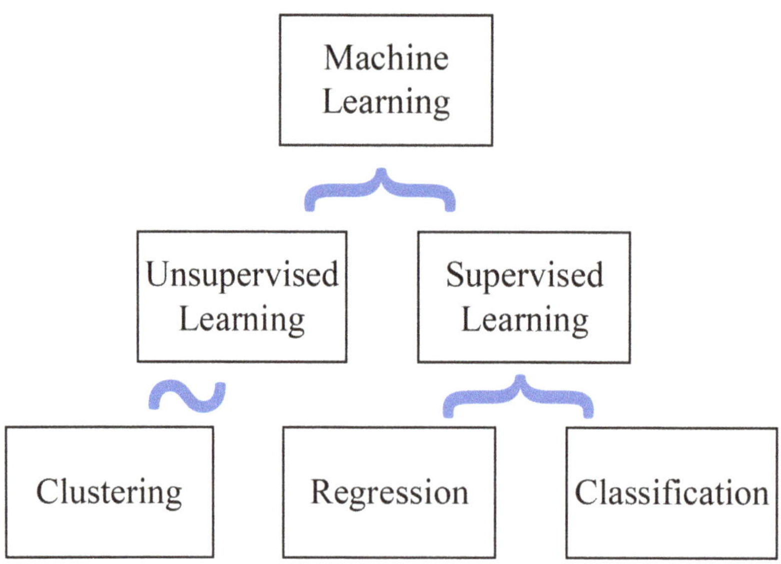

Figure 5.13. Types of classification.

To evaluate the performance of the system, a SVM classification method has been employed.

A popular and useful way to classify medical images is to use a SVM. A backup vector machine SVM looks for the best hyperplane to act as a multipart data separator (here two parts) in the input space. To achieve the constraints of the optimization problem, the SVM is used to evaluate the natural vector w in the hyperplane, the bias b, and the slack variable η, which is defined for incorrect training patterns that support generalization, as follows:

$$y = \min\frac{\| w \|^2}{2} + C \times \sum_{i=1}^{n} \eta_i, \tag{5.45}$$

with the separator function:

$$y_i(q \times x_i + b) \geqslant 1 - \eta_i. \tag{5.46}$$

The feature space is greatly affected by the separator function in the equation. So, to produce the desired output, it is necessary to make the right choice of function. Accordingly, the vector device uses kernel support, which is used to change the data into feature space. In this study, four different kernels, including linear, polynomial, radial basis function (RBF), and sigmoid, have been used. Figure 5.14 shows a typical SVM.

For numerical analysis of the classification in this study, three popular measurement indicators in classification problems have been used. These criteria are accuracy (ACC), precision (PR), and sensitivity (SN). By comparing the actual

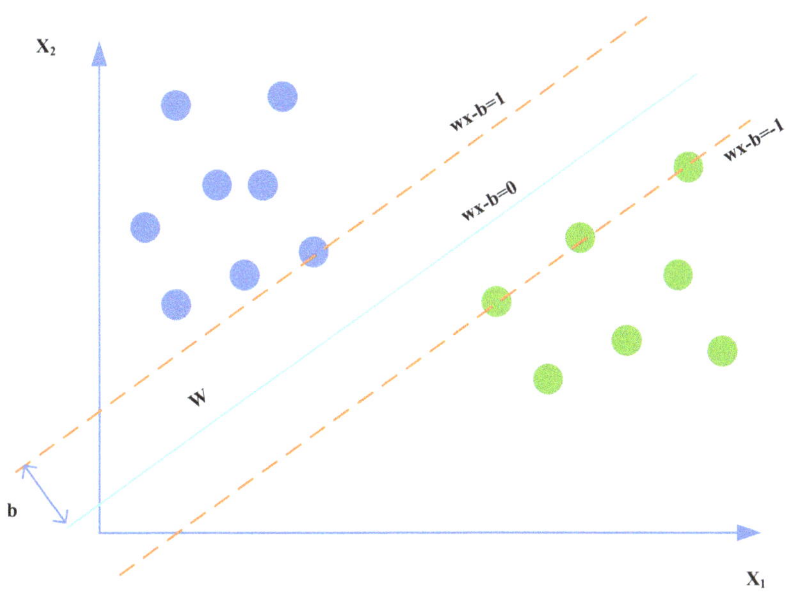

Figure 5.14. A basic model of a support vector machine.

Table 5. 4. Database classification results based on the different kernels of a support vector machine.

Data set	Kernel	ACC (%)	PR (%)	SN (%)
DermIS	Linear	89.20	90.35	89.20
	RBF	59.16	60.22	59.16
	Polynomial	67.58	59.07	67.58
	Sigmoid	62.57	62.34	62.57
Dermquest	Linear	78.14	79.62	78.14
	RBF	48.32	51.49	48.32
	Polynomial	45.38	38.25	45.38
	Sigmoid	39.47	34.92	39.47

result with the amount obtained from the classification, the following classification indicators were evaluated:

$$\text{ACC} = \frac{\text{TP} + \text{TN}}{\text{TP} + \text{TN} + \text{FP} + \text{FN}} \times 100, \tag{5.47}$$

$$\text{PR} = \frac{\text{TP}}{\text{TP} + \text{FP}} \times 100, \tag{5.48}$$

$$\text{SN} = \frac{\text{TP}}{\text{TP} + \text{FN}} \times 100. \tag{5.49}$$

where TP, TN, FP, and FN represent true positive, true negative, false positive and false negative, respectively.

Therefore, by analyzing the efficiency of the proposed method and considering different kernels based on the above indicators, table 5.4 has been achieved.

From table 5.4, it can be seen that the proposed linear kernel, in addition to simplicity, has obtained the best values for all indicators. Therefore, this kernel is used here to classify the features.

5.8 Final evaluation

To comprehensively evaluate the efficiency of the proposed method, five measurement indicators, including specificity (SP), positive predictive value (PPV), negative predictive value (NPV), F1 score, and Matthew's correlation coefficient (MCC), are considered. Their mathematical model is shown below:

$$\text{SP} = \frac{\text{TN}}{\text{FP} + \text{TN}}, \tag{5.50}$$

$$\text{PPV} = \frac{\text{TP}}{\text{TP} + \text{FP}}, \tag{5.51}$$

Table 5.5. Comparison result of the proposed method with several other recent methods.

Method	MCC (%)	SP (%)	PPV (%)	NPV (%)	F1 score (%)
Proposed method	88.64	88.81	79.53	89.19	78.24
Astorino's [28]	68.59	86.06	75.52	83.10	65.46
Hassan's [29]	75.52	83.11	67.16	87.54	64.29
Barros's [30]	84.73	62.59	66.37	87.38	70.15
Santos's [31]	85.29	65.36	69.38	87.26	76.65

$$\mathrm{NPV} = \frac{\mathrm{TN}}{\mathrm{TN} + \mathrm{FN}}, \tag{5.52}$$

$$\mathrm{F1score} = \frac{2 \times \mathrm{TP}}{2 \times \mathrm{TP} + \mathrm{FP} + \mathrm{FN}}, \tag{5.53}$$

$$\mathrm{MCC} = \frac{\mathrm{TP} \times \mathrm{TN} - \mathrm{FP} \times \mathrm{FN}}{\sqrt{(\mathrm{TP} + \mathrm{FP})(\mathrm{TP} + \mathrm{FN})(\mathrm{TN} + \mathrm{FP})(\mathrm{TN} + \mathrm{FN})}}. \tag{5.54}$$

The proposed general method is compared with five other recent methods, and the comparison results are shown in table 5.5. The compared methods are as follows: Astorino's [28], based on multi-sample learning; Hassan's [29], based on a simple image pre-processing method; Barros's [30], based on a hardware design by a MLP; and Santos's [31], based on neural networks and fuzzy logic.

As can be observed from table 5.5, the F1 score, which defines the accuracy and retrieval of test data, for the proposed method was 78.24%, the highest among all methods compared. Further, the MCC value in the proposed method is the highest among all cases, at 88.64%, and since it uses all the terms of analysis, the proposed method shows higher efficiency than other methods. Also, the proposed method exhibits higher values of NPV and PPV, with 89.19% and 79.53%, respectively, compared to other methods, which indicates the existence of better conditions in the proposed method of controlling the probability of cancer detection test than the other methods. Finally, a higher SP value according to the proposed method reports results independent of the occurrence of the algorithm.

5.9 Conclusions

Skin cancer is one of the most dangerous cancers in the world. The skin, as the first cell layer of the body that is exposed to the external environment, can suffer from many injuries and diseases including cancer, which occurs in the tissues of the largest part of the skin. Skin cancer is the most common cancer type in the United States.

If skin cancer is diagnosed early, it can be treated, while late diagnosis can lead to death. Only experienced physicians can diagnose melanoma in a timely manner using appropriate tools and histological reports. One of the devices used to diagnose skin cancer is the dermatoscope. Using this tool, pigment changes in skin lesions in diseases can be evaluated. With the advancement of science in recent years, digital dermatoscopes have replaced conventional dermatoscopes capable of capturing and storing skin images. With the development of digital dermatoscopes, researchers have developed algorithms for detecting melanoma, as well as other methods which have been proposed to increase the accuracy of inspecting skin lesions. Based on the mentioned cases, in this project, due to the aforementioned necessity of early and timely diagnosis of skin cancer, a new method based on medical image processing and intelligent algorithms was presented, which was used to diagnose and determine the exact location of cancerous areas. According to the proposed method in this study, the masses are completely separated from other parts of the image and their quality and brightness are increased to clearly determine the location and size of the mass in a desired image with high accuracy. The proposed method is very effective in reducing human errors in detecting cancerous masses in images. Numerous images accessed from public databases were analyzed by the proposed model, the results of which are very acceptable and the reported accuracy high. Specifically, the proposed model algorithm was applied to images taken from the Dermquest and DermIS databases. In the developed algorithm, after receiving an image, additional noise is removed from the images using image pre-processing. The filtered output image is segmented by a threshold method. Then, a number of image properties are extracted from the resulting image to reduce the complexity of the work. Finally, several different classification methods were used to diagnose the target cancer. The proposed method is a safe, accessible, effective, and noninvasive method with high accuracy and reasonable price. With the proposed method, ordinary people will be able to initially diagnose their skin lesions without consulting a doctor, and, in principle, specialists will will be able to use it as an intelligent, fast, and accurate diagnostic assistant.

References

[1] Siegel R L, Miller K D and Jemal A 2019 Cancer statistics, 2019 *Cancer J. Clinicians* **69** 7–34

[2] WCRF 2019 Skin cancer statistics https://wcrf.org/dietandcancer/cancer-trends/skin-cancer-statistics

[3] Bansal P, Kumar S, Srivastava R and Agarwal S 2021 Using transfer learning and hierarchical classifier to diagnose melanoma from dermoscopic images *Int. J. Healthcare Information Systems and Informatics (IJHISI)* **16** 73–86

[4] Emre Celebi M *et al* 2008 Border detection in dermoscopy images using statistical region merging *Skin Res. Technol.* **14** 347–53

[5] Razmjooy N, Mousavi B S, Soleymani F and Khotbesara M H 2013 A computer-aided diagnosis system for malignant melanomas *Neural Comput. Appl.* **23** 2059–71

[6] Rashid Sheykhahmad F, Razmjooy N and Ramezani M 2015 A novel method for skin lesion segmentation *Int. J. Inf. Security Syst. Manage.* **4** 458–66

[7] Razmjooy N, Sheykhahmad F R and Ghadimi N 2018 A hybrid neural network—World Cup optimization algorithm for melanoma detection *Open Medicine* **13** 9–16

[8] Jadhav A R, Ghontale A G and Shrivastava V K 2019 Segmentation and border detection of melanoma lesions using convolutional neural network and SVM *Computational Intelligence:*

Theories, Applications and Future Directions - Volume I vol 798 ed N K Verma and A K Ghosh (Berlin: Springer) pp 97–108

[9] Pennisi A *et al* 2016 Skin lesion image segmentation using Delaunay triangulation for melanoma detection *Comput. Med. Imaging Graph.* **52** 89–103

[10] Heller N, Bussman E, Shah A, Dean J and Papanikolopoulos N 2018 Computer aided diagnosis of skin lesions from morphological features *Technical Report* TR 18-014 Unviersity of Minnesota, Computer Science & Engineering

[11] Somfai E *et al* 2021 Minimizing false negative rate in melanoma detection and providing insight into the causes of classification arXiv:2102.09199

[12] Vocaturo E and Zumpano E 2021 Useful features for computer-aided diagnosis systems for melanoma detection using dermoscopic images *Handbook of Research on Automated Feature Engineering and Advanced Applications in Data Science* (Hershey, PA: IGI Global) pp 48–71

[13] Sreelatha T, Subramanyam M and Prasad M G 2019 Early detection of skin cancer using melanoma segmentation technique *J. Med. Syst.* **43** 190

[14] Dey N, Rajinikanth V, Lin H and Shi F 2021 A study on the bat algorithm technique to evaluate the skin melanoma images *Applications of Bat Algorithm and Its Variants* ed N Dey and V Rajinikanth (Berlin: Springer) pp 45–60

[15] Tschandl P *et al* 2019 Expert-level diagnosis of nonpigmented skin cancer by combined convolutional neural networks *JAMA Dermatology* **155** 58–65

[16] Fan T *et al* 2021 Identification of skin melanoma based on microscopic hyperspectral imaging technology *20th Int. Conf. on Signal Processing Systems* **11719** 1171908

[17] Hekler A *et al* 2019 Superior skin cancer classification by the combination of human and artificial intelligence *Eur. J. Cancer* **120** 114–21

[18] Tan T Y, Zhang L, Neoh S C and Lim C P 2018 Intelligent skin cancer detection using enhanced particle swarm optimization *Knowl.-Based Syst.* **158** 118–35

[19] Abedinpourshotorban H, Shamsuddin S M, Beheshti Z and Jawawi D N A 2016 Electromagnetic field optimization: a physics-inspired metaheuristic optimization algorithm *Swarm and Evolutionary Computation* **26** 8–22

[20] Song S, Jia H and Ma J 2019 A chaotic electromagnetic field optimization algorithm based on fuzzy entropy for multilevel thresholding color image segmentation *Entropy* **21** 398

[21] Bouchekara H, Zellagui M and Abido M A 2017 Optimal coordination of directional overcurrent relays using a modified electromagnetic field optimization algorithm *Appl. Soft Comput.* **54** 267–83

[22] Bouchekara H 2020 Solution of the optimal power flow problem considering security constraints using an improved chaotic electromagnetic field optimization algorithm *Neural Comput. Appl.* **32** 2683–703

[23] Razmjooy N, Khalilpour M and Ramezani M 2016 A new meta-heuristic optimization algorithm inspired by FIFA world cup competitions: theory and its application in PID designing for AVR system *J. Control, Automation and Electrical Systems* **27** 419–40

[24] Wang G-G, Deb S, Gao X-Z and Dos Santos Coelho L 2016 A new metaheuristic optimisation algorithm motivated by elephant herding behaviour *Int. J. Bio-Inspired Computation* **8** 394–409

[25] Dhiman G and Kumar V 2018 Emperor penguin optimizer: a bio-inspired algorithm for engineering problems *Knowl.-Based Syst.* **159** 20–50

[26] Database D 2019 Dermquest database https://derm101.com/dermquest/

[27] Xu H and Mandal M 2015 Epidermis segmentation in skin histopathological images based on thickness measurement and k-means algorithm *EURASIP J. Image and Video Processing* **2015** 18

[28] Astorino A, Fuduli A, Veltri P and Vocaturo E 2020 Melanoma detection by means of multiple instance learning *Interdisciplinary Sciences: Computational Life Sciences* **12** 24–31

[29] Mohamed S H, Tarek A and May H E 2019 Detection of melanoma using image processing techniques driven TDS index *J. Environmental Science* **46** 1–46

[30] Barros W K *et al* 2020 Proposal of the CAD system for melanoma detection using reconfigurable computing *Sensors* **20** 3168

[31] Santos D F and Espitia H E 2020 Detection of uveal melanoma using fuzzy and neural networks classifiers *Telkomnika* **18** 2213–23

Chapter 6

Evaluation of COVID-19 lesion from CT scan slices: a study using entropy-based thresholding and DRLS segmentation

Hong Lin

Pneumonia is one of the primary lung diseases in humans, causing mild to severe respiratory problems. Timely screening and treatment execution is essential to control and cure the disease. Recently, pneumonia caused due to severe acute respiratory syndrome coronavirus-2 (SARS-CoV-2, referred to from here in shortened form as COVID-19) affected a broad population globally. This chapter proposes a hybrid image-processing system to evaluate pneumonia infection in the lungs with the help of CT scan slices (CTSs). This scheme implements a two-step procedure: (i) an elephant herding optimization (EHO) algorithm and entropy-based thresholding, and (ii) a distance regularized level set (DRLS) using single-/double-well segmentation. Furthermore, this work provides a comparative assessment of entropy functions, such as Shannon's, Tsallis's, and Kapur's, in order to establish the most acceptable threshold practice. In addition, this study investigates the axial, coronal, and sagittal planes of the lung CTSs, to identify the best two-dimensional slice orientation. The experimental outcome confirms that (i) thresholding based on Shannon's entropy offers a better outcome than other entropy functions, and (ii) the axial plane of a CTS presents enhanced results. The proposed research helps to achieve better mean values of Jaccard index (82.74 ± 3.17), Dice (89.42 ± 4.18), and accuracy (98.14 ± 1.13) when tested using clinical-grade lung CTSs infected with COVID-19.

6.1 Introduction

In recent years, the spread of disease in humankind has been gradually rising for various reasons. Subsequently, appropriate detection and control are necessary when an infectious disease begins to spread. Usually, infectious diseases are caused due to viruses or bacteria, which are also known as communicable diseases since

doi:10.1088/978-0-7503-4012-0ch6

they spread from one infected individual to another healthy person. Infectious diseases caused by viruses are considered more harmful than those by bacteria; infections can be controlled/cured with the help of appropriate medication. Early diagnosis and treatment will support speedy recovery, and also helps to temporarily/permanently stop the disease's spread [1–4].

In recent years, respiratory tract infection caused by SARS-CoV-2 (COVID-19) has emerged as a global threat, being the chief contributor to a significant disease rate worldwide [5–7]. Even though several vaccines are now available, the disease's spread is gradually rising due to continuous mutations in the virus. Earlier research works on COVID-19 detection have detailed the protocol followed in hospitals, which includes the following:

- *Sample collection and execution of reverse transcription-polymerase chain reaction (RT-PCR) tests* [8–11].
  RT-PCR is the laboratory practice of uniting reverse transcription of ribonucleic acid (RNA) into deoxyribonucleic acid (DNA) to enhance the exact DNA targets with the PCR technique. When this technique presents a negative result, the tested individual is not infected with COVID-19. However, if the result is positive, then bioimaging-supported screening is necessary to detect the presence of respiratory tract infection due to COVID-19.
- *Image-supported diagnosis* [12–14].
  Image-supported disease diagnosis plays a significant role in detecting disease/infection in internal body organs. The detection of COVID-19 infection involves recording the respiratory tract using a chosen radiological method and then inspecting the disease with the help of a skilled doctor or with a chosen computer algorithm. Earlier works establish that chest radiographs (x-rays) and computed tomography (CT) are widely deployed to detect COVID-19 infection. Then, treatment planning and execution are performed to aid the patient's recovery based on a disease score. If the infection score is high and the infected individual cannot breathe naturally, artificial ventilation is provided until the patient's condition returns to normal.

Due to its significance, a great deal of research work has been undertaken to detect COVID-19 infection in the chosen medical imaging modalities. The disease's visibility in lung CT scans is good compared to x-rays. Further, the lung CT is obtainable as a three-dimensional (3D) image, which can subsequently be examined in two-dimensional (2D) form using a chosen 3D to 2D conversion [15, 16].

Earlier works substantiate that CT scan slices (CTSs) provide better COVID-19 detection. Hence, a considerable number of segmentation [17–25] and classification [26–29] works have reported done with different artificial intelligence (AI) methods, such as machine-learning (ML) and deep-learning (DL) techniques. Furthermore, as recent work has discussed, the infection score plays a significant role in the treatment execution [30–32]. Hence, several segmentation works are employed to mine and evaluate the infection from the 2D CTS of a chosen plane.

This research aims to implement an AI-supported joint thresholding and segmentation technique to mine and analyze COVID-19 infection in 2D CTS.

The various phases involved in this research include (i) image collection and 3D to 2D conversion, (ii) artifact removal to extract the lung section to be examined, (iii) maximal-entropy-based thresholding to improve the visibility of the infected section, (iv) distance regularized level set (DRLS) segmentation to mine the infection using a single-/double-well technique, and (v) comparison of the mined region with ground truth (GT) and performance validation.

The mined COVID-19 infection is taken from the CTS's axial, coronal, and sagittal planes with a semi-automatic DRLS scheme. The DRLS is a bounding-box-based methodology executed to extract the infected section with superior accuracy. Further, this work presents a detailed assessment of the well-known entropy-based thresholding schemes, such as Shannon's, Tsallis's, and Kapur's. Finding the optimal threshold with the chosen entropy function is performed automatically using an elephant herding optimization (EHO) algorithm. The test images for this study are collected from [33], and the 3D to 2D conversion is achieved using ITK-Snap [17, 34]. The experimental task of this research is executed using MATLAB®, and the achieved results are separately presented for the different 2D CTSs considered in this work.

The main contributions of this work include the following:

(i) Artifact removal to enhance visibility of the lung section.
(ii) EHO and entropy-based thresholding to enhance the infection and single-/double-well DRLS implementation to mine the infection.
(iii) Development of a simple procedure to examine the various planes of a 2D CTS.

6.2 Context

Recently, a considerable number of AI-based COVID-19 detection techniques have been discussed in the literature. Processes such as segmentation and classification are widely implemented with 2D CTSs. The COVID-19 infection is mined during the segmentation phase using a chosen conventional and/or deep-learning scheme. After the extraction, the mined section is compared and verified against a binary image, known as a GT, supplied by a disease expert. Table 6.1 presents a summary of the recent COVID-19 mining procedures found in the literature.

The earlier works presented in table 6.1 confirm that deep-learning schemes are widely adopted in mining the disease section from 2D CTSs. This research employs a simple and effective procedure to extract the COVID-19 infection from the different planes of a 2D CTS.

6.3 Methodology

The performance of an AI-supported disease detection scheme depends on the methodology employed. This work employs a heuristic algorithm, entropy-based thresholding, and DRLS-based segmentation to mine the COVID-19 infection in chosen 2D CTSs. The proposed scheme is depicted in figure 6.1. Initially, the necessary test pictures are collected from an image database. Every collected CT is in 3D form; hence, 3D to 2D conversion is implemented using ITK-Snap. This helps to

Table 6.1. Summary of COVID-19 segmentation schemes.

Reference	Methodology implemented
Qayyum *et al* [17]	Implementation of multiscale deep-learning procedure (DLP) is discussed to mine COVID-19 infection.
Kesavan *et al* [19]	Res-UNet-based segmentation and examination of COVID-19 lesions is presented using 2D CTS with axial-plane images.
Amin *et al* [20]	Ensemble DLP is employed to achieve microscopic segmentation and categorization of COVID-19 infection.
Satapathy *et al* [21]	Automatic mining of COVID-19 lesions in 2D CTSs is discussed using Kapur's/Otsu's thresholding and a cuckoo search algorithm. This work presented a segmentation accuracy >90%.
Arunmozhi *et al* [22]	Detection of COVID-19 lesions using VGG-UNet is presented and a classification of healthy/disease class lung CT is presented using handcrafted features.
Kadry *et al* [23]	Machine-learning-based automatic classification of 2D CTSs into healthy/COVID-19 is presented.
Rajinikanth *et al* [17]	This work implemented a joint thresholding and segmentation scheme to extract COVID-19 lesions from 2D CTSs. This work utilizes a threshold filter to mine the artifact, Otsu's thresholding to enhance the image, and watershed segmentation to extract the lesion.
Kadry *et al* [24]	UNet-supported segmentation of COVID-19 lesions in lung CT is presented.
Yao *et al* [25]	This work presented a novel label-free segmentation of COVID-19 lesions from 2D CTSs.
Dey *et al* [26]	Implementation of conventional segmentation and classification is presented using 2D CTSs.

get axial-, coronal-, and sagittal-plane 2D slices, and from these images any artifacts are then extracted using the threshold filter discussed in prior works. The pre-processed 2D CTSs are then considered for thresholding-based enhancement and DRLS-based segmentation. Based on the requirement, the DRLS scheme implements a single-well or double-well bounding-box technique to mine the COVID-19 infection. Finally, the mined binary image is compared with the GT and the necessary image metrics are computed. Based on the computed image metrics, the merit of the proposed scheme is verified. In this work, the different entropy functions, such as Shannon's, Tsallis's, and Kapur's, are considered. The experimental outcome confirms that the Shannon-based thresholding offers a superior outcome compared to Tsali's and Kapur's.

6.3.1 COVID-19 database

The selection of a database to test an AI-supported disease detection technique plays a vital role. Therefore, clinical-grade images are widely adopted to test the

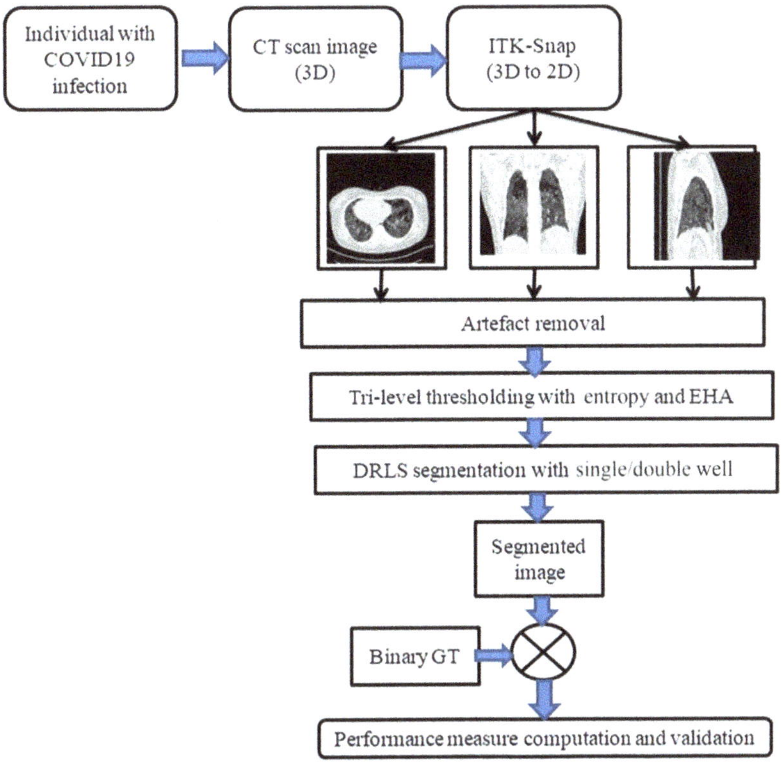

Figure 6.1. Pictorial representation of the COVID-19 lesion evaluation scheme.

performance of AI-based examination systems under development. In this work, the COVID-19 image database available in [33] is considered for the examination. In this database, 20 patient images are available along with their associated GTs, and every image is recorded from actual COVID-19 patients. Earlier works based on this database can be accessed from [24–26].

All the images (test pictures and GTs) are recorded in 3D form. After collecting the images, ITK-Snap (an open-source software widely used to process medical images) 3D to 2D conversion is executed, as depicted in figure 6.2, and extracted 2D slices of the axial, coronal, and sagittal planes are considered for assessment. Figure 6.3 presents sample test pictures for patients 1 to 5 in this study. This dataset consists of 20 patient images, with 10 2D slices being extracted from every patient. Therefore, for every 2D plane, 200 test images are considered for assessment.

6.3.2 Image conversion and pre-processing

After extracting the 2D slices of the particular modality, every image and its GT are resized to 512×512×1 pixels, and this converted image is then considered for the examination. Initially, the artifacts from each test picture are removed using the threshold filter discussed in [35–37]. The threshold filter is a binary thresholding procedure typically considered to remove the skull region from MRI scans [37] and

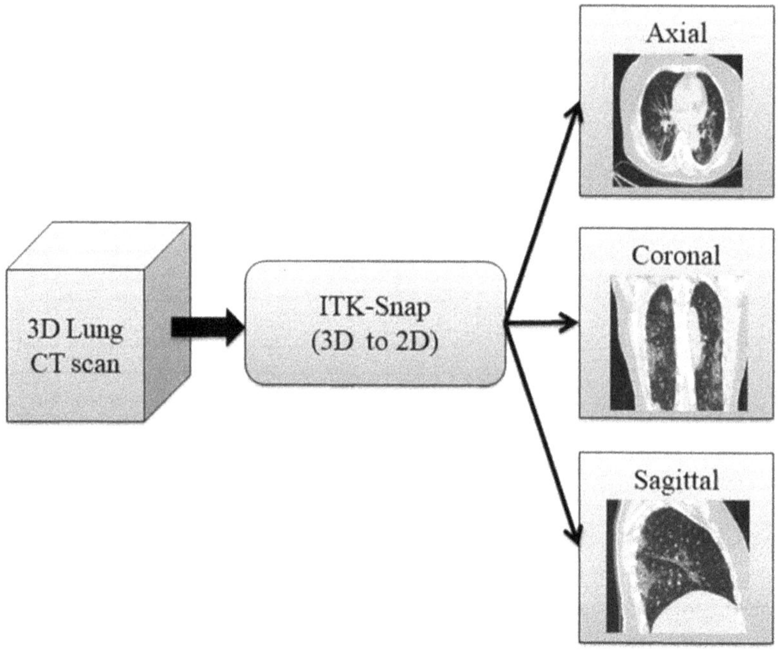

Figure 6.2. 3D to 2D conversion with ITK-Snap.

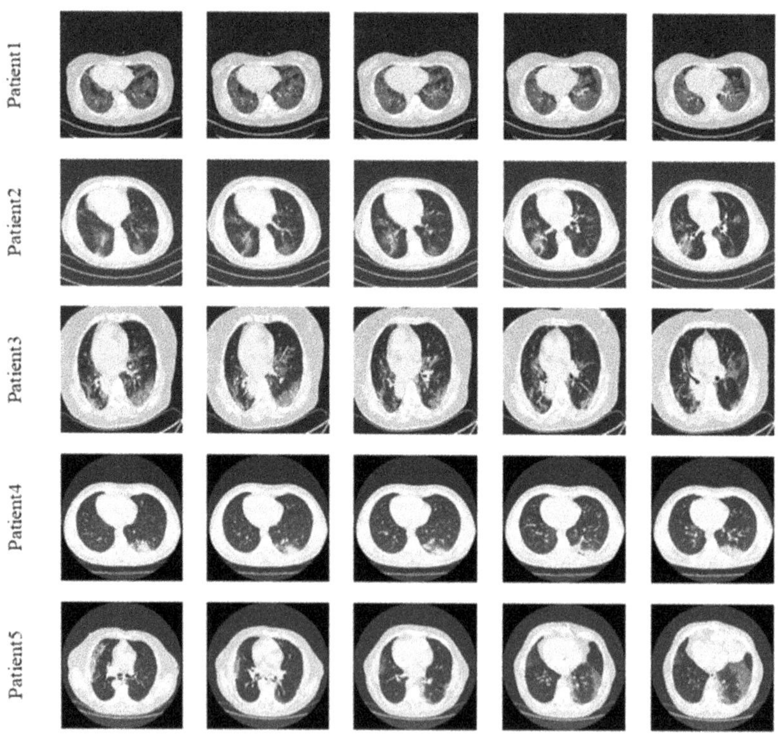

Figure 6.3. Sample test images of dimension 512×512×1 pixels considered in this research.

unwanted sections from the CT scans. After implementing the threshold filter, a 2D CTS with a clear lung section is available for assessment, which is then considered for further enhancement and mining of the targeted COVID-19 section.

6.3.3 Image thresholding

Conventional and soft-computing-based multi-thresholding is a recognized pre-processing practice broadly adopted in the image-processing literature to augment the visibility of abnormalities in different test imagery. For example, a threshold can be observed by plotting a histogram for a test picture of the gray/red-green-blue (RGB) scale. A histogram is a graphical expression of the diagram's pixel distribution (x-axis) with a threshold value (y-axis). For each picture, the threshold is predetermined, and the pixel allocation will differ based on the size and information obtainable for the medical image. Thresholding is one of the commonly adopted pre-processing schemes, in which a chosen methodology is employed to find an appropriate threshold to enhance a specific section of a given image. Many bi-level and multilevel thresholding schemes have already been discussed sufficiently in the literature to enhance gray/RGB scale pictures [37–40].

In this work, a tri-level thresholding procedure is employed to improve the visibility of the COVID-19 section from the test image. The concept of tri-level thresholding is commonly adopted in image segmentation methods. This helps to separate the image into three sections: (i) a background, (ii) a normal image region, and (iii) an abnormal image section, which contains the disease information. Therefore, the research presented here employs a tri-level thresholding process to improve the disease section in the considered 2D CTSs.

6.3.3.1 Entropy function

The entropy of an image is defined as the measure of the degree of randomness, and this scheme helps improve the visibility of the abnormality present in a digital picture. Entropy-supported image thresholding is widely discussed in the literature [41, 42] and is primarily implemented to improve the presentation of abnormalities in biomedical images.

Based on the mathematical expression, the entropy functions vary. In this research, entropy functions, such as Shannon's, Tsallis's, and Kapur's, are adopted. These functions are considered to improve the visibility of the COVID-19 infection in 2D CTSs. In the literature, entropy-based assessment can be found in [43]; each earlier work considered the maximization of the entropy function, which helps to get better values of the abnormality detection. Earlier work on entropy-based medical image thresholding can be found in [44], which implemented thresholding using the chosen entropy value. The optimal threshold is identified with the help of an EHO algorithm. The experimental outcome of the study confirmed that Shannon's function helps to better enhance such medical images compared to other entropies.

The expression for Shannon's entropy was clearly discussed in the work of Kannappan [45]. Let us decide a test picture of size $A \times B$. The pixel relationship in the test picture (x,y) is defined as $F(x,y)$, for $x \in \{1,2,..., A\}$ and $y \in \{1,2,..., B\}$. Let L

be the total gray level of the 2D CTS, and the set of all gray values $\{0, 1, 2, \ldots, L-1\}$ can be denoted as O, in such a way that

$$F(X, Y) \in O \,\forall\, (x, y) \in \text{Image}. \tag{6.1}$$

Then, the standardized histogram will be

$$S = (t_0, t_1, \ldots, t_{L-1}). \tag{6.2}$$

For a bi-level thresholding case, equation (6.1) becomes

$$S(T) = a_0(T_1) + a_1(T_2), \tag{6.3}$$

$$E(T) = \max_T \{S(T)\}, \tag{6.4}$$

where $T = \{T_1, T_2, \ldots, T_L\}$ is the threshold value, $S = \{a_0, a_1, \ldots, a_{L-1}\}$ is the normalized histogram, and $E(T)$ is the optimal threshold.

6.3.3.2 Elephant herding optimization algorithm

Heuristic-algorithm-based methods help to solve a variety of engineering optimization tasks as well as to provide appropriate solutions for complex real-world problems. In this work, the optimal threshold selection process is achieved using an EHO, as proposed by Wang *et al* in 2015 [46]. Due to its optimization accuracy, it is widely adopted to solve various engineering optimization problems [47, 48, 49].

An EHO stipulates the following considerations:

- Every clan consists of a fixed number of elephants in a herd.
- During every generation, a fixed number of adult male elephants will leave the herd and live alone.
- Each clan is led by an older and intelligent elephant, known as a matriarch, responsible for leading the herd toward food and water sources.

This research considered a traditional EHO, which consists of the following stages.

Stage 1: Clan-updating operator.

A matriarch guides every clan; during a search, the new position of every elephant in the clan is adjusted based on the position of the matriarch.

In a clan, the new position of each elephant is denoted as

$$X_{\text{new}, ci, j} = X_{ci, j} + a^*\left(X_{\text{best}, ci} - X_{ci, j}\right)^* r,$$

where ci is the matriarch of the clan, $X_{ci, j}$ is the old position, $X_{\text{new}, ci, j}$ is the new position, j is the total number of elephants in the clan, and a and r are random values in the range

$$\in [0,1]. \tag{6.5}$$

During each operation, the new position can also be denoted as

$$X_{\text{new},\, ci,\, j} = \beta^{*} X_{\text{center},\, ci}, \tag{6.6}$$

$$X_{\text{center},\, ci,\, d} = \frac{1}{n_{ci}} \times \sum_{j=1}^{n_{ci}} X_{ci,\, j,\, d}, \tag{6.7}$$

where $X_{\text{center},\, ci,\, d}$ is the central elephant in the clan and d is the search dimension.
The discussed scheme is represented with an appropriate picture in figure 6.4.

Stage 2: Separating process
As the number of generations increases, male elephants are discarded from the group and permitted to roam independently. This process is denoted in figure 6.5, and the mathematical expression for this process is depicted in equation (6.8):

$$X_{\text{worst},\, ci} = x_{\min} + (x_{\max} - x_{\min} + 1)^{*}\text{rand}. \tag{6.8}$$

In every generation, an adult male elephant is discarded from the group and, if necessary, the herd is guided by a new matriarch. In the proposed work the following values are assigned for the EHO: number of elephants = 25; number of generations = 5; dimensions of search = 3; objective value = maximization of entropy; number of iterations = 2000; and algorithm termination = maximum iterations. Other related works on this algorithm can be found in [47].

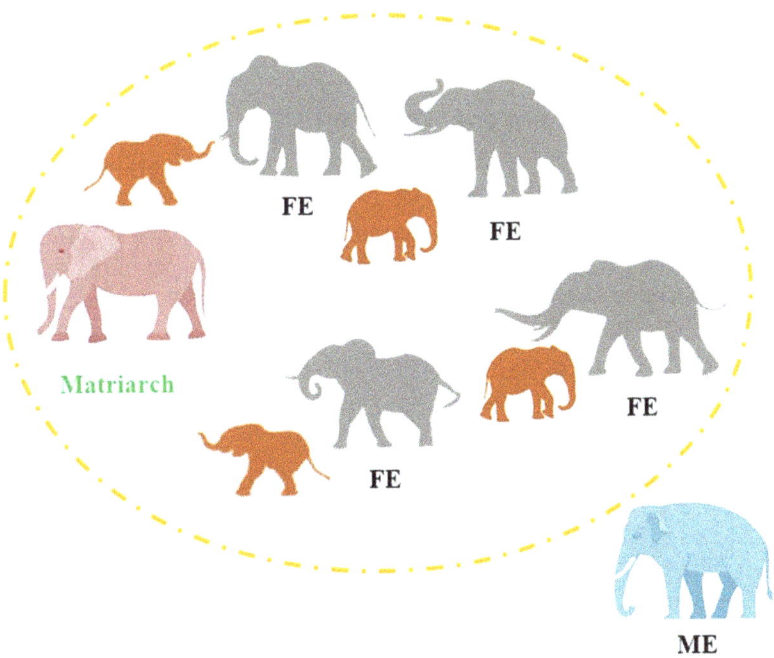

Figure 6.4. Pictorial representation of clan-updating process.

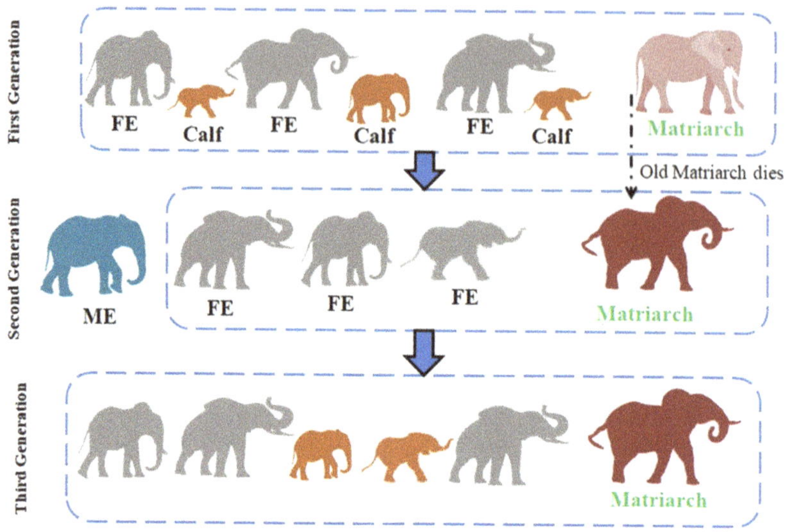

Figure 6.5. Change in the clan with respect to the generations.

6.3.4 Distance regularized level set segmentation

In image-processing applications, segmentation is considered to extract a particular region from an image for further analysis. In this work, a DRLS scheme, widely adopted in medical image evaluation tasks, is considered. This scheme can be implemented in single-well (single box) and double-well (two bounding box) versions, and this approach is also known as the level set segmentation. Earlier works on this scheme can be found in [47].

6.3.5 Performance computation and validation

This scheme initially employs a joint thresholding and segmentation scheme to mine COVID-19 infection from 2D CTSs. The implemented approach helps to mine said COVID-19 infection in the form of a binary image, which is then compared with the GT to compute the performance metrics. This comparison primarily computes the metrics such as true positive (TP), fals negative (FN), true negative (TN), and false positive (FP). From these values, other metrics, like Jaccard index (JA), Dice index (DI), accuracy (AC), precision (PR), sensitivity (SE), specificity (SP), and negative predictive value (NPV), are computed.

These measures can be mathematically expressed as in equations (6.8)–(6.14):

$$JA = \frac{TP}{TP + FP + FN}, \tag{6.8}$$

$$DI = \frac{2TP}{2TP + FP + FN}, \tag{6.9}$$

$$AC = \frac{TP + TN}{TP + TN + FP + FN}, \tag{6.10}$$

$$\mathrm{PR} = \frac{\mathrm{TP}}{\mathrm{TP} + \mathrm{FP}}, \tag{6.11}$$

$$\mathrm{SE} = \frac{\mathrm{TP}}{\mathrm{TP} + \mathrm{FN}}, \tag{6.12}$$

$$\mathrm{SP} = \frac{\mathrm{TN}}{\mathrm{TN} + \mathrm{FP}}, \tag{6.13}$$

$$\mathrm{NPV} = \frac{\mathrm{TN}}{\mathrm{TN} + \mathrm{FN}}. \tag{6.14}$$

6.4 Results and discussions

This research section presents the experimental results achieved with the proposed scheme. All the achieved results are obtained with MATLAB®.

Initially, the entropy-based optimal thresholding is implemented using the EHO, and the infected section from this image is mined using the DRLS. Figure 6.6 presents a sample test image and its GT for the axial, coronal, and sagittal planes. These images are then treated with the threshold filter to remove any artifacts. The artifact-removed images are then considered for thresholding with EHO+entropy, and the enhanced image is then treated with DRLS segmentation. The results achieved with this methodology for the axial plane are presented in figure 6.7. A similar task for the other 2D planes and its achieved outcomes are depicted in figure 6.8. Figure 6.7(a) presents the thresholded image, figures 6.7(b) and (c) show the initial and converged bounding box, and figure 6.7(d) presents the mined binary COVID-19 infection.

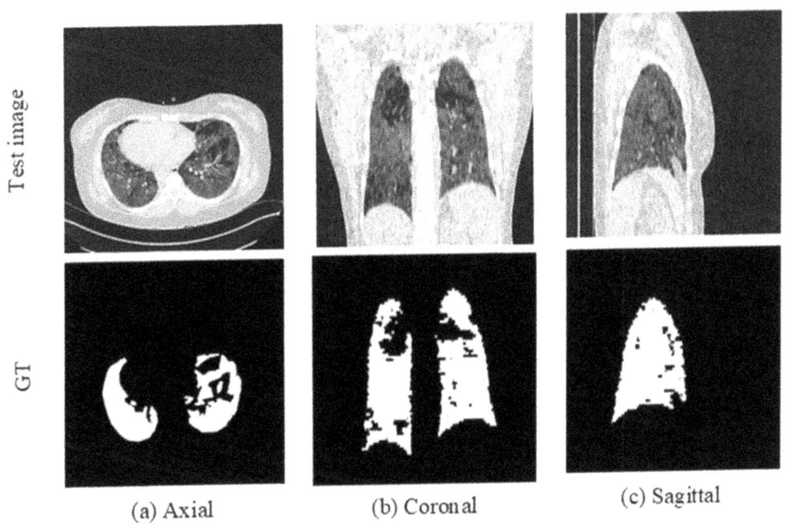

Figure 6.6. Sample test images with different 2D slices.

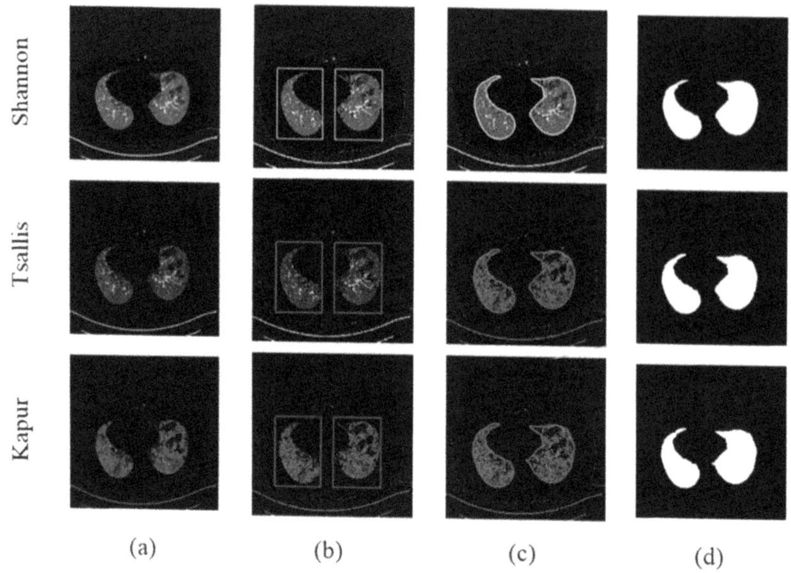

Figure 6.7. Results attained using axial-view CT scan slices. (a) Thresholded image, (b) bounding box, (c) converged DRLS contour, and (d) extracted COVID-19 lesion.

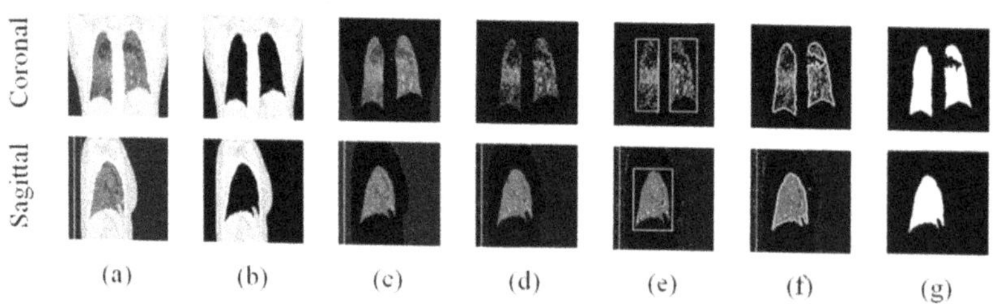

Figure 6.8. Results attained with coronal- and sagittal-view CT scan slices.

Table 6.2. Performance metrics achieved for a chosen test image with various entropy values.

	TP	FP	TN	FN							
Image	Total number of pixels				JAI	DIC	ACC	PRE	SEN	SPE	NPV
Axial Shannon's	11320	101	229558	2018	0.8423	0.9144	0.9913	0.9912	0.8487	0.9996	0.9913
Tsallis's	11327	94	229405	2135	0.8356	0.9104	0.9908	0.9918	0.8414	0.9996	0.9908
Kapur's	11311	110	229306	2124	0.8351	0.9101	0.9908	0.9904	0.8419	0.9995	0.9908
Coronal	22182	728	204697	7516	0.7290	0.8433	0.9649	0.9682	0.7469	0.9965	0.9646
Sagittal	28414	990	230408	2319	0.8957	0.9450	0.9874	0.9663	0.9245	0.9957	0.9900

After mining the necessary section from the test image, a comparison is implemented between the mined binary image and the GT. This comparison helps to acquire the necessary metrics discussed in section 6.3.5; these values are presented in table 6.2. This table confirms that the performance measure achieved with Shannon's function is better than Tsallis's and Kapur's. Hence, the sagittal and coronal planes are thresholded only with Shannon's entropy. The performance values in table 6.2 are then graphically analyzed, as in figure 6.9, showing a glyph plot representation. Figure 6.9(a) presents the results achieved with various entropies for the axial-plane image; this comparison confirms that the overall merit of Shannon+DRLS is better than other methods. Figure 6.9(b) compares the results achieved for the axial, coronal, and sagittal planes. The outcome of this study verifies that the proposed scheme provides better results for axial 2D CTSs than the alternatives.

The planned scheme is then implemented on the remaining test images (200 images) using the axial plane with different entropy functions, and the necessary performance metrics are then computed. Following this, the mean ± standard deviation for every measure is computed; these values are presented in table 6.3. This confirms the merit of the proposed scheme on the chosen test images. Finally, a graphical comparison is performed to identify the proposed scheme's performance; the achieved results are depicted in figure 6.10.

The results of figure 6.10 confirm that the performance achieved with Shannon's entropy is better than other entropies. Also, the overall segmentation accuracy

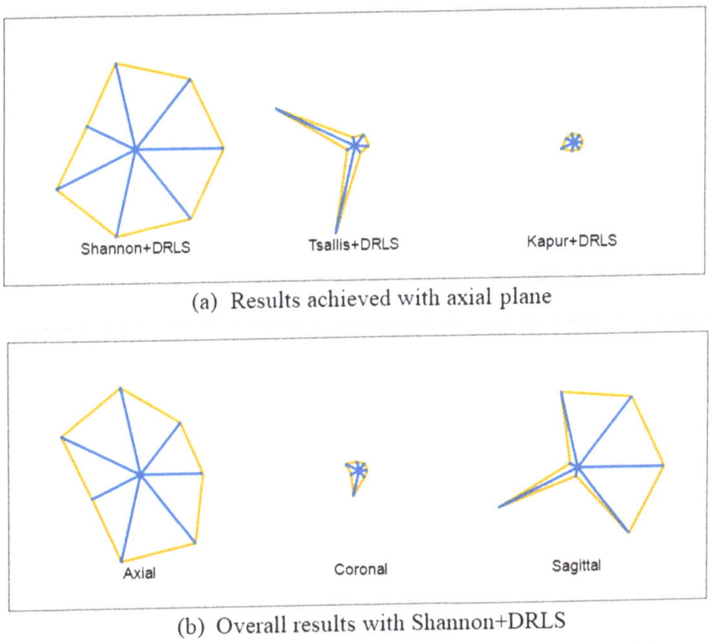

Figure 6.9. Glyph plot comparing the performance of the implemented schemes.

Table 6.3. Overall segmentation performance for the axial-plane 2D CTS.

Entropy	JAI	DIC	ACC	PRE	SEN	SPE	NPV
Shannon's	82.74 ± 3.17	89.42 ± 4.18	98.14 ± 1.13	83.61 ± 4.28	84.25 ± 3.94	99.18 ± 0.13	99.08 ± 0.17
Tsallis's	82.16 ± 2.94	89.16 ± 3.75	97.93 ± 2.04	83.55 ± 4.14	83.64 ± 3.96	99.23 ± 0.19	98.96 ± 0.31
Kapur's	81.93 ± 3.24	88.86 ± 3.92	97.86 ± 2.16	83.51 ± 4.06	82.81 ± 4.17	99.11 ± 0.21	98.93 ± 0.26

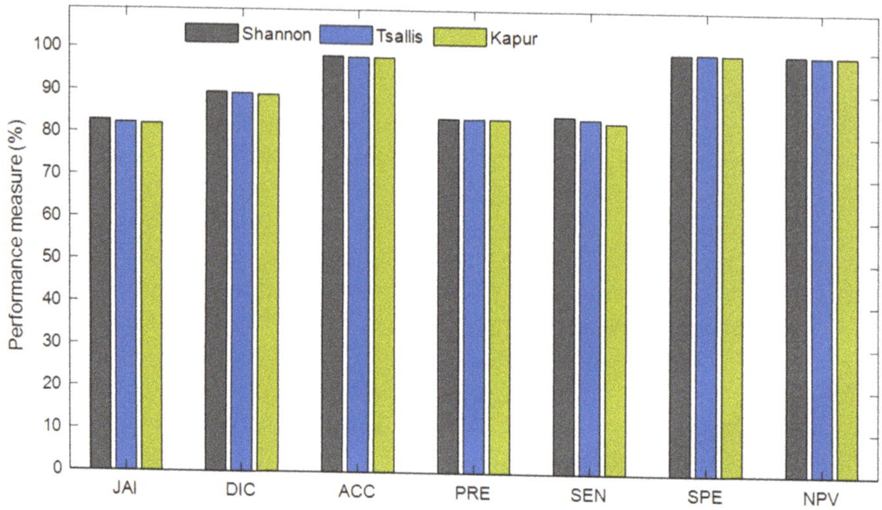

Figure 6.10. Assessment of performance measures with different entropy values.

achieved with the proposed scheme is better (98.14% ± 1.13%), confirming that the proposed technique can be considered to examine clinical-grade 2D CTSs. Thus, in the future, the proposed technique can be considered to examine clinically collected COVID-19 images. Further, the result of this study can be verified with other segmentation schemes available in the literature.

6.5 Conclusion

Computerized medical image assessment plays a vital role in evaluating disease, using standard procedures such as segmentation and classification. COVID-19 is a serious disease which causes severe lung infection; untreated, the disease can lead to death. Hence, appropriate detection is necessary to implement treatment in order to cure the disease. This work implemented a joint thresholding and segmentation scheme to extract and evaluate COVID-19 infection from 2D CTSs. First, (tri-level) thresholding was implemented with an entropy function, in which identification of the optimal threshold was achieved with a traditional EHO. Then, the infected sections in the thresholded images were mined using single-/double-well DRLS. The extracted binary image was then compared with the GT and the performance metrics computed. The experimental investigation of this study verifies that Shannon's entropy helps achieve a better performance than other entropies. Further, this scheme helps to achieve a segmentation accuracy of >97%, which confirms its clinical significance.

References

[1] Adeola H A, Bello I O, Aruleba R T, Francisco N M, Adekiya T A, Adefuye A O and Musaigwa F 2022 The practicality of the use of liquid biopsy in early diagnosis and treatment monitoring of oral cancer in resource-limited settings *Cancers* **14** 1139

[2] Varesi A, Pierella E, Romeo M, Piccini G B, Alfano C, Bjørklund G and Pascale A 2022 The potential role of gut microbiota in Alzheimer's disease: from diagnosis to treatment *Nutrients* **14** 668

[3] Bakiya A, Kamalanand K, Rajinikanth V, Nayak R S and Kadry S 2020 Deep neural network assisted diagnosis of time-frequency transformed electromyograms *Multimedia Tools Appl.* **79** 11051–67

[4] Thivya Roopini I, Vasanthi M, Rajinikanth V, Rekha M and Sangeetha M 2018 Segmentation of tumor from brain MRI using fuzzy entropy and distance regularised level set *Computational Signal Processing and AnalysisLecture Notes in Electrical Engineering* vol 490 (Singapore: Springer) pp 297–304

[5] Cascella M, Rajnik M, Aleem A, Dulebohn S C and Di Napoli R 2022 Statpearls: Features, evaluation, and treatment of coronavirus (COVID-19) https://www.ncbi.nlm.nih.gov/books/NBK554776/

[6] Xie Y, Xu E, Bowe B and Al-Aly Z 2022 Long-term cardiovascular outcomes of COVID-19 *Nat. Med.* **28** 583–90

[7] WHO 2022 WHO Coronavirus (COVID-19) dashboard https://covid19.who.int/

[8] Tahamtan A and Ardebili A 2020 Real-time RT-PCR in COVID-19 detection: issues affecting the results *Expert Rev. Mol. Diagn.* **20** 453–4

[9] van Kasteren P B, Veer van D, van den Brink B, Wijsman S, de Jonge L, van den Brandt J A and Meijer A 2020 Comparison of seven commercial RT-PCR diagnostic kits for COVID-19 *J. Clin. Virol.* **128** 104412

[10] Lan L, Xu D, Ye G, Xia C, Wang S, Li Y and Xu H 2020 Positive RT-PCR test results in patients recovered from COVID-19 *JAMA* **323** 1502–3

[11] Khatami F, Saatchi M, Zadeh S S T, Aghamir Z S, Shabestari A N, Reis L O and Aghamir S M K 2020 A meta-analysis of accuracy and sensitivity of chest CT and RT-PCR in COVID-19 diagnosis *Sci. Rep.* **10** 1–12

[12] Subramanian N, Elharrouss O, Al-Maadeed S and Chowdhury M 2022 A review of deep learning-based detection methods for COVID-19 *Comput. Biol. Med.* **143** 105233

[13] Alyasseri Z A A, Al-Betar M A, Doush I A, Awadallah M A, Abasi A K, Makhadmeh S N and Zitar R A 2022 Review on COVID-19 diagnosis models based on machine learning and deep learning approaches *Expert Syst.* **39** e12759

[14] Fuhrman J D, Gorre N, Hu Q, Li H, El Naqa I and Giger M L 2022 A review of explainable and interpretable AI with applications in COVID-19 imaging *Med. Phys.* **49** 1–14

[15] Yushkevich P A, Piven J, Hazlett H C, Smith R G, Ho S, Gee J C and Gerig G 2006 User-guided 3D active contour segmentation of anatomical structures: significantly improved efficiency and reliability *Neuroimage* **31** 1116–28

[16] itk-SNAP 2018 itk-SNAP software application www.itksnap.org/pmwiki/pmwiki.php

[17] Kesavan S M, Al Naimi I, Al Attar F, Rajinikanth V and Kadry S 2021 Res-UNet supported segmentation and evaluation of COVID-19 lesion in lung CT *2021 Int. Conf. on System, Computation, Automation and Networking (ICSCAN)* pp 1–4

[18] Amin J, Anjum M A, Sharif M, Rehman A, Saba T and Zahra R 2022 Microscopic segmentation and classification of COVID-19 infection with ensemble convolutional neural network *Microsc. Res. Tech.* **85** 385–97

[19] Satapathy S C, Hemanth D J, Kadry S, Manogaran G, Hannon N M and Rajinikanth V 2022 Microscopic segmentation and classification of COVID-19 infection with ensemble convolutional neural network *Microscopy Res. Tech.* **85** 385–97

[20] Kadry S, Rajinikanth V, Rho S, Raja N S M, Rao V S and Thanaraj K P 2020 Development of a machine-learning system to classify lung CT scan images into normal/COVID-19 class arXiv:2004.13122

[21] Arunmozhi S, Sarojini V S S, Pavithra T, Varghese V, Deepti V and Rajinikanth V 2021 Automated detection of COVID-19 lesion in lung CT slices with VGG-UNet and handcrafted features *Digital Future of Healthcare* (Boca Raton, FL: CRC Press) pp 185–200

[22] Rajinikanth V, Dey N, Raj A N J, Hassanien A E, Santosh K C and Raja N 2020 Harmony-search and otsu based system for coronavirus disease (COVID-19) detection using lung CT scan images arXiv:2004.03431

[23] Kadry S, Al-Turjman F and Rajinikanth V 2020 Automated segmentation of COVID-19 lesion from lung CT images using U-net architecture *Int. Summit Smart City 360°* (Cham: Springer) pp 20–30

[24] Dey N, Rajinikanth V, Fong S J, Kaiser M S and Mahmud M 2020 Social group optimization–assisted Kapur's entropy and morphological segmentation for automated detection of COVID-19 infection from computed tomography images *Cognitive Computation* **12** 1011–23

[25] Ahuja S, Panigrahi B K, Dey N, Rajinikanth V and Gandhi T K 2021 Deep transfer learning-based automated detection of COVID-19 from lung CT scan slices *Appl. Intel.* **51** 571–85

[26] Syed H H, Khan M A, Tariq U, Armghan A, Alenezi F, Khan J A and Rajinikanth V 2021 A rapid artificial intelligence-based computer-aided diagnosis system for COVID-19 classification from CT images *Behav. Neurol.* **2021** 2560388

[27] Kumar S N, Ahilan A, Fred A L and Kumar H A 2021 ROI extraction in CT lung images of COVID-19 using fast Fuzzy C means clustering *Biomedical Engineering Tools For Management For Patients with COVID-19* ed V E Balas, O Geman and G Wang *et al* (New York: Academic) pp 103–19

[28] Kumar A, Tripathi A R, Satapathy S C and Zhang Y D 2022 SARS-Net: COVID-19 detection from chest X-rays by combining graph convolutional network and convolutional neural network *Pattern Recognit.* **122** 108255

[29] Kogilavani S V, Prabhu J, Sandhiya R, Kumar M S, Subramaniam U, Karthick A and Imam S B S 2022 COVID-19 detection based on lung CT scan using deep learning techniques *Comput. Math. Methods Med.* **2022** 7672196

[30] Jalali S M J, Ahmadian M, Ahmadian S, Hedjam R, Khosravi A and Nahavandi S 2022 X-ray image based COVID-19 detection using evolutionary deep learning approach *Expert Syst. Appl.* **201** 116942

[31] Dey N, Zhang Y D, Rajinikanth V, Pugalenthi R and Raja N S M 2021 Customized VGG19 architecture for pneumonia detection in chest x-rays *Pattern Recognit. Lett.* **143** 67–74

[32] Rajinikanth V, Sivakumar R, Hemanth D J, Kadry S, Mohanty J R, Arunmozhi S and Nhu N G 2021 Automated classification of retinal images into AMD/non-AMD class—a study using multi-threshold and gassian-filter enhanced images *Evolutionary Intelligence* **14** 1163–71

[33] Nazar U, Khan M A, Lali I U, Lin H, Ali H, Ashraf I and Tariq J 2020 Review of automated computerized methods for brain tumor segmentation and classification *Current Medical Imaging* **16** 823–34

[34] Rajinikanth V, Priya E, Lin H and Lin F 2021 *Hybrid Image Processing Methods for Medical Image Examination* (Boca Raton, FL: CRC Press)

[35] Kaur N and Kaur R 2011 A review on various methods of image thresholding *Int. J. Comp. Sci. Eng.* **3** 3441

[36] Pare S, Kumar A, Singh G K and Bajaj V 2020 Image segmentation using multilevel thresholding: a research review *Iranian J. Science and Technology, Trans. of Electrical Engineering* **44** 1–29

[37] Narkhede H P 2013 Review of image segmentation techniques *Int. J. Sci. and Mod. Eng.* **1** 54–61

[38] Abualigah L, Diabat A, Sumari P and Gandomi A H 2021 A novel evolutionary arithmetic optimization algorithm for multilevel thresholding segmentation of COVID19 CT images *Processes* **9** 1155

[39] Hasan A M, Al-Jawad M M, Jalab H A, Shaiba H, Ibrahim R W and AL-Shamasneh A A R 2020 Classification of COVID-19 coronavirus, pneumonia and healthy lungs in CT scans using Q-deformed entropy and deep learning features *Entropy* **22** 517

[40] Jumiawi W A H and El-Zaart A 2022 Improving minimum cross-entropy thresholding for segmentation of infected foregrounds in medical images based on mean filters approaches *Contrast Media and Molecular Imaging* **2022** 9289574

[41] Kannappan P L 1972 On Shannon's entropy, directed divergence and inaccuracy *Zeitschrift Für Wahrscheinlichkeitstheorie Und Verwandte Gebiete* **22** 95–100

[42] Wang G G, Deb S and Coelho L D S 2015 Elephant herding optimization *2015 3rd Int. Symp. on Computational and Business Intelligence (ISCBI)* pp 1–5

[43] Li J, Lei H, Alavi A H and Wang G G 2020 Elephant herding optimization: variants, hybrids, and applications *Mathematics* **8** 1415

[44] Duan Y, Liu C, Li S, Guo X and Yang C 2022 Gradient-based elephant herding optimization for cluster analysisApplied Intelligence **52** 11606–37

[45] Alhassan A M *et al* 2022 Enhanced fuzzy elephant herding optimization-based OTSU segmentation and deep learning for Alzheimer's disease diagnosis *Mathematics* **10** 1259

[46] Li C, Xu C, Gui C and Fox M D 2010 Distance regularized level set evolution and its application to image segmentation *IEEE Trans. Image Process.* **19** 3243–54

[47] Ma J *et al* 2020 COVID-19 CT lung and infection segmentation dataset (version 1.0) zenodo https://doi.org/10.5281/zenodo.3757476

[48] Qayyum A, Lalande A and Meriaudeau F 2022 Effective multiscale deep learning model for COVID-19 segmentation tasks: a further step towards helping radiologist *Neurocomputing* **499** 63–80

Chapter 7

Automated classification of brain tumors into LGG/HGG using concatenated deep and handcrafted features

J Sivakumar, S Rajesh Kannan and K Suresh Manic

The brain is an essential internal organ in human physiology, and any abnormality in the brain will have a significant impact on an individual's daily activities. Furthermore, untreated brain abnormalities can result in a variety of conditions, including, ultimately, death. This chapter will make use of a pre-trained convolutional neural network (CNN) scheme to implement an automated brain tumor detection system. This study is divided into two sections: (i) the implementation of a U-Net scheme to extract the tumor division from 2D MRI slices, and (ii) the classification of the tumor sections into low-grade glioma/high-grade glioma using concatenated deep features and handcrafted topographies. Approaches such as local binary patterns and gray-level cooccurrence matrixes are used to extract the essential handcrafted features. The performance of well-known CNN schemes, such as VGG16, is evaluated in the proposed work. The proposed study's results confirm that AlexNet with a *k*-nearest neighbor classifier assists in achieving improved classification accuracy (96%) when compared to similar studies carried out in this area.

7.1 Introduction

The brain is among the most vital internal organs in the human body, and any abnormality in the brain poses an important medical emergency. Patient recovery can be improved if the abnormality is diagnosed and managed as quickly as possible [1–3]. Clinical-level assessment of brain conditions is typically performed using biosignal-based methods [4, 5], although imaging-based approaches can help to obtain clearer information in comparison to signal-based techniques. Furthermore, bioimages can be captured using a variety of imaging procedures such as computed tomography (CT), magnetic resonance imaging (MRI), and functional magnetic

doi:10.1088/978-0-7503-4012-0ch7

resonance imaging (fMRI) in different modes, namely diffusion weighting (DW), T1, T1C, T2, and flair [6–10].

Each modality has its own merits, and the results of each technique will provide useful information for diagnosis. According to previous research, flair and T2 modality brain MRI slices are widely used due to their high visibility. A number of researchers have recently discussed a range of brain condition examination procedures based on MRI, utilizing hybrid methods combining machine learning (ML) and deep learning (DL) with binary and multi-class classifiers.

When a brain abnormality is clearly evaluated from collected images from the patient, then the doctor will review the results and plan for essential treatment procedures, such as chemotherapy and/or surgery to cure the patient. In specialist hospitals, the number of patients requiring advanced screening is more, and hence a higher volume of images will be collected from each patient for further assessment. Conventionally, radiologists and doctors perform their initial assessments and provide opinions as a result. The mass screening processes involved create higher volumes of MRI slices, and their evaluation can thus become a time-consuming process.

As a result, a large number of MRI-based brain abnormality assessment procedures are being developed in order to detect abnormalities to a high degree of accuracy. The majority of previous work on this topic has utilized a classification task to separate abnormal MRI images from normal MRI images; in this, the classification of high-grade glioma (HGG) along with low-grade glioma (LGG) is quite complex compared to existing methods. As particularly severe forms of brain tumor, crucially, if LGG and HGG are clearly identified then the appropriate treatment for the patient can be implemented.

The proposed work aims to create and implement a hybrid image-processing methodology that combines DL and ML features in order to examine these classes of brain tumor (LGG/HGG) with greater accuracy using a binary classifier. The proposed work includes the following image-evaluation frameworks: (i) implementation of a pre-trained VGG16 structure to excerpt deep features (DFs), and (ii) implementation of a U-Net structure to extract the tumor section from the MRI slice as well as chosen handcrafted features (HFs). Following feature extraction, the essential feature vector of the specified dimension is obtained using a principal-component-analysis-based feature concatenation method, as discussed in [10]. Finally, the binary MRI slices are classified into LGG/HGG using a binary classifier with tenfold cross-validation.

The SoftMax classifier is used for DL-based categorization, and the performance of DL methods such as VGG16, VGG19, AlexNet, ResNet18, and ResNet50, is evaluated. The collected ML features are then combined with the DL features, and the proposed work is repeated. The overall outcomes of this research affirm that AlexNet with a a *k*-nearest neighbor (*k*-NN) classifier outperforms other methods on the considered MRI data set.

The proposed work includes the following contributions: (i) implementation of a pre-trained DL structure to classify MRI segments into LGG/HGG classes, (ii) implementation of U-Net segmentation, and (iii) feature concatenation and validation. In this study, T2 modality MRI slices were used to collect test images from the The Cancer Imaging Archive (TCIA) and BRaTS2015 databases, and the overall results obtained with the proposed technique helped improve classification accuracy during the classification of LGG/HGG-class images.

The remaining sections of this chapter are as follows. The research context is given and explained in section 7.2, the methodology is presented in section 7.3, and the outcomes are discussed in sections 7.4 and 7.5.

7.2 Context

MRI-assisted brain condition monitoring is among the most commonly used clinical methodologies, in which an experienced doctor manually evaluates axial-view slices of MRI scans to detect any existing abnormalities. However, when the number of images to be examined is large, this process can become time consuming. As a result, researchers have devised a large number of brain MRI evaluation procedures, a few selected approaches to which are summarized in table 7.1.

Table 7.1 shows previous methods which have used either ML or DL techniques to examine neurological symptoms from a chosen MRI modality. Further, earlier works [22–27] provide us with a detailed assessment of the available modalities of MRI.

Throughout this work, LGG/HGG-class tumors are detected using a DL scheme using integrated, combined DL and ML characteristics; the outcomes obtained are accessible using various binary classifiers from the literature. The results obtained from the considered MRI databases confirm that the proposed scheme aids in the achievement of better classification results.

7.3 Methodology

A common approach to the diagnosis of neurological conditions is imaging-assisted assessment, and to this end a variety of techniques have been proposed and implemented in the literature. This chapter utilizes a hybrid technique to enhance the accuracy of tumor detection; the stages used in this scheme are depicted in figure 7.1.

This scheme is made up of two distinct pipelines to extract key features from brain MRI scans. It consists of the following stages: collection of three-dimensional (3D) brain MRI test images from a selected database; the conversion of 3D images to two-dimensional (2D) images using ITK-Snap, and resizing of the 2D MRI slices for further assessment, feature extraction, and serial fusion concatenation; and implementation of a binary classifier to classify the considered MRI images into LGG and HGG classes. The first pipeline, employing a U-Net CNN, is utilized to extract the tumor sections from the 2D MRI slice [11]. Following this step, gray-level cooccurrence matrix (GLCM) features are extracted from the binary image [12]. Then local binary pattern (LBP)-based features are extracted; in the present study, the HFs are defined as the combination of the GLCM and the LBP. The second pipeline extracts the essential components using a pre-trained DL scheme. Finally, these two characteristics are integrated to create a vector with one-dimensional (1D) features which is used to train and validate binary classifiers. The proposed work considers a number of classification models, and the performance is confirmed based on the achieved overall results.

Table 7.1. Summary of brain tumor examination with MRI slices.

Reference	Methodology	Abnormality and database
Amin *et al* [1]	Extraction and evaluation of brain tumors is achieved using a chosen heuristic algorithm.	Brain tumor and BRaTS
Dey *et al* [3]	This research employed a hybrid image-examination scheme by combining a thresholding and segmentation technique.	
Qureshi *et al* [13]	Tumor extraction with joint thresholding and segmentation is implemented and HF-based classification is implemented.	
Satapathy and Rajinikanth [14]	A Jaya-algorithm-assisted thresholding and segmentation technique is implemented to mine the tumor region from a brain MRI slice.	
Rajeshkannan *et al* [15]	Implementation of fuzzy-entropy-based tumor enhancement and level-set supported segmentation is implemented.	
Menze *et al* [16]	This work employed Kapur's entropy thresholding for MRI enhancement, and Chan–Vese segmentation-based extraction and evaluation is discussed.	
Rajinikanth *et al* [17]	To examine the CT/MRI brain slices, a hybrid image-processing scheme is used.	
Rajinikanth *et al* [18]	This work implemented Kapur's threshold and Markov random-field-based evaluation for brain abnormality detection.	
Bauer *et al* [2]	A detailed summary of various tumor segmentation and evaluation methods is offered.	
Rajinikanth *et al* [19]	Feature extraction and feature-based classification of brain abnormalities is discussed using a random forest classifier.	
Manic *et al* [20]	Implementation of a DL scheme is discussed and abnormalities in the brain are recognized with enhanced accuracy.	
Louis *et al* [21]	This work presents a through survey on the brain MRI assessment techniques found in the literature.	

7.3.1 Image databases

The proposed technique's performance must be validated using clinical-grade images. The brain MRI images used in this study were obtained from image databases such as the TCIA [28, 29] and BRaTS2015 [30]. Both are well-known image data sets that have been widely used in the literature to assess the performance

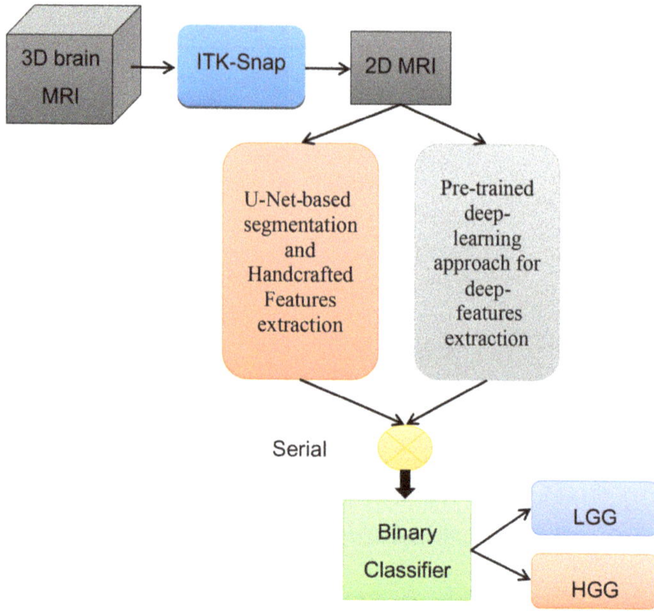

Figure 7.1. Proposed scheme for brain MRI assessment.

Table 7.2. Test images considered in the proposed disease-detection scheme.

Image Class	Dimensions	Database	Total images	Training images	Validation images
LGG	256 × 256 × 3	TCIA	300	200	100
		BRaTS2015	300	200	100
HGG	256 × 256 × 3	TCIA	300	200	100
		BRaTS2015	300	200	100

of image-processing-based disease-detection systems. The TCIA database contains images that include skull sections, whereas the BRaTS2015 database contains MRI slices that do not include skull sections. ITK-Snap [31] is used in this work to extract 2D slices from a 3D image, and the extracted images are then evaluated. Table 7.2 depicts details of the experimental data sets, while figure 7.2 depicts sample test images from the TCIA database.

7.3.2 Handcrafted feature extraction

The essential HFs are extracted from the sample test slices utilizing the proposed GLCM and LBP, the methodologies of which is here given in this section.

7.3.2.1 U-Net scheme

One of the most important tasks is the segmentation and evaluation of the abnormal sections of brain MRIs; various approaches available in the literature can be found

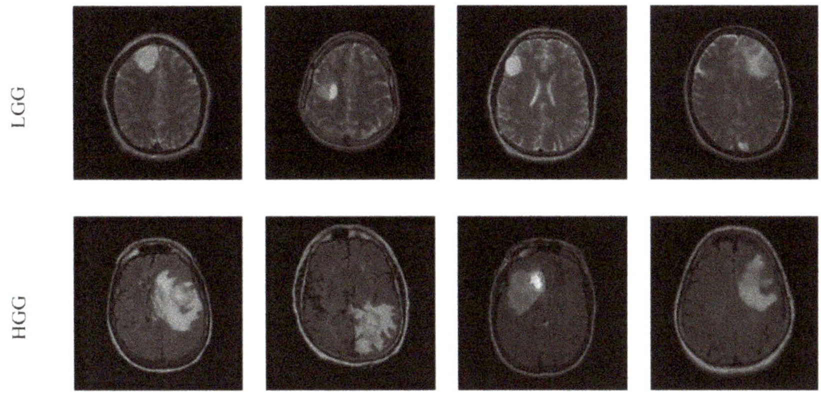

Figure 7.2. Sample brain MRI slices from the TCIA database.

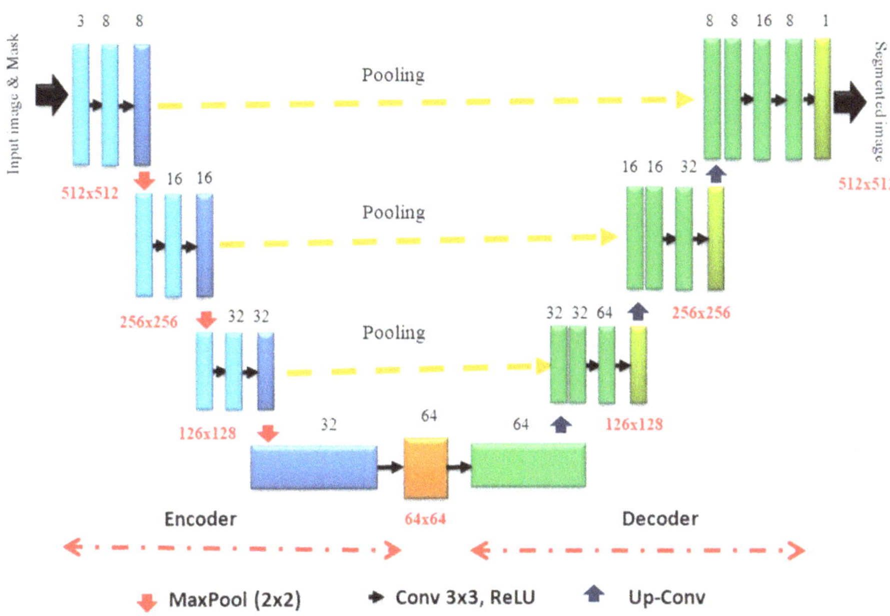

Figure 7.3. U-Net architecture considered to extract the tumor section.

in [32, 33]. In this work, tumor sections from MRI scans are segmented using a U-Net scheme, which consists of encoder-decoder sections. The required information can be extracted from the U-Net, which aids in achieving a binary form of the tumor section as the final outcome. Figure 7.3 depicts the U-Net scheme used in this study.

The above U-Net is a pre-trained scheme, in which the considered test images (original and augmented) are used to train and validate the CNN architecture for the selected image database. After the essential training process, a SoftMax layer comprising the final layer of the U-Net separates the tumor section from the background. In this work, the final image is given in binary form, in which binary 1 denotes the tumor section and binary 0 represents the background.

7.3.2.2 Feature extraction

The execution of the automated disease-detection system is primarily determined by the extracted features, which guide the system through the disease-detection task. A number of procedures have been considered in the prior literature to extract the critical image features from grayscale/red-green-blue class images. GLCM characteristics, extracted from a gray/binary image of specific dimensions, play an important role in a number of image-based disease-detection schemes. Earlier research provides detailed information on such GLCM features [34–39]. In this proposed work, the GLCM characteristics, with dimensions $1 \times 1 \times 25$, are obtained from the binary tumor slices, and mathematically represented as shown in equation (7.1):

$$\text{F1}_{\text{GLCM}}\ (1 \times 25) = \text{GLCM}_{(1,1)},\ \text{GLCM}_{(1,2)},\ \ldots,\text{GLCM}_{(25,1)}. \tag{7.1}$$

Later, the LBP features are extracted based on the technique discussed by Gudigar *et al* [7]. In this work, a weighted LBP is considered for the experimental investigation and the weights (W) are assigned with a value of 1–4. From every image, a 1D feature vector of size $1 \times 1 \times 59$ is attained, and the total features collected will accordingly be $4^*(1 \times 1 \times 59) = 1 \times 1 \times 236$. These values are depicted mathematically as in equation (7.2):

$$\begin{aligned}\text{F2}_{\text{LBP}}\ (1 \times 236) = \text{LBP}_1\ (1 \times 59) + \text{LBP}_2\ (1 \times 59) + \text{LBP}_3\ (1 \times 59) \\ + \text{LBP}_4\ (1 \times 59).\end{aligned} \tag{7.2}$$

Equation (2) shows that each image aids in obtaining an essential binary pattern as its information, and the collected LBP features will help to specify the complete information about the tumor. This concept is then integrated along with the GLCM to produce the HF vector, specified in equation (7.3):

$$\text{HF}_{(1\times 261)} = \text{F1}_{\text{GLCM}}\ (1 \times 25) + \text{F2}_{\text{LBP}}\ (1 \times 236). \tag{7.3}$$

7.3.3 Deep feature extraction

The extraction of the DFs is a key process. In this study, pre-trained architectures are evaluated. Resized images with dimensions of $224 \times 224 \times 3$ (VGGs and ResNets) and $227 \times 227 \times 3$ (AlexNet) are considered for the training and validation operations based on the chosen architecture. Essential information regarding the considered schemes can be found in [40–42]; these procedures helped to achieve a feature vector of dimensions $1 \times 1 \times 1024$ features.

7.3.4 Feature concatenation

Previous research in the literature confirms that combining HFs with DFs improves the overall outcomes, as, for example, presented by Rajinikanth *et al* [19]. This work provides extensive information on this process. In this method, the HFs and DFs are sorted and both features are serially combined to form a feature vector, as shown in equation (7.4):

$$\text{FV}_{(1\times 1285)} = \text{HF}_{(1\times 261)} + \text{DF}_{(1024)}. \tag{7.4}$$

This vector can then be used to process and validate a binary classifier's performance. SoftMax, decision tree (DT), *k*-NN, random forest (RF), and support vector machine-radial basis function (SVM-RBF) classifiers are chiefly used in this work.

7.3.5 Performance measure computation and validation

The final step in the proposed system's scheme is to evaluate and validate its disease-detection performance. The effectiveness of this scheme in disease diagnosis is demonstrated by computing key procedures such as true positive (TP) rate, true negative (TN) rate, false positive (FP) rate, and false negative (FN) rate. Other information can be calculated from these values, such as accuracy (Acc), precision (Pre), sensitivity (Sen), specificity (Spe), F1 score (F1S), and negative predictive value (NPV), the mathematical representations of which can be found in [43–50].

A tenfold cross-validation is performed on each classifier, and the best performance among the obtained results is considered. To demonstrate the overall performance, a glyph plot is constructed, and the performance is validated based on the dimensions of this plot.

7.4 Results and discussion

This section of the chapter contains the investigational results and findings. MATLAB® software is used to conduct all of the experimental research. The test images shown in table 7.2 are used for evaluation during this investigation.

The U-Net system is trained several times using both the original and augmented images of the brain MRI data set considered in this work. Following flawless training, the tumor section in each test image is extracted using the final layer of U-Net's decoder section (SoftMax), and the extracted image is saved as a binary image. Figure 7.4(a) shows the results of a test image obtained with the U-Net. Figures 7.4(b) and (c) show test images with the initial and final values of the encoder and decoder, respectively, and figure 7.4(d) shows the binary version of the

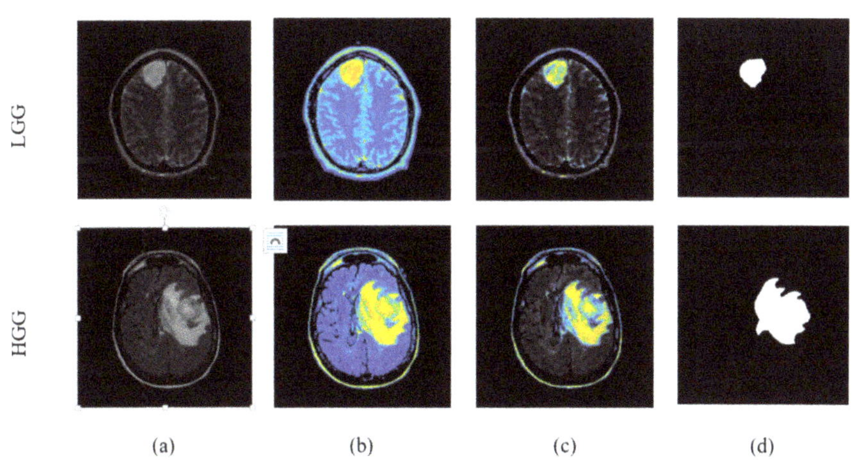

Figure 7.4. Result attained with U-Net scheme.

extracted tumor. After the binary image is extracted, the essential GLCM values of the LGG and HGG classes are extracted. The test images are then processed using the LBP with $W = 1–4$; the results are shown in figures 7.5(a)–(d), respectively. A feature value of 1×59 is extracted from each image, and the overall HFs are a composite of the GLCM and the LBP, which are considered to have been acquired without any decline or alteration.

Following the extraction of the HFs from the MRI database, the DFs are extracted using various pre-training architectures. During this process, the SoftMax classifier is used to perform a binary classification to identify the best pre-trained scheme and the results compared. During these procedures, 200 MRI slices (100 from the TCIA and 100 from the BRaTS database) are used to evaluate the proposed system, with the results presented in table 7.3. This table shows that AlexNet achieves better classification accuracy than other schemes. Figure 7.6 shows the AlexNet's overall performance as a glyph plot, along with comparisons, and this result further affirms AlexNet's superiority on the considered image database.

Finally, sequential nested loops of the DFs and HFs are implemented to build a single melded feature vector, with a dimensions of 1×1285 features, to improve the performance of the AlexNet's disease-detection classifier. These characteristics are then used to evaluate the performance of the binary classifiers used in this

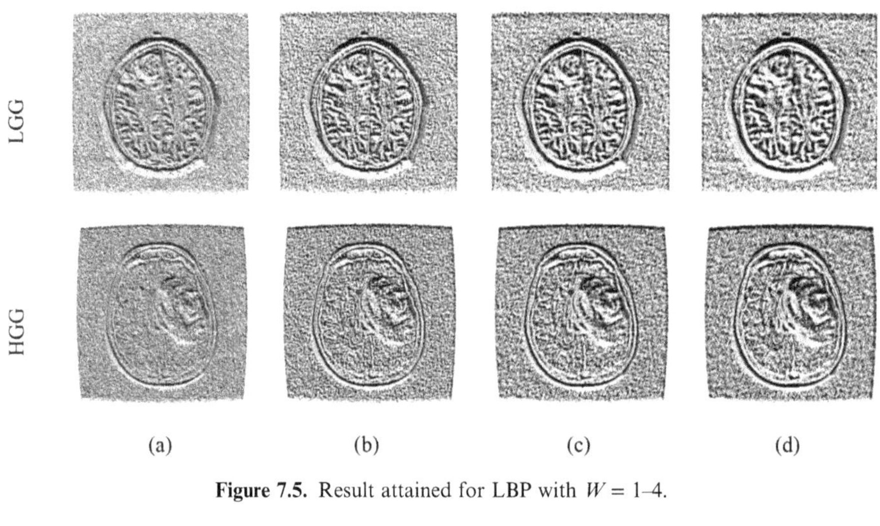

Figure 7.5. Result attained for LBP with $W = 1–4$.

Table 7.3. Experimental outcome attained with pre-trained deep-learning schemes.

Scheme	TP	FN	TN	FP	Acc	Pre	Sen	Spe	NPV	F1S
VGG16	183	17	185	15	92.00	92.42	91.50	92.50	91.58	91.96
VGG19	184	16	185	15	92.25	92.46	92.00	92.50	92.04	92.23
AlexNet	**182**	**18**	**189**	**11**	**92.75**	**94.30**	**91.00**	**94.50**	**91.30**	**92.62**
ResNet18	183	17	181	19	91.00	90.59	91.50	90.50	91.41	91.04
ResNet50	181	19	184	16	91.25	91.88	90.50	92.00	90.64	91.18

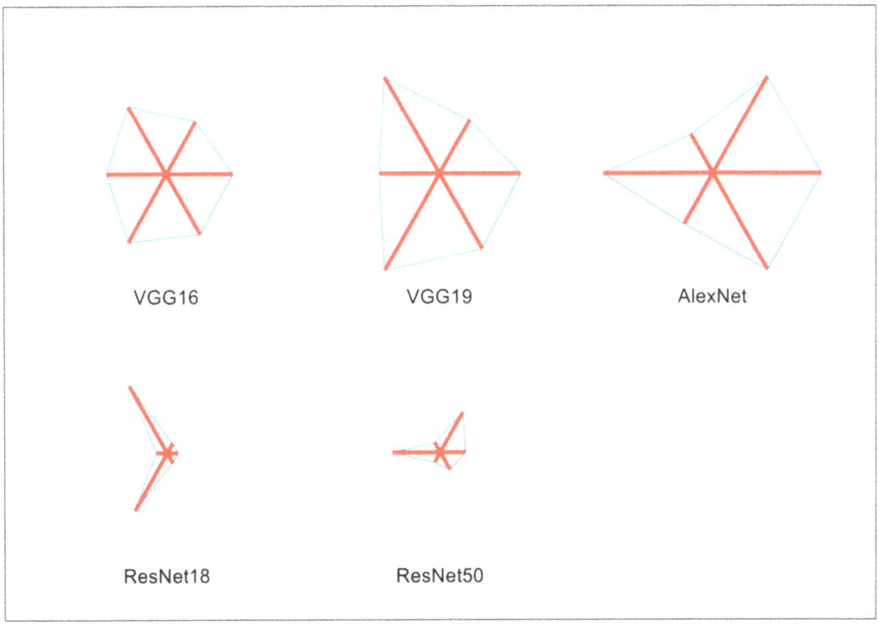

Figure 7.6. Glyph plots for the overall results of deep-learning performance.

Table 7.4. Experimental results obtained with concatenated HF and DF.

Classifier	TP	FN	TN	FP	Acc	Pre	Sen	Spe	NPV	F1S
SoftMax	186	14	190	10	94.00	94.89	93.00	95.00	93.14	93.94
DT	185	15	186	14	92.75	92.96	92.50	93.00	92.54	92.73
***k*-NN**	**193**	**7**	**191**	**9**	**96.00**	**95.54**	**96.50**	**95.50**	**96.46**	**96.02**
RF	184	16	188	12	93.00	93.88	92.00	94.00	92.16	92.93
SVM-RBF	188	12	192	8	95.00	95.92	94.00	96.00	94.12	94.95

investigation; table 7.4 lists the experimental data demonstrated with various classifiers.

This table confirms that the detection performance demonstrated by the AlexNet classifier in conjunction with a *k*-NN classifier is superior to that of other binary classifiers. Figure 7.7 depicts the obtained convergence graph for the accuracy and error rate of AlexNet with a *k*-NN classifier, which confirms that the proposed scheme aids in classification with a simulation time of 185 s (3 min 5 s) using a chosen workstation utilizing a core i5 processor, 16 GB RAM, and 2 GB graphics card. Figure 7.7 further details all of the necessary information on iteration, epoch, error rate, and so on. The glyph plots in figure 7.8 confirm the superiority of *k*-NN over SoftMax, DT, RF, and SVM-RBF.

Thus, the proposed method will classify brain MRI slices into LGG/HGG using a combined HF and DF scheme utilizing a CNN-based method. The proposed program's performance has been validated exclusively using the TCIA and BRaTS

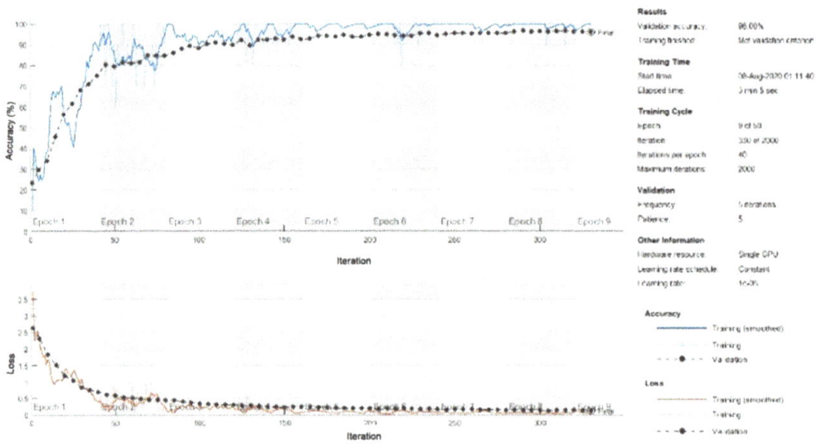

Figure 7.7. Accuracy and error rate attained for the pre-trained AlexNet.

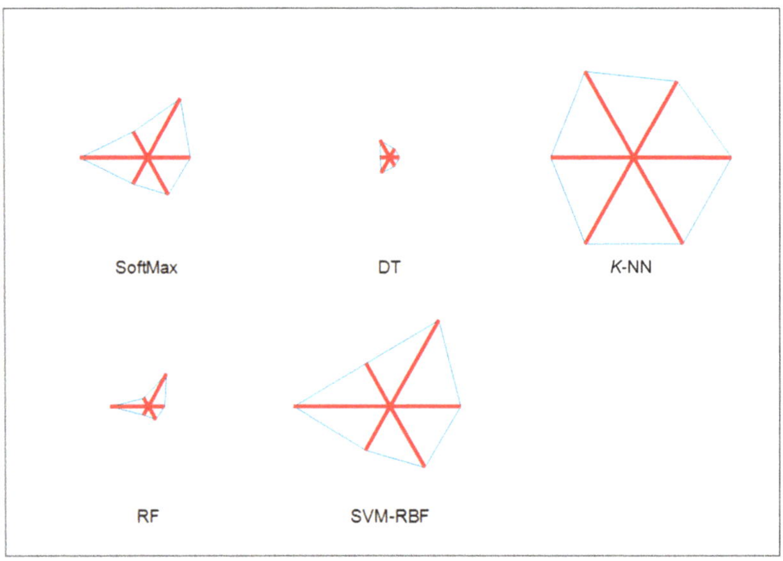

Figure 7.8. Glyph plots of the overall results attained using the combined HF and DF.

data sets. The research detailed here can be improved in future work as follows: (i) clinically collected images could be used to evaluate the AlexNet's performance, and (ii) a feature-reduction approach could be proposed to minimize the characteristics to a lower value. In addition to the here used GLCMs and LBPs, other HFs found in the literature can be integrated to enhance the scheme's outcome.

7.5 Conclusion

The use of brain MRI scans for disease detection is a well-established procedure. Brain tumors in this chapter were analyzed using a CNN-based technique. In this work, sample images from the TCIA and BRaTS databases were used for experimental investigation, and tumors observed in the images were identified using a binary classifier unit. The proposed work (i) implemented DF-based LGG/HGG classification with a pre-trained architecture, and discovered that AlexNet performed better than the alternatives; and (ii) concatenated together HFs and DFs, which were then deemed to evaluate the performance of the AlexNet with various classifiers, and additionally discovered that the accuracy attained using a k-NN (96%) classifier was better than other methods. High-precision diagnosis appears to be achievable in future by taking into consideration the other HFs that underpinned this study.

References

[1] Amin J, Sharif M, Yasmin M and Fernandes S L 2018 Big data analysis for brain tumor detection: deep convolutional neural networks *Future Generation Computer System* **87** 290–7

[2] Bauer S, Wiest R, Nolte L P and Reyes M 2013 A survey of MRI-based medical image analysis for brain tumor studies *Med. Image Process. Anal.* **58** R97

[3] Dey N *et al* 2019 Social-group-optimization based tumor evaluation tool for clinical brain MRI of flair/diffusion-weighted modality *Biocybern Biomed Eng* **39** 843–56

[4] Acharya U R *et al* 2019 Automated detection of Alzheimer's disease using brain MRI images—a study with various feature extraction techniques *J. Med. Syst.* **43** 302

[5] Hemanth D J 2020 EEG signal based modified Kohonen neural networks for classification of human mental emotions *J. Artificial Intel. Syst.* **2** 1–13

[6] Fernandes S L, Tanik U J, Rajinikanth V and Karthik K A 2019 A reliable framework for accurate brain image examination and treatment planning based on early diagnosis support for clinicians *Neural Comput. Appl.* **32** 15897–908

[7] Gudigar A *et al* 2019 Global weighted LBP based entropy features for the assessment of pulmonary hypertension *Pattern Recognit. Lett.* **125** 35–41

[8] Bhandary A *et al* 2020 Deep-learning framework to detect lung abnormality—a study with chest x-ray and lung CT scan images *Pattern Recognit. Lett.* **129** 271–78

[9] He T, Pamela M B and Shi F 2016 Curvature manipulation of the spectrum of a valence—arousal-related fMRI dataset using a Gaussian-shaped fast fourier transform and its application to fuzzy KANSEI adjective modeling *Neuro Computing* **174** 1049–59

[10] Hemanth D J *et al* 2021 Image fusion practice to improve the ischemic-stroke-lesion detection for efficient clinical decision making *Evolutionary Intelligence* **14** 1089–1099

[11] Balakrishna C, Dadashzadeh S and Soltaninejad S 2018 Automatic detection of lumen and media in the IVUS images using U-Net with VGG16 encoder arXiv:1806.07554

[12] El-Dahshan E S A, Mohsen H M, Revett K and Salem A-B M 2014 Computer-aided diagnosis of human brain tumor through MRI: a survey and a new algorithm *Expert Syst. Appl.* **41** 5526–554

[13] Qureshi S, Karilla S and Vanichayobon S 2019 GACNN sleep TuneNet: a genetic algorithm designing the convolutional neural network architecture for optimal classification of sleep stages from a single EEG channel *Turkish J. Electrical Eng. Comput. Sci.* **27** 4203–19

[14] Satapathy S C and Rajinikanth V 2018 Jaya algorithm guided procedure to segment tumor from brain MRI *J. Optimization* **2018** 3738049

[15] Rajeshkannan S, Sivakumar J and Ezhilarasi P 2021 Automatic detection of COVID-19 in chest radiographs using serially concatenated deep and handcrafted features *J. X-Ray Sci. Technol.* **30** 231–44

[16] Menze B *et al* 2015 The multimodal brain tumor image segmentation benchmark (BRATS) *IEEE Trans. Med. Imaging* **34** 1993–2024

[17] Rajinikanth V, Satapathy S C, Dey N and Lin H 2018 Evaluation of ischemic stroke region from CT/MR images using hybrid image processing techniques *Intelligent Multidimensional Data And Image Processing* ed S De, S Bhattacharyya and P Dutta (Hershey, PA: IGI Global) pp 194–219

[18] Rajinikanth V, Raja N S M and Kamalanand K 2017 Firefly algorithm assisted segmentation of tumor from brain MRI using Tsallis function and Markov random field *J. Control Eng. Appl. Inform* **19** 97–106

[19] Rajinikanth V, Joseph Raj A N, Thanaraj K P and Naik G R 2020 A customized VGG19 network with concatenation of deep and handcrafted features for brain tumor detection *Applied Sciences* **10** 3429

[20] Manic K S, Hasoon F A, Shibli N A, Satapathy S C and Rajinikanth V 2019 An approach to examine brain tumor based on Kapur's entropy and Chan–Vese algorithm *AISC* **797** 901–9

[21] Louis D N *et al* 2016 The 2016 World Health Organization classification of tumors of the central nervous system: a summary *Acta Neuropathol.* **131** 803–20

[22] Kanmani P and Marikkannu P 2018 MRI brain images classification: a multi-level threshold based region optimization technique *J. Med. Syst.* **42** 62–72

[23] Khan M A *et al* 2020 Multimodal brain tumor classification using deep learning and robust feature selection: a machine learning application for radiologists *Diagnostics* **10** 565

[24] Kovalev V and Kruggel F 2007 Texture anisotropy of the brain's white matter as revealed by anatomical MRI *IEEE Trans. Med. Imaging* **26** 678–85

[25] Leandrou S, Petroudi S, Kyriacou P A, Reyes-Aldasoro C C and Pattichis C S 2018 Quantitative MRI brain studies in mild cognitive impairment and Alzheimer's disease: a methodological review *IEEE Rev. Bio.-Med. Eng.* **11** 97–111

[26] Liu M, Zhang J, Nie D, Yap P-T and Shen D 2018 Anatomical landmark based deep feature representation for MR images in brain disease diagnosis *IEEE J. Biomed. Health.* **22** 1476–85

[27] Lu S, Lu Z and Zhang Y D 2019 Pathological brain detection based on AlexNet and transfer learning *J. Computational Science* **30** 41–7

[28] Scarpace L *et al* 2016 The Cancer Imaging Archive: Radiology data from The Cancer Genome Atlas Glioblastoma Multiforme [TCGA-GBM] collection https://wiki.cancerimagingarchive.net/pages/viewpage.action?pageId=1966258

[29] Pedano N *et al* 2016 The Cancer Imaging Archive: Radiology data from The Cancer Genome Atlas Low Grade Glioma [TCGA-LGG] collection https://wiki.cancerimagingarchive.net/pages/viewpage.action?pageId=5309188

[30] https://sites.google.com/site/braintumorsegmentation/home/brats

[31] www.itksnap.org/pmwiki/pmwiki.php

[32] Jiao L, Huo L, Hu C and Tang P 2020 Refined UNet V2: end-to-end patch-wise network for noise-free cloud and shadow segmentation *Remote Sens.* **12** 3530

[33] Oktay O, Schlemper J, Folgoc L L, Lee M and Heinrich M 2018 Attention U-Net: learning where to look for the pancreas arXiv:1804.03999

[34] Pugalenthi R, Rajakumar M P, Ramya J and Rajinikanth V 2019 Evaluation and classification of the brain tumor MRI using machine learning technique *Control Eng. Appl. Inform.* **21** 12–21

[35] Pugalenthi R, Sheryl Oliver A and Anuradha M 2020 Impulse noise reduction using hybridneuro-fuzzy filter with improved firefly algorithm from x-ray bio-images *Int. J. Imaging Syst. Technol.* **30** 1119–31
[36] Jafarpour S, Sedghi Z and Amirani M C 2012 A robust brain MRI classification with GLCM features *Int. J. Computer Applications* **37** 1–5
[37] Vlis V D T A *et al* 2017 Impact of the revised WHO classification of diffuse low-grade glioma on clinical decision making: a case report *Surgical Neurology Int.* **8** 223
[38] Nazar U *et al* 2020 Review of automated computerized methods for brain tumor segmentation and classification *Current Medical Imaging* **16** 823–34
[39] Dey N, Zhang Y-D, Rajinikanth V, Pugalenthi R and Sri Madhava Raja N 2021 Customized VGG19 architecture for pneumonia detection in chest x-rays *Pattern Recognit. Lett.* **143** 67–74
[40] Toğaçar M, Cömert Z and Ergen B 2020 Classification of brain MRI using hyper column technique with convolutional neural network and feature selection method *Expert Syst. Appl.* **149** 113274
[41] Hussain U N *et al* 2020 A unified design of ACO and skewness based brain tumor segmentation and classification from MRI scans *J. Control Eng. Appl. Inform.* **22** 43–55
[42] Iandola F N, Han S, Moskewicz M W, Ashraf K, Dally W J and Keutzer K 2016 SqueezeNet: AlexNet-level accuracy with 50x fewer parameters and <0.5 MB model size arXiv:1602.07360
[43] Ma C, Luo G and Wang K 2018 Concatenated and connected random forests with multiscale patch driven active contour model for automated brain tumor segmentation of MR images *IEEE Trans. Med. Imaging* **37** 1943–54
[44] Palani T K, Parvathavarthini B and Chitra K 2016 Segmentation of brain regions by integrating meta heuristic multilevel threshold with Markov random field *Current Medical Imaging Reviews* **12** 4–12
[45] Rajinikanth V, Fernandes S L, Bhushan B and Sunder N R 2018 Segmentation and analysis of brain tumor using Tsallis entropy and regularised level set *Proc. 2nd Int. Conf. Micro-Electronics, Electromagnetics and Telecommunications* vol **434** pp 313–21
[46] Rampun A, Strange H and Zwiggelaar R 2013 Texture segmentation using different orientations of GLCM features *Proc. 6th Int. Conf. on Computer Vision/Computer Graphics Collaboration Techniques and Applications* p 17
[47] Rehman A *et al* 2020 Microscopic brain tumor detection and classification using 3D CNN and feature selection architecture *Microsc. Res. Tech.* **84** 133–49
[48] Ronneberger O, Fischer P and Brox T 2015 U-Net: convolutional networks for biomedical image segmentation *Medical Image Computing and Computer-Assisted Intervention* vol 9351 ed N Navab, J Hornegger, W Wells and A Frangi (Cham: Springer)
[49] Roopini T I, Vasanthi M, Rajinikanth V, Rekha M and Sangeetha M 2018 Segmentation of tumor from brain MRI using fuzzy entropy and distance regularized level set *Computational Signal Processing and Analysis* vol 490 ed A Nandi, N Sujatha, R Menaka and J Alex (Cham: Springer) pp 297–304
[50] Rajeshkannan S and Korah R 2016 Improved CRC based disparity estimation of vision system using local adapative hue census and mean shift clustring *Natl Acad. Sci. Lett.* **39** 35–8

Chapter 8

Detection of brain tumors in MRI slices using traditional features with AI scheme: a study

K Suresh Manic, Ali Saud Al-Bimani and Uma Suresh

Assessment of brain tumors using three-dimensional (3D) magnetic resonance imaging (MRI) is computationally multifaceted. In real time, a two-dimensional (2D) MRI is used in hospitals to assess irregularities, with a personal confirmation by a knowledgeable doctor followed by a computerized diagnostic tool (CDT). This research aims to develop a CDT to examine tumors with superior accuracy. This CDT is implemented to examine the axial, coronal, and sagittal views of MRI scans. This study implements examination procedures such as categorizing chosen MRIs with/without segmented tumors. In these cases, a Shannon's entropy and firefly algorithm (SE+FA)-based threshold is implemented to pre-process the chosen MRIs. The CDT consists of pre-processing, post-processing, feature-extraction, feature-selection, and categorization phases. Furthermore, this research investigates tumor segmentation techniques, like active contour, level set, watershed, and region growing. In addition, a comparative study is also presented using the classification procedures such as support vector machines, adaptive neuro-fuzzy inference systems, *k*-nearest neighbors, random forests, and AdaBoost. The experiment is realized using the BRaTS 2016 and a real-time 2D MRI database. The outcome of the CDT confirms that the implemented practice helps accomplish a standard classification accuracy of >95% when executing tumor-based categorization.

8.1 Introduction

In the medical field, acute disease diagnosis involves (i) initial screening by a skillful doctor, (ii) confirmation using biosignaling and bioimaging procedures, (iii) evaluation of the results by a doctor and a dedicated computerized diagnostic tool (CDT), and (iv) planning the probable treatment according to the observations [1–4].

In most acute cases, such as abnormality in the brain, lungs, spinal cord, and other sensitive internal organs, image-based assessment plays a crucial role in sickness

doi:10.1088/978-0-7503-4012-0ch8

detection and treatment planning in contrast to signal-based approaches [5–8]. Most imaging techniques are noninvasive and help to acquire two-dimensional (2D) and three-dimensional (3D) views of the abnormal section. With the help of these images, the infection rate and the orientation of the infected region can be easily computed, which plays a crucial function in treatment handling and implementation [9, 10].

Because of their merits, image-based examinations are extensively adopted to diagnose different diseases. This chapter considers inspection of brain tumors based on magnetic resonance imaging (MRI). MRI is a noninvasive technique that essentially adopts imaging procedures to better analyze abnormalities in the human brain compared to the related, widely adopted imaging procedure, computed tomography (CT).

MRI is documented using a preferred modality, and the reconstructed image is made available in 3D form for inspection. Evaluation of tumors in 3D MRI is quite tricky. In hospital scenarios, 2D brain MRIs, converted to various views for inspection, as in the axial, coronal, and sagittal planes, is adopted due to its simplicity. To capture MRI scans for a given patient, a physician will recommend a particular modality after conferring with a radiologist. The two most basic types of imaging rely on the relaxation times of the brain tissue, which are distinguished as longitudinal resting time (T1) and transverse resting time (T2) imaging.

Along with T1 and T2, a modality called fluid-attenuated inversion recovery (FLAIR) is also widely utilized in neurology. The characteristics of FLAIR is approximately similar to the T2 images. These modalities are adopted to capture vital aspects of the brain's physiology, like cerebrospinal fluid, gray matter, white matter, cortex, fat within the bone marrow, and inflammation. In this proposed work, examining brain tumors using the FLAIR and T2 modalities is adopted for the investigation [9].

Due to its importance in medicine, many custom and soft-computing-based image examination events have been proposed and implemented [11, 12]. For example, the recent works of Rajinikanth *et al* [8] and Rajinikanth and Satapathy [13] confirm that soft-computing-based methods help to realize better accuracy compared to traditional procedures. Further, recent hybrid works (i.e. threshold+segmentation) discussed widely in the literature confirm that soft-computing procedures can offer better results in various MRI cases [14].

This study aims to develop a soft-computing CDT to examine brain tumors based on 2D slices of FLAIR and T2 modality MRIs. The proposed work implements two procedures: (i) classification of brain MRIs according to the tumor grade, and (ii) classification of brain MRIs into normal and tumor cases. In both cases, the test images are initially enhanced using a pre-processing technique, which considers a threshold based on a firefly algorithm (FA) and Shannon's entropy (SE), hereafter referred to as SE+FA. In the first case, the tumor section from the pre-processed MRI is mined using a chosen segmentation procedure. Later, the gray-level co-occurrence matrix (GLCM) features are mined, the dominant features are then selected with the FA, and a chosen classification procedure is implemented to categorize the brain MRIs. In the second case, skull-stripped normal and abnormal brain MRIs are considered for assessment. This part of the work implements the pre-processing based on SE+FA, feature extraction based on a discrete wavelet transform (DWT) and GLCM, feature selection with FA, and, finally, the classification into normal and tumor cases using a selected classifier.

This work collects benchmark normal and abnormal brain MRIs from the BRaTS 2016 [15] and Brain-Web [16] databases. Further, normal and abnormal clinical images are obtained from Pro-Scans Diagnostics Pvt Ltd [17]. The experimental outcomes confirm that the tumor-based classification of 2D brain MRI offers better accuracy compared to the previous alternative procedures implemented in this work.

The main contributions of the proposed work include the following:

i) Detailed analysis of existing segmentation methods.
ii) Implementation of machine-learning-based disease-detection techniques to examine 2D MRI slices of sagittal, coronal, and axial views.

8.2 Context

MRI is comprehensively deployed in the healthcare sector to analyze the regular functioning and any irregularities of the interior organs. Recent progress in MRI scanners has expanded upon the capabilities of reconstruction and estimation of 3D imagery. Accessible review plans for this imagery can be further composited and require elevated computing plans due to their bulky information volume. Generally, to reduce the difficulty during the MRI assessment, the modernized 3D imagery is transformed into a meaningful selection of 2D imagery, i.e. slices, in order to utilize a suitable image-inspection method. Former studies on brain MRI have considered both 3D and 2D imagery for diagnosis of abnormalities. However, 3D brain MRI appraisals are still challenging due to their computational complexity. Jiang *et al* recommended population-based 3D brain tumor segmentation using real-time MRI scans [14, 18–20]. Song *et al* proposed a comparison study on clinical brain segmentation using 3D MRI [21]. Maria *et al* discussed the registration of 3D fetal MRI [20].

CDT-maintained 2D brain slice assessment is generally preferred because of its simplicity, quicker run times, and improved accuracy. Recently, computerized and semiautomated MRI assessment schemes have been employed to find brain abnormalities from different MRI modalities. Palani *et al* presented a two-step technique with Otsu's thresholding and a Markov random field (MRF) system to inspect brain imagery with and without skull fragments [22]. An alike approach with MRF was extended with a FA by Rajinikanth *et al* [7] and implemented to mine tumor fragments from FLAIR, T1, and T2 modalities. The work of Rajinikanth *et al* provides a detailed assessment of a diversity of entropy-based threshold approaches with BRaTS2015 data, and confirmed that Shannon's scheme offers superior results for tumor enhancement [1]. Rajinikanth *et al* proposed a cuckoo search approach to examine 2D MRI using Tsallis's entropy and distance-regularized level set (DRLS) segmentation [10]. The work of Rajinikanth and Satapathy [13] implemented a hybrid approach based on a social group optimization (SGO) algorithm and fuzzy-Tsallis entropy to examine stroke regions from the ISLES database. Their work also supplied a thorough relative evaluation of different existing cancer-segmentation methods. Fernandes *et al* discussed a picture fusion method to improve the results during MRI inspection [14]. In their work, the BRaTS data set was used during testing and a fusion approach was considered to generate FLAIR+T1, FLAIR+T2, FLAIR+T1C, and FLAIR+T2+T1C images. Their study confirmed that a picture-blending approach facilitates better picture performance in contrast with MRI using a solitary modality. Kanmani and Marikkannu implemented a tumor mining and classification approach, which obtained better statistical measures [4]. The research of Usman and Rajpoot [23] gives a detailed discussion on extracting tumor sections from multimodal MRI. Their work considered the BRaTS 2013 data set and achieved a performance of 88% for the Dice coefficient. Further brain tumor examination procedures can be found in [23].

8.3 Methodology

The methodology executed in this chapter is depicted in figure 8.1. The main aim of this research is to develop a CDT to classify 2D brain MRIs based on their tumor

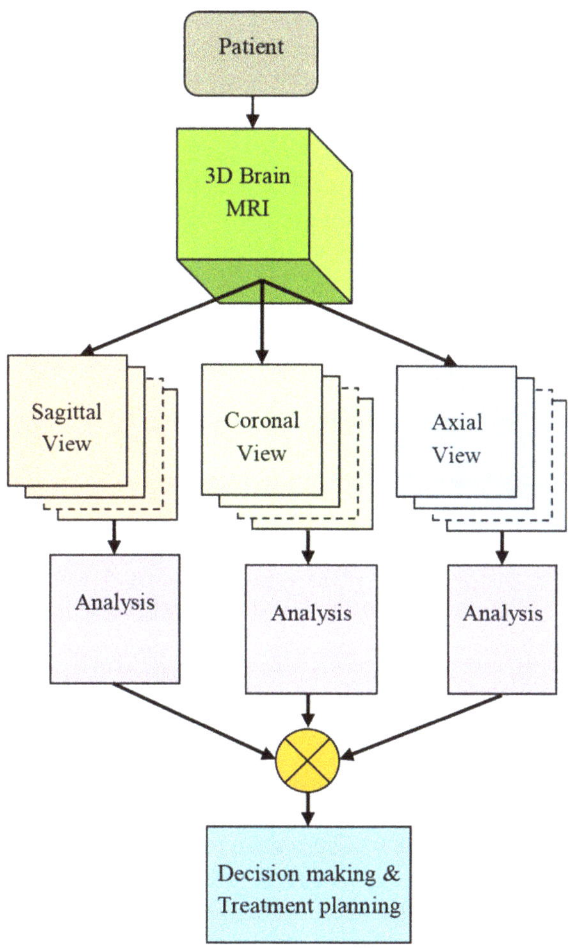

Figure 8.1. Outline of the proposed CDT considered to examine brain MRIs.

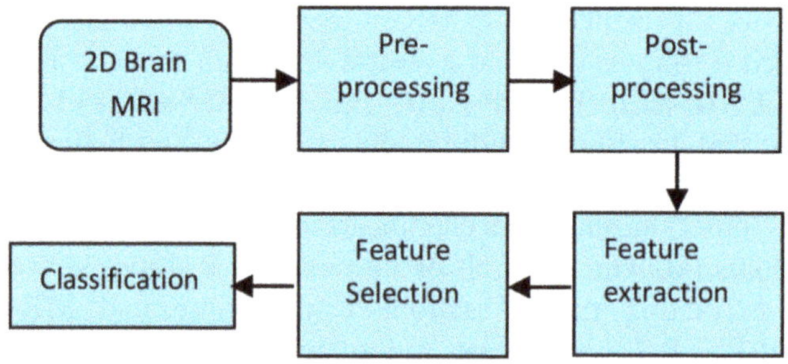

Figure 8.2. Various procedures implemented to analyze brain MRIs.

size. The proposed CDT is implemented for two cases: (i) classification of the tumor images according to their grade (based on the area covered by the tumor core and edema), and (ii) classification of test images into normal and tumor cases. In the initial technique the tumor grades are classified based on the GLCM features, and in the latter case the MRI images are classified based on the features of the DWT.

Figure 8.1 shows that a 3D brain MRI is initially obtained after screening the patient. Due to its complexity, the 3D MRI is divided into various 2D slices of the various views, such as in the axial, coronal, and sagittal planes. Then, the 2D slices are considered for analysis. The analysis stage (figure 8.2) consists of a pre-processing section, post-processing, feature extraction, and classification. The results of the axial, coronal, and sagittal views are then collected together to get the opinion of a doctor, who can recommend and implement possible treatment procedures based on the results obtained from the CDT.

8.3.1 Image data sets

The essential brain MRI 2D test images are collected from various databases (benchmark and clinical). In this work, 512 × 512 pixel-sized images are considered for examination. The clinical images are associated with the skull section. Before implementing the multi-thresholding based on SE+FA, a skull-stripping procedure is implemented for these images to remove the outer skull. The BRaTS 2016 database consists of reconstructed 3D images recorded with T1, T1C, T2, and FLAIR modalities along with a 3D ground-truth (GT) image. The itk-SNAP tool [24] is then utilized to extract 2D slices of the axial, coronal, and sagittal views along with their associated GTs. In this work, FLAIR and T2 modality test images are considered for the assessment because of their better visibility in comparison to the T1 and T1C modalities. In the initial examination case, 500 images (200 low-grade and 300 high-grade tumors) are considered for the classification task. Later, the features of the images are collected using the GLCM feature-mining procedures described in the literature [25, 26]. The dominant features are then identified using the FA-based feature-selection procedure. Finally, a chosen classifier unit is implemented to categorize the test pictures based on their features, and the essential values of the processes are computed. Similar pre-processing and feature-based classification is then implemented on normal and abnormal brain MRIs to classify the considered test pictures into routine and abnormal cases, with and without SE +FA-based thresholding. The experimental outcome confirms that the classification with a chosen classifier helps achieve better results.

8.3.2 Pre-processing

Image pre-processing is an essential procedure widely deployed to enhance the contents of test MRIs before implementing other tasks, such as segmentation, feature extraction, and classification. Pre-processing techniques can be used for noise removal, fixing errors during the reconstruction task, skull stripping, and multilevel thresholding. The later segmentation accuracy relies mainly on implementing accurate pre-processing techniques to enhance the test images [14]. Some pre-processing procedures are here given.

Skull stripping. Brain scans obtained from MRI usually include the skull section. Modalities such as FLAIR, T1, T1C, and T2 have noticeable skull sections in their axial, coronal, and sagittal views. In FLAIR and T2 MRIs, the strength of the skull section is almost similar to the tumor since the picture threshold levels are equal. In order to develop an efficient CDT, a skull-stripping step is necessary to eradicate the skull section from the brain MRI. Various skull-removing procedures implemented by researchers can be found in [7–9].

Thresholding. Recent bioimaging processing works have confirmed that a multi-level threshold is an essential pre-processing work to enhance the visibility of tumors and edemas. These earlier works suggest the need for a thresholding technique in the image-processing domain [1, 3]. This work implements a tri-level threshold based on SE+FA, as discussed in [7].

Firefly algorithm. FA is a swarm-based heuristic technique, first proposed by Yang [27]. It is formed by constructing a mathematical model for flashing patterns of fireflies. The various actions of a firefly in a search field and its other necessary information can be found in [28–31]. Tansformation in soft power and attraction with adjacent fireflies are the main limitations in FA's optimization accuracy.

This limitation can be expressed as

$$\text{Change in light intensity} = Y(l) = Y_0 e^{-\gamma l^2}, \tag{8.1}$$

where Y_o represents early light strength, Y represents the updated light strength, γ is the absorption coefficient with a value $\gamma \in [0,10]$, which varies in steps of 0.01, and l denotes the distance:

$$\text{Attraction among adjacent fireflies} = \phi(l) = \phi_0 e^{-\gamma l^2}, \tag{8.2}$$

where φ is the attraction parameter and φ_0 denotes attractiveness among fireflies when the distance $l = 0$.

Let us choose i and j as two random fireflies with a situation H, accessible in m-dimensional search space. Then, the Cartesian distance between i and j will be

$$l_{ij} = \| H_i - H_j \| = \sqrt{\sum_{k=1}^{m} \left(H_{i,k} - H_{j,k}\right)^2}, \tag{8.3}$$

where $H_{i,k}$ and $H_{j,k}$ are the kth factor of the spatial coordinate in the ith and jth fireflies, respectively.

In the m-dimensional space, the movement of the ith firefly toward a brighter firefly j can be expressed as follows:

$$H_i' = H_i + \phi_0 e^{-\gamma l_{ij}^2}\left(H_j - H_i\right) + \psi, \tag{8.4}$$

where H_i' is the updated location of the ith firefly, H_i denotes the earlier location of the ith firefly, H_j specifies the present location of the jth firefly, and ψ represents the motivating operator. In this study, a Brownian distribution (BD)-based FA is implemented to execute the pre-processing task, the related details of which can be found in the literature [32]. The mathematical expression of a FA driven by BD can be expressed as follows:

$$H_i' = H_i + \phi_0 e^{-\gamma l_{ij}^2}\left(H_j - H_i\right) + BD. \tag{8.5}$$

The tuning of the FA parameters plays a major role in the optimization task. In the proposed work, the FA algorithm parameters implemented in Raja *et al* [33] are adopted since the considered brain MRI is also a grayscale picture. The FA algorithm parameters are assigned as follows: number of fireflies = 30; search dimensions = 3; number of iterations = 2000; stopping criterion = maximized entropy value. In this work, the initial algorithm parameters are tuned as discussed by the aforementioned work of Raja *et al* [32, 33], and the BD-based search offers better results on the selected brain MRIs.

Shannon's entropy. Recently, SE-based multi-thresholding has been used to pre-process medical images [34]. In order to explain SE, let us consider an image with measurement $A \times B$. The gray-level pixel organization of image (h,v) is expressed as $G(h,v)$, for $h \in \{1,2,..., A\}$ and $v \in \{1,2,..., B\}$. Let L be the number of gray levels of the test image and the set of all gray values $\{0, 1, 2,\ldots, L-1\}$ be symbolized as Z, in such a way that

$$\mathrm{G}(h, v) \in \mathrm{Z}\ \forall\ (h, v) \in \text{image}. \tag{8.6}$$

Then, the normalized histogram will be $X = \{x_0, x_1,\ldots,x_{L-1}\}$.

For the tri-level thresholding case, equation (8.6) becomes

$$X(T) = x_0(t_1) + x_1(t_2) + x_2(t_3), \tag{8.7}$$

$$f(T) = \max_T \{\mathrm{X(T)}\}, \tag{8.8}$$

where $T = \{t_1, t_2,\ldots, t_L\}$ is the threshold value, $X = \{x_0, x_1,\ldots, x_{L-1}\}$ is the normalized histogram, and $f(T)$ is the optimal threshold.

In this study, the best possible SE for the chosen test image is attained using the FA. This work identifies the tri-level threshold by maximizing the SE function $f(T)$, as discussed in [1]. The proposed SE+FA threshold enhances the FLAIR and T2 modality brain MRIs, and their abnormal regions, such as the tumor core and edema sections, can easily be extracted with the chosen segmentation procedures.

8.3.3 Post-processing

This step is adopted to mine the tumor section from the pre-processed brain MRI. The extracted region consists of the abnormal brain sections, such as the tumor core and edema. First, this section is compared with the GT to confirm the merits of the proposed pre- and post-processing techniques. Then, this section's texture and area features are computed based on a GLCM procedure, as discussed in [25, 26]. The mined abnormal section varies based on the adopted segmentation approaches existing in the literature, and these techniques are discussed below.

Watershed algorithm. The watershed agorithm (WSA) is one of the simple and efficient procedures used to mine the abnormal section from a thresholded picture. This algorithm implements procedures such as edge detection, color fill based on the detected edge, morphological dilation, and section extraction. The accuracy of the WSA depends on the marker's pixel value considered in the morphological dilation. According to Rajinikanth and Satapathy [13], this algorithm falls under the category of automated segmentation. The experimental outcome of this approach also confirms that the execution time of the WSA is comparatively quicker than the other approaches considered in this study. Further details regarding the WSA can be found in [35].

Active contour. The active contour (AC) procedure implemented in this work is based on the adjustable snake model, which modifies its direction to track identical pixel clusters existing in pre-processed images based on energy minimization theory. Details on the AC technique implemented in this work can be found in [13]. The essential operations of the AC procedure involve the following:

- Edge discovery.
- Initial contour production based on the edges.
- Correcting the snake's track to identify the pixel group until the energy function reaches a minimal value according to a gradient descent criterion.
- Ending contour creation, and extraction of the tumor section which lies inside the contour.

The merit of AC is that, like other segmentation methods, it does not need any initiation process; hence, it is widely adopted in automated image-processing tools.

Chan–Vese. The Chan–Vese (VS) technique is also a kind of AC segmentation, proposed in 2001 by Chan and Vese [36]. The CV technique requires the initiation of a bounding box (BB) based on the tumor region to be extracted. The CV technique is widely considered to be a semiautomated image-processing tool because it requires this initiation of a BB whose edges will be adjusted continuously based on the assigned iteration number. When all pixel grouping is completed, the section within the contour is extracted and displayed.

Distance-regularized level set. Since the 1990s, the level set (LS) technique has been extensively considered to examine chosen sections from test images [37]. An advantage of the LS technique in contrast to AC is that it creates contours of a multipart topology to handle its splitting and merging actions through the image outline examination [38]. This study implements a recent iteration of a LS, known as a DRLS.

A single-well DRLS is implemented to mine the tumor section from the chosen MRI. DRLS also requires a BB initialization like CV, as widely used in semiautomated examination procedures [39].

Region growing. Region mining is a well-known practice based on seed initiation, generally a point or a pixel that decides the region of the image to be extracted. Starting with a seed value at a specified location, the region will be cultivated by attaching similar neighboring pixels. Researchers have also adopted this procedure to develop a semiautomated image-processing tool, the relevant information of which can be found in [40].

8.3.4 Feature extraction

This step extracts the essential information from the test image under study. The extracted features' size is usually significant, and includes dominant and straightforward features. In this work, feature-mining processes, such as GLCM and DWT, are considered to acquire the necessary disease information. As discussed in earlier works, the GLCM feature is initially considered to extract the texture and shape features from the brain tumor section. The extracted features are then considered to train and test the classifier section. If the entire feature set is considered to train and test the classifier, then the complexity will increase. Hence, a feature-selection procedure based on a FA is implemented to identify the dominant features from the extracted GLCM features, which can help classify the tumor based on its grade. Later, the integration of DWT and GLCM is then implemented to extract the feature from the whole brain MRI. The extracted features are then considered to categorize the brain MRIs into normal and tumor classes. Finally, the selection of the dominant image features is achieved with the FA-based feature-selection procedure. An example of dominant feature selection based on an heuristic algorithm can be found in [38].

Gray-level co-occurrence matrix. A surface report of the tumor is extracted initially with the Haralick texture analysis system, which is lengthily recognized as the gray-level co-occurrence matrix (GLCM). Former research works utilizing GLCMs have established that texture descriptions can frequently be adopted to gather essential information from tumors. These features are then considered to train, test, and confirm the classifier units, which are deployed to classify the brain tumor under analysis into benign and malignant classes, which may then support the doctor in making the right decision in recommending an appropriate treatment method to cure or regulate the brain abnormality.

In this work, the GLCM is considered to extract around 20 texture features from the tumor. After extracting these features, it is necessary to choose the key features from among them in order to minimize the complexity of constructing the disease classifier units. In the literature, proper guidelines have been proposed to select the main features of a GLCM, as in [25, 26]. Accordingly, in this work, features such as contrast, correlation, cluster prominence, energy, entropy, sum entropy, informational measure of correlation (IMC), are selected using the FA, and these values are then considered to train the classifier system.

Discrete wavelet transform. Earlier works have demonstrated that a wavelet technique can be considered to evaluate the various frequencies of a given test picture via different scales. A DWT is a widely adopted procedure to extract features from test pictures. In this work, a DWT is adopted to extract the coefficient of wavelets from the 2D MRI slices. A 2D DWT is considered in this work, which works in four sub-bands such as low-low (LL), high-low (HL), low-high (LH), and high-high (HH). A 2D level decomposition of an image displays an approximation with detailed 3D images representing the low-level and high-level frequency contents in an image, respectively. The features obtained with a DWT are dominant, and the level of complexity in its implementation is comparatively low.

Let $p(t)$ denote the square integral utility. $\psi(t)$ is their continuous wavelet transform, represented as follows:

$$W_\psi(x, y) = \int_{-\infty}^{\infty} p(t)\psi_{x,\,y}(t)dt, \tag{8.9}$$

$$\psi_{x,\,y}(t) = \frac{1}{\sqrt{2}}\psi\left(\frac{t-x}{y}\right). \tag{8.10}$$

The $\Psi_{x,y}(t)$ wavelet is computed from $\psi(t)$ based on procedures such as dilation and translation, where their features are x and y, respectively. In every point, four sub-bands (LL, LH, HL, HH) are extracted as the DWT features. Further details on DWTs can be found in [9].

8.3.5 Classification

Classification is the most essential procedure in disease diagnosis. In this section of the chapter, a detailed discussion of the classification procedures executed on an existing database is discussed.

Support vector machine. A support vector machine (SVM) is one of the most widely adopted types of classifier in the image-processing domain. The data are split into a decision surface, which signifies a hyperplane. The main purpose is to maximize the margins between two classes using the data in nonlinear fashion. Various SVM kernels are used to choose the existing classifiers, like linear kernels, radial basis function kernels, polynomial kernels, and sigmoid kernels. In this case, a SVM with a linear kernel is used to classify the brain MRI slices based on the selected features.

The decision function of a SVM is as follows:

$$C(a) = Sgn\left[\sum_{i=1}^{Nv} b_i \in i.\ K(s_i, a) + y\right], \tag{8.11}$$

where $\in i$ is the Lagrange coefficient obtained during the optimization process. The separating plane is generated from those Nv input vectors for which $\in i \neq 0$. Related information on a (linear) SVM can be found in [41].

Adaptive neuro-fuzzy inference system. An adaptive neuro-fuzzy inference system (ANFIS)-based classifier is implemented to categorize the brain MRI slices. ANFIS is a familiar classifier scheme built based on the neural network framework and Takagi–Sugeno fuzzy inference configuration. The work of Manickavasagam *et al* [41] verified that ANFIS has the potential to present the best categorization results compared to other neural-network-supported classifiers due to its hybrid nature. The inference structure in ANFIS is based on a set of fuzzy 'If–Then' rules, which have learning potential to approximate nonlinear functions. Due to its competence, ANFIS is generally adopted by researchers to classify signals and images [42–45].

The ANFIS classifier's training is realized in two trials, such as a forward and reverse trial.

In the forward training session, a least-squares approach is applied, and during the backward training session, minimization of the overall quadratic cost value is adopted. While executing these procedures, the training algorithm determines the optimal set of parameters, which can be used to assist the testing process. The initial parameters for the ANFIS classifier were assigned as follows: initially, a generalized bell-shaped membership function was chosen for the fuzzy system; iteration number = 250; parameter adaptation step size = 0.01; error acceptance = 0.005.

k-nearest neighbor. From the literature, it is noted that the examination capability of a CDT system mainly depends on the type and quality of the classifier system. Quite a few classifier systems exist in the field of brain MRI examination, but in this work only the well-known k-nearest neighbor (k-NN) technique was implemented to classify the brain MRI into normal versus abnormal [46]. Like other classifiers, k-NN also needs training and testing based on image features.

k-NN extrapolates the distance from a range of new data to all training data points, and finds the shortest distance as the best neighbor. The k-value is empirically determined using the training sample's sorting error.

The mathematical expression of the k-NN implemented in this work is as follows.

Let there exist two feature vectors of D dimensions, $M = (M_1, M_2, \ldots, M_n)^T$ and $N = (N_1, N_2, \ldots, N_n)^T$. Then the Euclidean distance can be shown as

$$\text{Euclidean distance}\left(\vec{M},\vec{N}\right)=\sqrt{\begin{matrix}(M_1 - N_1)^2 + (M_2 - N_2)^2 \\ +, \ldots, (M_D - N_1)^2\end{matrix}}. \tag{8.12}$$

Random forest. This technique is an enhanced technique, which is robust to noise and competent with huge data sets. It is modeled as a set of tree predictors. Each tree relies on arbitrary vector values, which are sampled separately and with the same distribution of all trees in the forest [47]. This technique is relatively quick and it is easy to implement.

A random forest (RF) function can be expressed as follows:

$$H(a) = \text{argmax}_b \sum^{k} I(h_1(x) = Y), \tag{8.13}$$

where $H(a)$ denotes the final combined classifier, k represents the decision tree number, $h_1(x)$ defines the decision tree, where the class label is illustrated by Y and $I(h_l(x) = Y)$ indicates x belongs to class Y.

AdaBoost. AdaBoost represents a new boosting plan that has been used with the goal of improving classification accuracy. It integrates weak classifiers with high error rates and generates a resulting classifier with a low error rate. This method is simple and very fast. This technique has been successfully applied to many classification problems [48].

8.3.6 Performance evaluation

The performance of the proposed CDT is authenticated by calculating well-known image performance measures. In order to enhance the assessment potential, pre-processing based on the SE+FA thresholding procedure is implemented. The performance measures adopted in this work are depicted in equations (8.2)–(8.6):

$$\text{Precision} = \text{PRE} = T_P/(T_P + F_P), \tag{8.14}$$

$$\text{Sensitvity} = \text{SEN} = T_P/(T_P + F_N), \tag{8.15}$$

$$\text{F1 Score} = 2T_P/(2T_P + F_P + F_N), \tag{8.16}$$

$$\text{Specificity} = \text{SPE} = T_N/(T_N + F_P), \tag{8.17}$$

$$\text{Accuracy} = ACC = (T_P + T_N)/(T_P + T_N + F_P + F_N), \tag{8.18}$$

where T_N, T_P, F_N, and F_P signifies true negative, true positive, false negative, and false positive, respectively [1, 7–10].

8.4 Results and discussion

This section presents the results achieved with the proposed CDT. The literature verifies the feasibility of the proposed MRI examination. This work implements a procedure to inspect benchmark brain MRI images as well as MRI images obtained from a clinical setting. As aforementioned, this work considers the assistance of a modern heuristic procedure combining a FA along with SE (i.e. SE+FA).

A detailed assessment of the existing segmentation procedures was also conducted. Finally, a tumor classification system was implemented based on a chosen classification, and trained and tested using the well-known texture features referred to as a GLCM. The developed CDT was executed in a workstation with an Intel Core i5 CPU with 8 GB of RAM and implemented in MATLAB®.

Initially, the FLAIR and T2 tumor data set was considered for evaluation. This data set contains MRI scans acquired from various data sets with pixel dimensions of 512 × 512. This data set also include GTs offered by an expert. It is a 3D data set and supports axial, coronal and sagittal views. Initially, 2D slices were extracted from the 3D images using a chosen tool (itk-SNAP). Throughout this study, the axial, coronal, and sagittal views are considered for evaluation [1].

Figures 8.3–8.5 depict the test images. The (a) panels denote the assigned pseudonym of the 2D brain MRI; the (b) panels the 2D test images; the (c) panels the GTs; and the (d) panels SE+FA threshold image. Initially, pre-processing based on three-level thresholding with SE+FA is executed on the chosen test image and the search is allowed to run until the entropy function of the test image is maximized. Later, the tumor section from the threshold picture is mined using a chosen segmentation procedure.

Initially, the axial view brain MRI (S_45) is considered for the examination. SE +FA-based three-level thresholding is implemented to enhance the tumor section, as discussed in [1, 7]. The pre-processed picture is then considered for the next level of the assessment.

Figure 8.6 depicts the outcome obtained with the WSA. Figure 8.6(a) shows the test image considered for the analysis, while figures 8.6(b) and (c) depict the detected

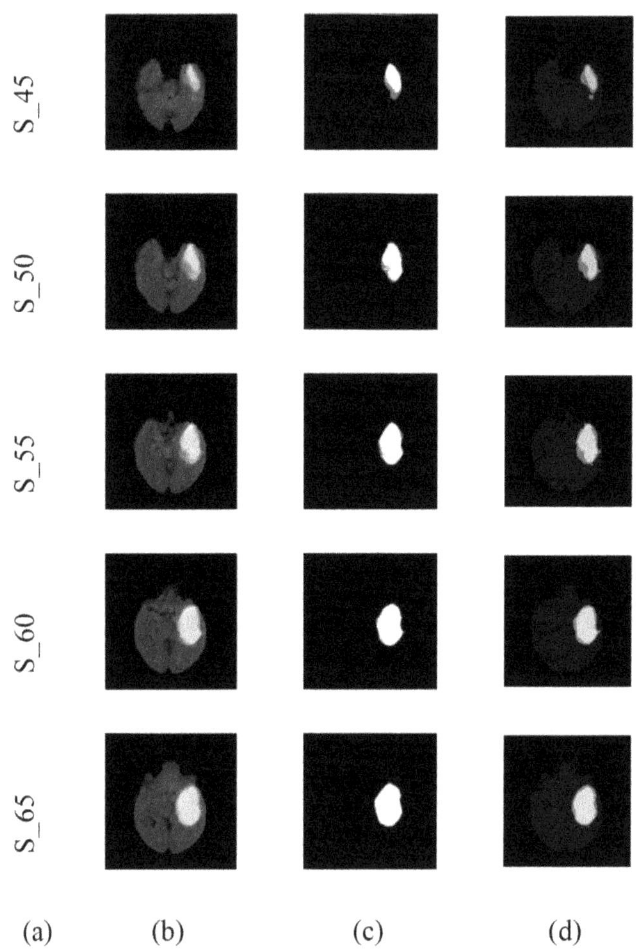

Figure 8.3. Sample BRaTS test image (axial). (a) Pseudonym, (b) test image, (c) GT, (d) thresholded picture.

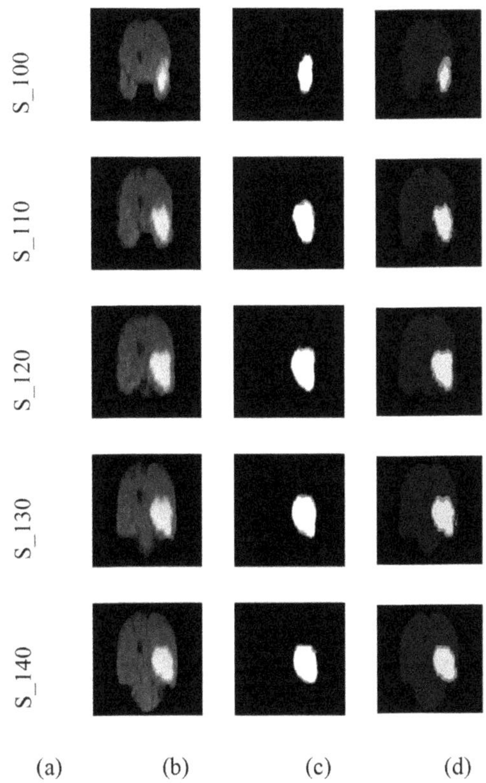

Figure 8.4. Sample BRaTS test image (coronal). (a) Pseudonym, (b) test image, (c) GT, (d) thresholded picture.

edge and the filled watershed sections, and figures 8.6(d) and (e) show the enhanced and the extracted tumor section, respectively.

Figure 8.7 represents the result obtained with the AC technique. Figure 8.7(a) shows the scaling of the test picture based on the threshold value, figure 8.7(b) presents the detected edges of the tumor section, and figures 8.7(c) and (d) depict the initial contour, final contour, and the extracted tumor, respectively.

Figure 8.8 shows the outcomes obtained with the CV technique. This figure depicts images of the test picture, initial BB, final contour, and the extracted tumor.

Figure 8.9 depicts the results of the DRLS procedure. Figure 8.9(a) depicts the initial BB, figures 8.9(b) and (c) present the converged LS and the extracted tumor section, respectively. Finally, figure 8.10 depicts the result obtained with the RF approach. From this experimental work, it can be noted that the WS algorithm's execution is relatively faster than the AC, CV, DRLS, and RF techniques.

After extracting the tumor section from the chosen test images (500 2D images with axial, coronal, and sagittal views), the extracted tumor sections are then compared with their related GTs, available in the chosen data set. A comparison between the extracted tumor and the GT can be used to obtain essential image similarity values. If these values show an improvement, then the proposed pre- and

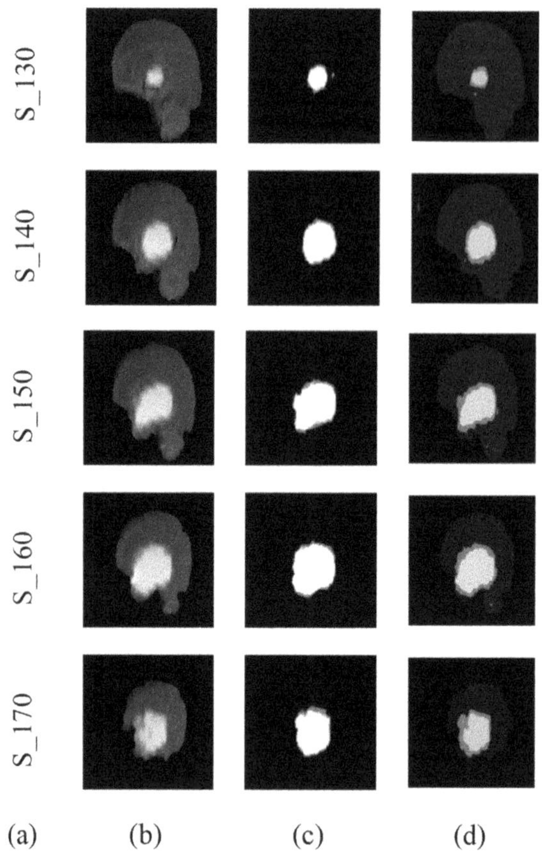

Figure 8.5. Sample BRaTS test image (sagittal). (a) Pseudonym, (b) test image, (c) GT, (d) thresholded picture.

post-processing procedures herein can be considered to extract tumor regions from clinical data sets in future.

Table 8.1 presents the performance measures obtained for the test image with pseudonym 'S_45' and the computed performance measures for the chosen segmentation procedures. For this image, the RF-based technique offered a better result compared to other methods. A similar procedure is then implemented for the remaining test images (500 in total) and its average performance measures are considered for evaluation, as presented in figure 8.11. This figure confirms that the proposed segmentation methods work well on the chosen data set and offer better values for the performance measures on the considered data set.

The extracted tumor section is mostly a combination of a tumor core and an edema section. When this section occupies a greater area in the picture frame of a test picture, then it is considered as a high-grade tumor; if it occupies a lesser section, then it falls under low-grade tumor categorization. Finally, the feature extraction is then implemented on the entire set of test images (200 low grade + 300 high grade = 500 in total) using the GLCM procedure, in which 20 features are then

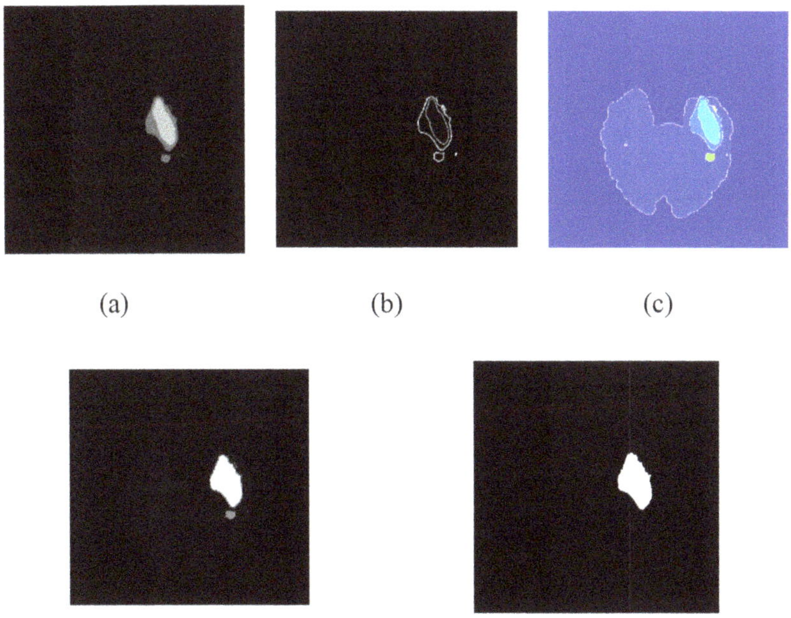

(a) (b) (c)

(d) (e)

Figure 8.6. Outcome of WSA. (a) Test image, (b) edge detection, (c) watershed implementation, (d) identified tumor section, and (e) mined tumor.

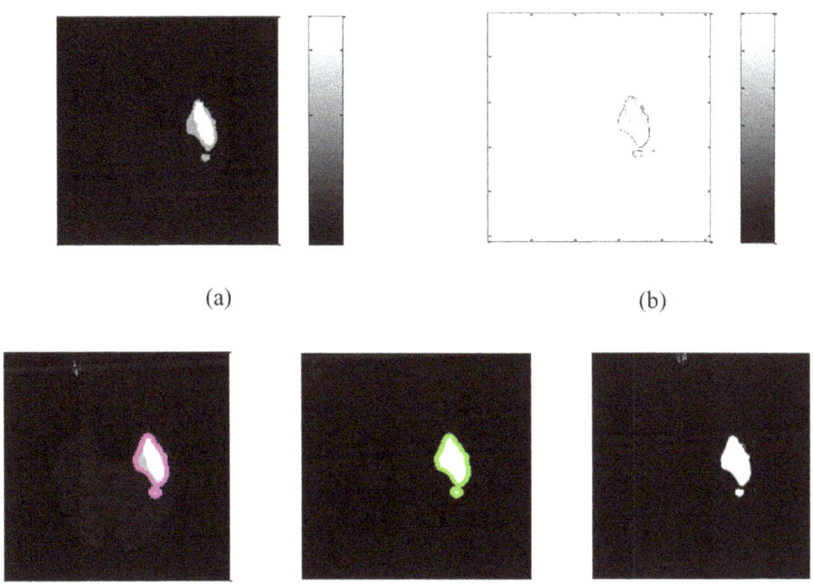

(a) (b)

(c) (d)

Figure 8.7. Outcome of AC technique. (a) Histogram evaluation, (b) tumor boundary, (c) initial and final contour, and (d) mined tumor.

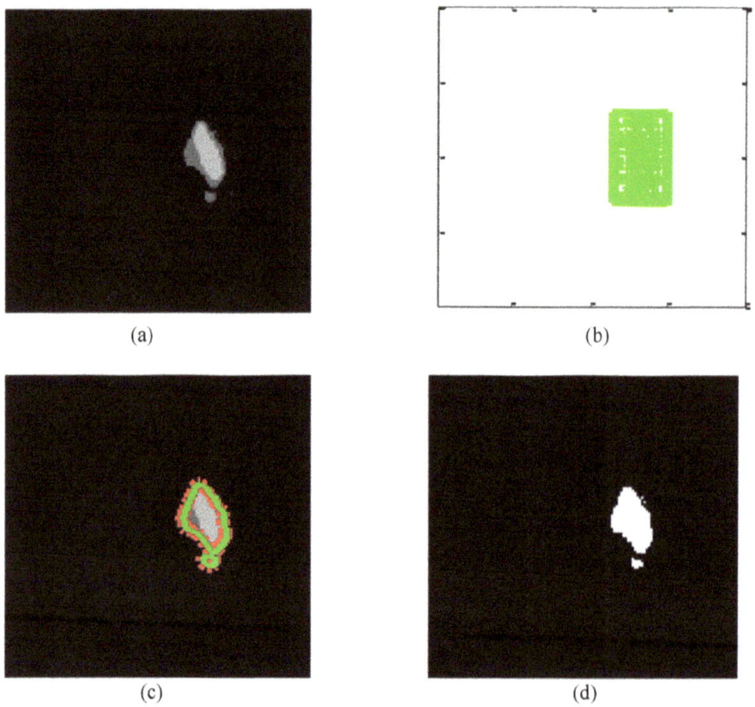

Figure 8.8. Outcome of AC technique with (a) chosen test image, (b) initial bounding box, (c), convered contour, and (d) mined tumor.

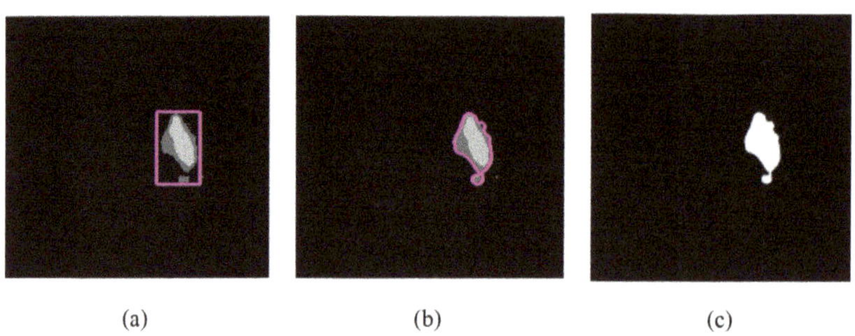

Figure 8.9. Outcome of DRLS approach. (a) Initial bounding box, (b) converged contour, and (c) mined tumor.

extracted from the considered tumors. The FA-based feature-selection procedure is then executed on these feature sets, and eight out of the extracted dominant features are then adapted to train, test, and validate the classifier section.

Table 8.2 presents the performance obtained with the various classifier units on the chosen data set. The average performance measures attained with the GLCM +*k*-NN extraction and classification method is better compared to other classifiers. The implementation of the *k*-NN is simple, and it is also a well-established and proven classifier unit according to extensive earlier research works. In addition to

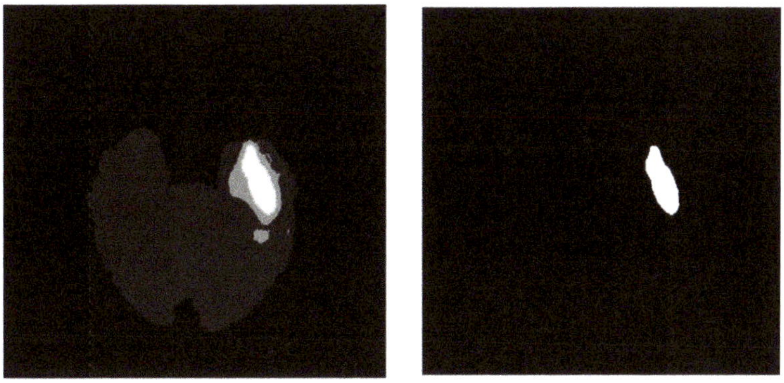

(a) (b)

Figure 8.10. Outcome of RF procedure. (a) Identified tumor and (b) mined tumor.

Table 8.1. Performance measures obtained by comparison of extracted tumor and GT images.

Method	ACC (%)	PRE (%)	SEN (%)	SPE (%)	F1 score (%)
WS	88.10	99.46	99.94	77.66	99.69
AC	90.01	99.54	99.89	81.09	99.72
CV	99.28	99.97	99.93	98.64	99.95
DRLS	96.21	99.83	99.99	92.57	99.91
RF	99.47	100	98.95	100	99.47

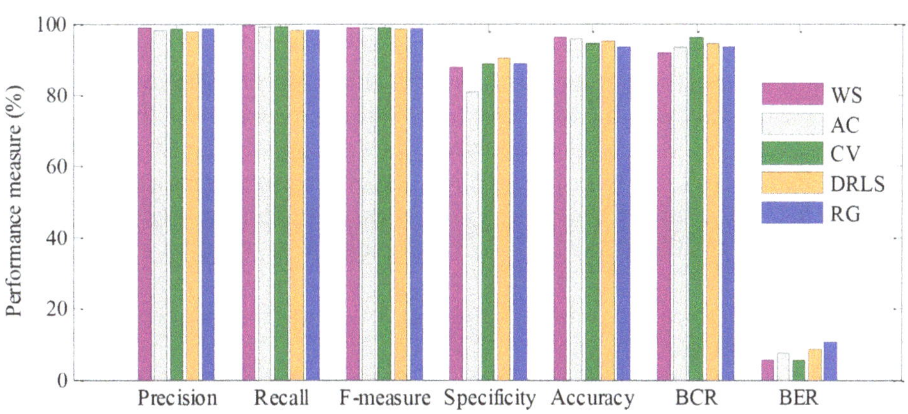

Figure 8.11. Performance evaluation of tumor mining procedures.

k-NN, the average results attained with the other classifiers was also better (>95%) on the BRaTS 2016 database pictures.

The clinical significance of the proposed CDT is then tested on clinical data as well as the benchmark images obtained from the BRaTS and Brain-Web databases [16]. Initially, normal and abnormal 2D MRI slices (axial plane) are collected from

Table 8.2. Classification accuracy obtained for the brain MRI data set based on tumor feature classification.

Feature extraction+classification	ACC (%)	PRE (%)	SEN (%)	SPE (%)	F1 score (%)	Average
GLCM+SVM	96.40	96.43	97.70	94.39	97.06	96.39
GLCM+ANFIS	95.00	95.69	96.58	92.13	96.14	95.13
GLCM+*k*-NN	96.20	97.61	95.97	96.53	96.79	96.72
GLCM+RF	96.20	96.52	96.85	95.33	96.68	96.34
GLCM+AdaBoost	95.00	96.47	96.19	92.45	96.33	95.36

Table 8.3. Clinical brain MRI data set considered in this study.

Class	Images
Normal case	150 images (100 clinical images + 50 benchmark images)
Brain tumor case	350 images (75 clinical images + 275 benchmark images)
Total	500

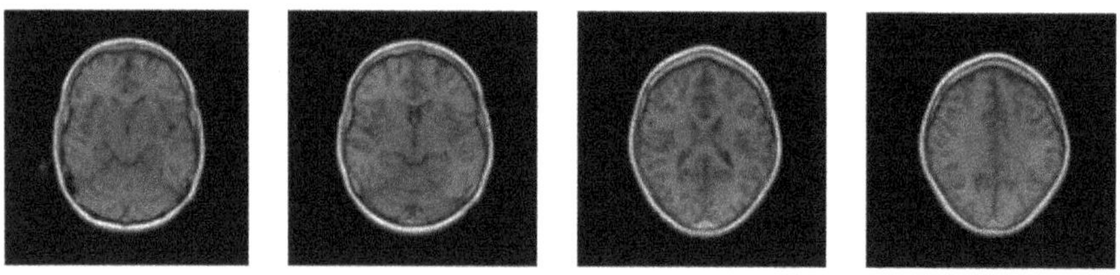

Figure 8.12. Normal test images.

the clinical data set (100 normal cases and 75 abnormal cases). Additionally, 325 brain MRI scans are then collected from a standard benchmark database. Table 8.3 presents the details of the images considered for the examination. Initially, before the examination, the skull sections of the test images are removed using a skull-stripping tool [1]. The skull-stripped test pictures are then considered to train and test the classifier section. In this work, the DWT technique is adopted to extract the key features from the pictures. This work is implemented as (i) direct implementation of the DWT and classification, and (ii) implementation of classification based on the pre- and post-extracted features.

Table 8.3 presents the number of test images collected and considered for this study. For this case, also, a total of 500 images are considered for the examination. Figure 8.12 depicts normal brain sections considered for demonstration, and figure 8.13 presents enhanced tumor sections from the benchmark MRI set after multilevel thresholding. Finally, the essential DWT-based technique is then implemented to extract the features in two cases: (i) without pre- and post-processing operations, and (ii) with the essential pre- and post-processing operations.

Figures 8.14 and 8.15 present some of the clinical MRIs considered to test the performance of the proposed CDT system. Initially, the skull-stripping task is

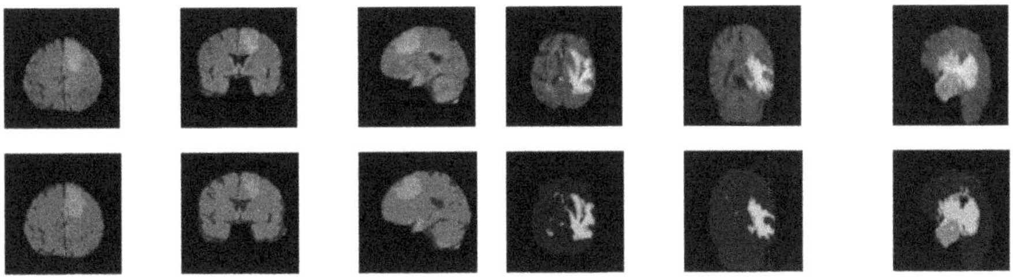

(a) (b) (c) (d) (e) (f)

Figure 8.13. Abnormal test images. (a), (d) Axial view; (b), (e) coronal view; (c), (f) sagittal view.

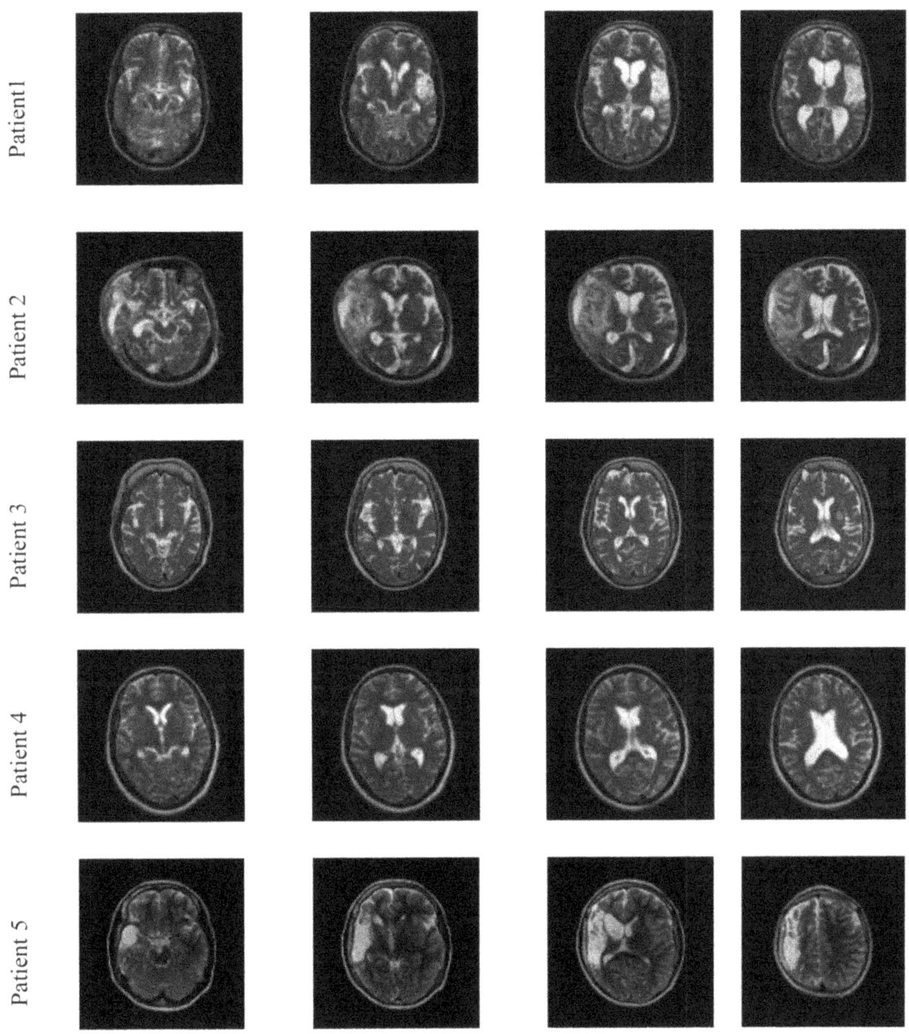

Figure 8.14. Abnormal test images from the clinical data set.

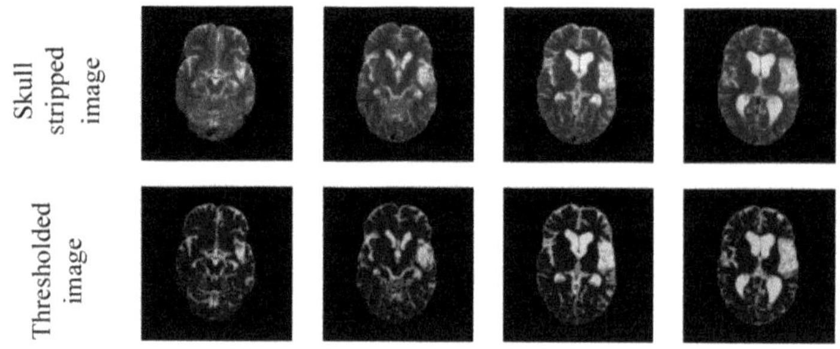

Figure 8.15. Pre-processed abnormal test.

Table 8.4. Classification accuracy obtained for the brain MRI data set (without the pre-processing task).

Feature extraction+classification	ACC (%)	PRE (%)	SEN (%)	SPE (%)	F1 score (%)	Average
DWT+SVM	89.75	88.06	91.24	88.35	89.62	89.32
DWT+ANFIS	85.25	86.13	88.74	80.47	87.42	85.69
DWT+*k*-NN	86.50	86.88	88.48	84.15	87.67	86.79
DWT+RF	86.75	88.48	91.54	77.86	89.98	86.97
DWT+AdaBoost	88.75	87.20	91.09	86.36	89.10	88.44

Table 8.5. Classification accuracy obtained for the brain MRI data set (with pre-processed images).

Feature extraction+classification	ACC (%)	PRE (%)	SEN (%)	SPE (%)	F1 score (%)	Average
DWT+SVM	93.80	93.52	96.81	88.77	95.13	93.56
DWT+ANFIS	92.40	91.99	94.62	89.59	93.29	92.37
DWT+*k*-NN	92.80	94.17	94.75	89.20	94.46	93.14
DWT+RF	93.60	93.99	96.31	88.57	95.14	93.50
DWT+AdaBoost	91.80	91.96	94.70	87.37	93.31	91.83

executed to increase visibility of the brain section. Later, the DW- based feature extraction is executed on the raw test images and the pre-processed images based on SE+FA. After extracting the essential features, the above discussed classifier systems are then implemented to test the performance of the CDT.

From tables 8.4 and 8.5, it can be noted that the average results displayed in table 8.5 are better than in table 8.4. This result also confirms that the SE+FA pre-processing technique helps to achieve better performance measures compared to test images without pre-processing. Thus, this result further confirms the merit of the proposed technique. The results of this study verify that tumor-based feature extraction and classification offers better performance measures in comparison to the other two cases. In future, this CDT can be enhanced by considering other facilities, such as entropy-measure-based analysis, and texture- and area-based methods.

8.5 Conclusion

This work proposed a CDT using pre-processing, post-processing, feature extraction, feature selection, and classification techniques. Pre-processing based on FA-assisted Shannon's tri-level thresholding enhanced the test images appropriately, and the segmentation or feature-extraction techniques implemented on these images offered enhanced results. This chapter used the BRaTS 2016 and Brain-Web databases as well as images collected from a medical clinic. Initially, the GLCM feature extraction and classification based on the tumor offered and enhanced performance measure. A similar procedure was then repeated on the test images with and without pre-processing and post-processing tasks, and the essential image features were then computed based on a DWT. The experimental outcome confirmed that the tumor-based classification provided better results compared to other approaches demonstrated in this work. Further, the classification results provided with SVM, ANFIS, *k*-NN, RF, and AdaBoost were relatively similar. In future, the merit of the proposed technique can be validated by considering more clinical image data sets. The experimental outcome of this work confirms that the proposed approach, based on pre- and post-processing, helped to achieve an average performance of >95%.

Acknowledgment

The authors of this chapter would like to acknowledge Pro-Scans Diagnostics Pvt Ltd, a leading scan center in Chennai, for providing the clinical brain MRI for experimental investigation.

References

[1] Rajinikanth V, Satapathy S C, Fernandes S L and Nachiappan S 2017 Entropy based segmentation of tumor from brain MR images—a study with teaching learning based optimization *Pattern Recognit. Lett.* **94** 87–95

[2] Pugalenthi R, Rajakumar M P, Ramya J and Rajinikanth V 2019 Evaluation and classification of the brain tumor MRI using machine learning technique *J. Control Eng. Appl. Inform.* **21** 12–21

[3] Raja N S M, Fernandes S L, Dey N, Satapathy S C and Rajinikanth V 2018 Contrast enhanced medical MRI evaluation using Tsallis entropy and region growing segmentation *J. Ambient Intell. Human Comput.* https://doi.org/10.1007/S12652-018-0854-8

[4] Kanmani P and Marikkannu P 2018 MRI brain images classification: a multi-level threshold based region optimization technique *J. Med. Syst.* **42** 62

[5] Tian Z *et al* 2018 Morphological segmenting and neighborhood pixel-based locality preserving projection on brain fMRI dataset for semantic feature extraction: an affective computing study *Neural Comput. Appl.* **30** 3733–48

[6] Moraru L *et al* 2018 Texture anisotropy technique in brain degenerative diseases *Neural Comput. Appl.* **30** 1667–77

[7] Rajinikanth V, Raja N S M and Kamalanand K 2017 Firefly algorithm assisted segmentation of tumor from brain MRI using Tsallis function and markov random field *J. Control Eng. Appl. Inform.* **19** 97–106

[8] Rajinikanth V, Dey N, Satapathy S C and Ashour A S 2018 An approach to examine magnetic resonance angiography based on Tsallis entropy and deformable snake model *Future Gener. Comput. Syst.* **85** 160–72
[9] Fernandes S L, Tanik U J, Rajinikanth V and Karthik K A 2019 A reliable framework for accurate brain image examination and treatment planning based on early diagnosis support for clinicians *Neural Comput. Appl.* **32** 15897–908
[10] Rajinikanth V *et al* 2018 Segmentation and analysis of brain tumour using Tsallis entropy and regularised level set *Proc. 2nd Int. Conf. on Micro-Electronics, Electromagnetics and Telecommunications* pp 313–21
[11] Edalati-rad A and Mosleh M 2019 Improving brain tumor diagnosis using mri segmentation based on collaboration of beta mixture model and learning automata *Arab. J. Sci. Eng.* **44** 2945–57
[12] Chakraborty R, Sushil R and Garg M L 2019 An improved PSO-based multilevel image segmentation technique using minimum cross-entropy thresholding *Arab. J. Sci. Eng.* **44** 3005–20
[13] Rajinikanth V and Satapathy S C 2018 Segmentation of ischemic stroke lesion in brain MRI based on social group optimization and Fuzzy-Tsallis entropy *Arab. J. Sci. Eng.* **43** 4365–78
[14] Acharya U R *et al* 2019 Automated detection of Alzheimer's disease using brain MRI images–a study with various feature extraction techniques *J. Med. Syst.* **43** 302
[15] Brain Tumour Database (BraTS-MICCAI) http://hal.inria.fr/hal-00935640 (Accessed: 05 February 2019)
[16] 2019 https://brainweb.bic.mni.mcgill.ca/brainweb/ (Accessed: 16 April 2019)
[17] 2017 https://proscans.in
[18] Maier O *et al* 2017 ISLES 2015 – a public evaluation benchmark for ischemic stroke lesion segmentation from multispectral MRI *Med. Image Anal.* **35** 250–69
[19] Menze B H *et al* 2015 The multimodal brain tumor image segmentation benchmark (BRATS) *IEEE Trans. Med. Imaging* **34** 1993–2024
[20] Chaddad A and Tanougast C 2016 Quantitative evaluation of robust skull stripping and tumour detection applied to axial MR images *Brain Informatics* **3** 53–61
[21] Song T, Angelini E, Mensh B and Laine A 2004 Comparison study of clinical 3D MRI brain segmentation evaluation *Conf. Proc. IEEE Eng. Med. Biol. Soc.* **3** 1671–4
[22] Palani T K, Parvathavarthini B and Chitra K 2016 Segmentation of brain regions by integrating meta heuristic multilevel threshold with markov random field *Current Medical Imaging Reviews* **12** 4–12
[23] Usman K and Rajpoot K 2017 Brain tumour classification from multi-modality MRI using wavelets and machine learning *Pattern Anal. Appl.* **20** 871–81
[24] itk-SNAP 2018 itk-SNAP software application tool www.itksnap.org/pmwiki/pmwiki.php
[25] Haralick R M, Shanmugam K and Dinstein I 1973 Textural features of image classification *IEEE Trans. on Systems, Man, Cybernetics* **SMC-3** 610–21
[26] Soh L and Tsatsoulis C 1999 Texture analysis of SAR sea ice imagery using gray level co-occurrence matrices *IEEE Trans. Geosci. Remote Sens.* **37** 780–95
[27] Yang X S 2008 *Nature-Inspired Metaheuristic Algorithms* (London: Luniver Press)
[28] Yang X S 2010 *Engineering Optimization: An Introduction with Metaheuristic Applications* (Hoboken, NJ: Wiley)
[29] Yang X S 2010 Firefly algorithm, Lévy flights and global optimization *Research and Development in Intelligent Systems* ed M Bramer, R Ellis and M Petridis vol 26 (London: Springer)

[30] Gandomi A H, Yang X S, Talatahari S and Alavi A H 2013 Firefly algorithm with chaos *Commun. Nonlinear Sci. Numer. Simul.* **18** 89–98

[31] Tilahun S L and Ngnotchouye J M T 2017 Firefly algorithm for discrete optimization problems: a survey *KSCE J. Civ. Eng.* **21** 535–45

[32] Raja N S M, Manic K S and Rajinikanth V 2013 Firefly algorithm with various randomization parameters: an analysis *SEMCCO 2013: Swarm, Evolutionary, and Memetic Computing* Lecture Notes in Computer Science vol 8297 ed B K Panigrahi, P N Suganthan and S Das *et al* (Cham: Springer) pp 110–21

[33] Raja N S M, Rajinikanth V and Latha K 2014 Otsu based optimal multilevel image thresholding using firefly algorithm *Model. Simul. Eng.* **2014** 794574

[34] Kannappan P L 1972 On Shannon's entropy, directed divergence and inaccuracy *Probability Theory and Related Fields* **22** 95–100 (in German)

[35] Roerdink J B T M and Meijster A 2000 The watershed transform: definitions, algorithms and parallelization strategies *Fundam. Inform.* **41** 187–228

[36] Chan T F and Vese L A 2001 Active contours without edges *IEEE Trans. Image Process.* **10** 266–77

[37] Malladi R, Sethian A and Vemuri B C 1995 Shape modeling with front propagation: a level set approach *IEEE Trans. Pattern Anal. Mach. Intell.* **17** 158–75

[38] Li C and Xu C 2010 Distance regularized level set evolution and its application to image segmentation *IEEE Trans. Image Process.* **19** 3243–54

[39] Kim D, Kim N, Lee S and Seo J B 2018 A fast and robust level set motion-assisted deformable registration method for volumetric CT guided lung intervention *Biocyber. Biomed. Eng.* **38** 439–47

[40] Panda R, Puhan N B and Panda G New binary Hausdorff symmetry measure based seeded region growing for retinal vessel segmentation *Biocyber. Biomed. Eng.* **36** 119–29

[41] Manickavasagam K, Sutha S and Kamalanand K 2014 Development of systems for classification of different plasmodium species in thin blood smear microscopic images *J. Advanced Microscopy Research* **9** 86–92

[42] Sarma K K 2009 Neural network based feature extraction for assamese character and numeral recognition *Int. J. Artificial Intelligence* **2** 37–56

[43] Pozna C *et al* 2010 New results in modelling derived from Bayesian filtering *Knowl.-Based Syst.* **23** 182–94

[44] Gil R P A, Johanyák Z C and Kovács T 2018 Surrogate model based optimization of traffic lights cycles and green period ratios using microscopic simulation and fuzzy rule interpolation *Int. J. Artificial Intelligence* **16** 20–40

[45] Albu A, Precup R-E and Teban T-A 2019 Results and challenges of artificial neural networks used for decision-making in medical applications *Facta Universitatis, Series: Mechanical Engineering* **17** 285–308

[46] Havaei M, Jodin P-M and Larochelle H 2014 Efficient interactive brain tumor segmentation as within-brain kNN classification *22nd Int. Conf. on Pattern Recognition* (Piscataway, NJ: IEEE)

[47] Lefkovits L, Lefkovits S and Szilágyi L 2016 Brain tumor segmentation with optimized random forest *Brainlesion: Glioma, Multiple Sclerosis, Stroke and Traumatic Brain Injuries* vol 10154 ed A Crimi, B Menze and O Maier *et al* (Cham: Springer) pp 88–99

[48] Hastie T, Tibshirani R and Friedman J 2009 *The Elements of Statistical Learning: Data Mining, Inference, and Prediction* 2nd edn (New York: Springer)

Chapter 9

Framework to classify EEG signals into normal/schizophrenic classes with machine-learning scheme

Venkatesan Rajinikanth and Seifedine Kadry

In the hospital setting, the brain's activity is generally studied with a chosen imaging/signaling method. Examination of the brain's functioning with an electroencephalogram (EEG) signal is one such approved method in hospitals. Evaluation of the EEG pattern can predict cerebral activities/brain abnormalities. The main aim of the proposed work is to develop a computerized tool to investigate and classify EEG signal patterns into normal and schizophrenic cases. This tool implements a sequence of procedures, such as EEG series splitting, nonlinear feature mining, Student's *t*-test-assisted feature selection, classification, and validation. This work also provides a detailed assessment of various classification techniques available in the literature. This study confirms that support-vector-machine-assisted classification offers superior results in EEG classification to other alternative practices implemented in this work.

9.1 Introduction

The brain is one of the crucial internal organs, and its malfunctioning/disordering or disease can affect normal human activities [1–3]. Abnormalities in the brain can be analyzed using a chosen imaging or signaling technique. However, imaging techniques, such as magnetic resonance imaging (MRI) and computed tomography (CT), are quite costly and require more recording and computation time compared to signaling procedures such as electroencephalograms (EEGs) [4–7]. However, an EEG signal recorded using appropriate electrode placement will reveal essential details regarding the brain's activity, and examining these signals may help reveal the condition of/abnormality in the brain [8–10]. Further, the availability of modern techniques (sensor arrays, recording systems, and analyzing systems) can help to

doi:10.1088/978-0-7503-4012-0ch9

predict abnormalities in the brain by examining its electrical activity (i.e. EEG patterns) under various conditions [11, 12].

Due to its clinical importance, several automated and semiautomated approaches have been widely proposed by researchers to examine the physiological signals of the brain [13–16]. EEG signals created due to neuronal activity are generally recorded by single or multichannel electrodes located on the scalp section. The EEG patterns are acquired during the clinical diagnosis by placing the electrodes at predefined scalp sections. EEG patterns have been extensively used to inspect syndromes such as dementia, Alzheimer's disease, sleep disorders, epilepsy, schizophrenia, and other related brain disorders [17–22].

The proposed research aims to develop an automated diagnostic tool (ADT) to identify schizophrenia by analyzing EEG patterns. Schizophrenia is a chronic brain abnormality and affects thinking ability and general behavior. Researchers have recently proposed and implemented numerous approaches to predict and categorize schizophrenia from normal class signals using multichannel EEG recorded in a controlled atmosphere [23, 24]. If schizophrenia is diagnosed in its early phases, then a possible treatment procedure can be implemented to cure the patient [25]. The diagnosis of schizophrenia is based on the history of the complaint and the presence of neurological and psychological features. The medical or behavioral record of the patient may be collected from the family and friends before any diagnosis is implemented [26, 27]. The age, diet pattern, use of drugs/medicines, and patient activities are also considered throughout screening for schizophrenia.

The clinical significance of schizophrenia and the accessibility of modern noninvasive recording procedures have attracted the research community to examine brain condition monitoring. Recently, researchers have proposed and employed various ADT schemes to inspect the occurrence and severity of schizophrenia [28, 29]. The standard structure of the ADTs employed for schizophrenia includes the following:

(i) Collection of raw EEG signals using a multichannel sensor array.
(ii) Implementation of signal pre-processing methods to improve the EEG signals.
(iii) Mining of nonlinear features with a preferred feature-mining technique.
(iv) Principal feature selection.
(v) Implementing a classifier structure to classify the EEGs into two classes.
(vi) Validation of the implemented ADT using a suitable EEG database.

In this work, an ADT method is constructed and executed to categorize the considered EEG signals into normal/schizophrenic classes. In this study, a multichannel (19-channel) EEG database, provided by Olejarczyk and Jernajczyk, is adopted for the assessment [30]. This data set consists of complex EEG patterns from 28 volunteers. It has already been prior assessed using a Gramian angular summation field (GASF). This technique helps to convert the signals into red-green-blue (RGB) class pictures [30, 31].

The proposed work initially executes a segmentation technique, which divides the complex EEG patterns into a simple EEG pattern with 6250 sample points. The simple EEGs are then grouped into two classes (normal/schizophrenic) and considered for further evaluation. After the segmentation, a feature-mining practice is employed to extract the nonlinear signal features from the EEGs. Around 157 features are extracted using the executed technique. Then, a Student's *t*-test is employed to choose a subset of features (16 numbers) based on the *p*-value for classification. Finally, a decision tree (DT), linear discriminant analysis (LDA), *k*-nearest neighbor (*k*-NN), probabilistic neural network (PNN), and support vector machines (SVMs) with various kernels are implemented to classify the EEG signals. The developed ADT is tested using 1142 reduced EEG patterns (516 normal and 626 schizophrenic cases). During the assessment, a threefold cross-validation is executed to authenticate the performance of the implemented ADT. The performance of the considered feature-extraction procedures is confirmed by computing the accuracy percentage; the positive predictive value (PPV), sensitivity, and specificity offered by the SVM with a radial basis function (RBF) kernel are superior to the other techniques considered in this study.

9.2 Related work

Detection and treatment of schizophrenia are essential in patients since it severely inconveniences human thinking, memory, and other living activities. Moreover, it is an unalterable process that damages human behavioral abilities in the later stages of life [6, 8]. Recently, researchers have proposed and implemented many works to diagnose brain abnormalities based on EEG signals.

Examination of EEG patterns with a well-chosen technique is essential to detect any abnormality/malfunction in the brain. The work of Acharya *et al* implemented a deep-learning technique to examine EEG signals to predict brain seizures [9]. Yuvaraj *et al* extracted the higher-order spectra features from a multichannel EEG to evaluate Parkinson's disease [10]. Acharya *et al* present a detailed review of focal EEG analysis [11]. Further, many recent works have proposed conventional and deep-learning techniques to evaluate EEG signals recorded in a controlled environment. They have proposed various disease-examination techniques based on EEG analysis [12–21].

Like other brain disorder evaluations, one can also implement assessment for schizophrenia with EEG signals. The work of Ibáñez-Molina *et al* implemented an examination for schizophrenia based on EEG signals. In this work, they concentrated on detecting multi-scale complexity with the EEG signals to predict abnormalities in patients. The work of Li *et al* implemented a technique to record and measure abnormal EEG patterns to identify cognitive disorders such as schizophrenia and depression [24]. The research by Kirsch *et al* discusses the dimensional complexity in multichannel EEG during examination for schizophrenia. This work also suggests possible implementation procedures to reduce the complexity [27]. Finally, the works of Jauhar *et al* and Saha *et al* propose a detailed review of the symptoms of schizophrenia, its therapeutic treatments, and rates of mortality, respectively [25, 26].

In the rest of this chapter, a sequence of techniques is implemented to examine normal and schizophrenic class EEG signals. Finally, the diagnostic accuracy is validated with chosen classifiers to develop the proposed ADT.

9.3 Methodology

The method employed in this work to examine the EEG signal is represented in figure 9.1. In addition, this research proposes an automated tool to process and classify the EEG signals into normal and schizophrenic cases with enhanced accuracy.

Initially, a 19-channel EEG signal is recorded in a controlled atmosphere; 14 normal and 14 schizophrenic case volunteers are considered for the evaluation [32]. The EEG signal patterns are highly complex, and the complexity will increase with the number of channels and their sequence duration. Other researchers have previously proposed and implemented many pre-processing methods to reduce the complexity of EEG signal assessment [33–36].

This work implements a sequence-splitting technique to segment a chosen sequence pattern from the raw EEG data in the database [32]. The implemented sequence-splitting procedure segments the entire raw signal data set (19 channels)

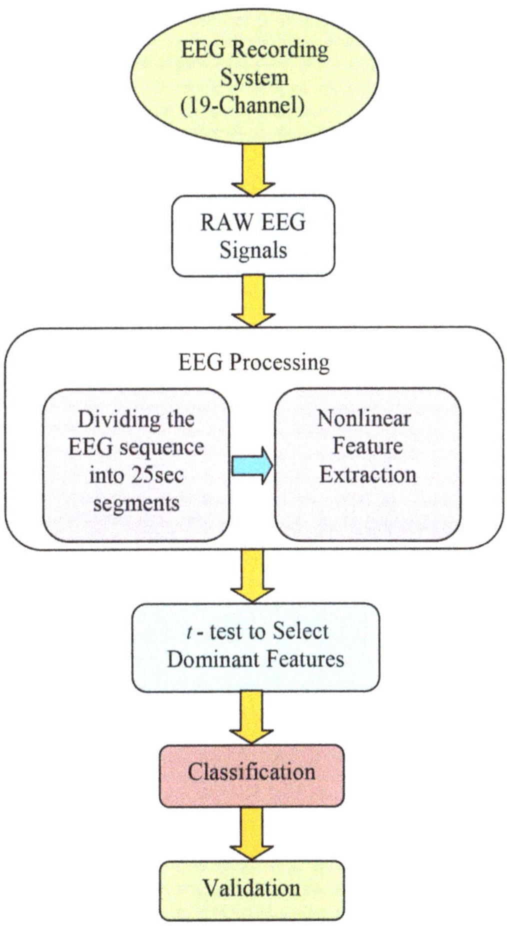

Figure 9.1. Organization of the proposed automated tool to detect schizophrenia.

into an uncomplicated EEG signal pattern with a sequence length of 25 s, with 6250 samples in each channel (total sampling points = 6250 × 19). The implemented splitting technique helps attain a sum of 1142 unique EEG signal patterns (516 normal and 626 schizophrenic cases), which can improve the performance of the proposed computerized tool. Furthermore, the examination of an image is relatively straightforward compared to a signal since the signal evaluation involves measuring amplitude, frequency, and pattern [37–43]. Hence, physiological signals have recently been transformed into pictures using various procedures to simplify task of assessment [30, 31, 44, 45]. In this work, the essential EEG features for both the normal and schizophrenic cases are extracted using the nonlinear feature-extraction methods discussed in [17].

Such nonlinear feature-extraction techniques help to attain 157 features, which can be further considered to train and test the classifier system. However, training and testing the classifier with many features will increase the complexity. Hence, it is essential to recognize the principal features to be accounted for during the classification task. A Student's t-test is then implemented to identify 16 such principal features from the 157 features based on the p-values achieved with an implemented test [46, 47]. Finally, a relative analysis of various classifiers existing in the literature is performed. The results confirm that the SVM-RBF [17, 48, 49] classifier offers a superior classification outcome with enhanced accuracy, PPV, sensitivity, and specificity on the considered EEG database compared to other classifiers employed in this work.

9.3.1 Electroencephalogram database

The EEG signals considered in this research work are adopted from the recent work of Olejarczyk and Jernajczyk [30]. The considered EEG data set includes signals recorded from 28 volunteers and is available in [32]. These signals were recorded using a 19-channel scalp EEG sensor array and separately stored for the normal and abnormal classes.

9.3.2 EEG pre-processing

The raw data coming out from the sensor normally require some early processing steps to smooth the measured variables by removing unwanted signals. Further, implenting a pre-processing step helps adjust the considered database values into a more accepted form. The pre-processing will help modify the existing data set in a more meaningful way.

9.3.2.1 Sequence extraction

The raw EEG is first pre-processed by a chosen method to reduce examination complexity. In this work, splitting of the raw EEG signal is implemented to modify the existing 19-channel EEG signal pattern sequence into a chosen 19-channel EEG pattern sequence of 6250 sample points. This procedure will help create more EEG patterns, which will help attain better results during the automated tool-based examination. The sequence-extraction technique helped attain 516 normal and 626 schizophrenic class EEG patterns from the 28 raw EEG signals.

9.3.3.2 Feature extraction

Feature extraction plays a major role in signal/image evaluation and classification [17]. Most real-time signal/images are nonlinear. Hence, it is essential to employ a suitable methodology that extracts the nonlinear features from the chosen raw/preprocessed data set. Previous researchers have widely discussed the extraction of linear/nonlinear features from EEG signals. In this work, a sum of 157 features is extracted from each EEG pattern using well-known parameters such as entropy (approximate, Kolmogorov–Sinai, permutation, Renyi, Tsallis, activity, wavelet, and Shannon), complexity (Lempel–Ziv, Kolmogorov, and Hjorth), Lyapunov exponent, cumulant, bispectrum, mobility, and other related features as discussed in the literature [17, 50]. The total number of features extracted in this work is quite large. If these features are considered as it is, it will increase the complexity of the classification task. Hence, a suitable feature-selection procedure is implemented to identify the dominant feature set from the unprocessed features.

9.3.3 Feature selection

In the proposed automated tool, feature selection plays a very important role during the classifier training and testing process. When optimally chosen features are considered, it is possible to attain better classification accuracy with a considerably reduced processing time [59]. Further, the optimally chosen features will reduce the complexity of the classifier system. In the literature, a range of conventional and heuristic feature-selection techniques are proposed to recognize the principal features from the extracted features of the individual group. In this work, a Student's t-test is employed to choose a subset of features based on their p-values. The related details on the feature-selection process can be found in [46, 47].

9.3.4 Classification

Classifiers are extensively adopted to maintain the automatic assessment of EEG signals. Firstly, the classifier system has to be trained based on its specific requirements. Subsequently, the classifier's performance has to be tested to confirm its efficiency. A classifier scheme is used to distinguish the considered EEG database in this work.

- A decision-tree (DT) method implements a tree-like configuration with a series of test series. A DT uses the characteristic test settings as the root and interior nodes and the class label from the terminal node. Once the DT configuration has been constructed, categorization is easily achieved based on the decision taken in each tree branch. Essential information on EEG classification using a DT can be found in [17, 51].
- Linear discriminant analysis (LDA) is one of the well-approved classifier systems. It identifies a matching category according to a set of values or findings based on the discovery of an optimal linear transformation, which maximizes the class reparability. LDA-based EEG signal classification details can be found in [50, 52].
- *K*-nearest neighbor (*k*-NN) is a widely considered classification procedure adopted to classify a range of medical data sets [17, 53]. In this work, a *k*-NN

is considered to classify the EEG signal. Like other classifiers, the k-NN needs training and testing based on available dominant features. A k-NN scheme assesses the distance between new features to each training feature and discovers the best neighbor [60]. The k-value is empirically identified with the training sample's sorting error. The arithmetical appearance of the k-NN is as follows.

Let there exist two feature vectors of D dimensions, $M = (M_1, M_2, \ldots M_n)^T$ and $N = (N_1, N_2, \ldots N_n)^T$; then, the Euclidean distance can be shown as

$$\text{Euclidean distance}\,(\overrightarrow{M}, \overrightarrow{N}) = \sqrt{(M_1 - N_1)^2 + (M_2 - N_2)^2 + , \ldots, (M_D - N_1)^2}. \tag{9.1}$$

- A probabilistic neural network (PNN) was initially proposed by Specht, in 1988, and uses a supervised neural network [54]. A PNN contains a feed-forward arrangement with multiple input, hidden, summing, and output layers. In a PNN, the hidden layer computes a probability density value and the summing layer accumulates the result. The output layer then produces a result class according to the implemented training process. An implementation of a PNN for EEG classification can be found in [55].
- Support vector machines (SVMs) are a commonly adopted classifier to separate data sets into two classes with the help of an attribute space by building a dividing hyperplane based on the features adopted during the training process [17]. Essential details on SVMs adopted to classify EEG signals can be found in earlier works [48, 49, 59]. The extracted nonlinear features, which are more complex to classify, are initially transformed into a higher-dimensional characteristic space with the help of chosen kernels. In this work, a SVM with a radial basis function (SVM-RBF) and a SVM with polynomial kernels with varied orders (SVM1, SVM2, and SVM3) are adopted to classify the normal/schizophrenic EEG signal data set.

9.3.5 Validation

The superiority of the proposed automated examination tool is authenticated by calculating common performance measures, such as accuracy (ACC), positive predictive value (PPV), sensitivity (SEN), and specificity (SPE) [2, 3, 47]. To enhance the assessment potential, a threefold cross-validation is executed. The performance measures implemented in this work are illustrated in equations (9.2)–(9.5):

$$\text{ACC} = (T_P + T_N)/(T_P + T_N + F_P + F_N), \tag{9.2}$$

$$\text{PPV} = \frac{\text{Amounts}}{\text{Amount of TPs} + \text{s}s}, \tag{9.3}$$

$$\text{SEN} = T_P/(T_P + F_N), \tag{9.4}$$

$$\text{s} = T_N/(T_N + F_P), \tag{9.5}$$

where TN, TP, FN, and FP denote true negative, true positive, false negative, and false positive, respectively.

9.4 Results and discussion

This work aims to implement an automated evaluation and classification technique to categorize normal/schizophrenic cases based on the patterns in EEG sequences.

This part of the chapter will demonstrate the experimental outcome and its discussions. Various processing, techniques presented in figure 9.1, are implemented to attain efficient results.

In this work, clinically collected EEG signals from normal/schizophrenic volunteers, as taken from [30, 32], are adopted for the investigation. The raw EEG data is complex due to its high dimensional channel numbers (19 channels) and the sequence length. Further, 28 EEG sequences (14 normal and 14 schizophrenic) are not sufficient to train and test the classifiers employed in most ADTs. Hence, in the proposed study, to increase the number of EEG signals, a frame-based extraction is implemented with a frame size of 25 s. This segmentation practice helped to acquire 516 normal EEG and 626 schizophrenic EEG patterns (516 + 626 = 1142 unique EEG patterns), which can help build a better diagnostic system. Due to the fixed frame size, the examination of pre-processed EEG is quite simple compared to the raw EEG.

Sample EEG signals of a normal and a schizophrenic case are depicted in figure 9.2. Figure 9.2(a) presents the EEG of a normal volunteer, which shows enhanced amplitude values in most of the channels compared to the schizophrenic case depicted in figure 9.2(b). From this, it is clear that examination of the EEG pattern will help diagnose the volunteer's mental condition. Table 9.1 shows the total number of EEG patterns considered in this study.

Figure 9.3 shows an approximate image of the normal/schizophrenic EEG signals obtained with the GASF, which can help evaluate the EEG signal in picture form. An application of a GASF in EEG analysis can be found in [30].

In this work, the nonlinear features of the pre-processed EEG pattern are extracted using the procedures discussed in earlier works [8, 10, 17, 19, 20]. The feature extraction implemented in this work helped to attain 157 features of various classes. Very few features show dominant performance, which can be identified and adopted to train and test the classifier. Table 9.2 illustrates the dominant features identified using Student's t-test. This test helped to identify 16 features out of 157 based on their p-values, as shown in table 9.2. This table further presents the t-values in addition to its analogous p-values, and statistical measures such as mean and standard deviation (SD) for both EEG cases. Further, a threefold cross-validation is executed to achieve an improved outcome during the EEG examination.

Figure 9.4 presents the association between the chosen dominant features with the EEG signals of the normal/schizophrenic classes. This figure also presents the measure of different features on the considered EEG signal database [56]. These features are then considered to train the classifier system, which helps to group the EEGs into two various classes.

Initially, the features extracted from the normal (516 cases) and schizophrenic (626) cases are considered to train and test the DT classifier system. To assess the classifier's performance, the feature size is varied from a minimum (two) to a

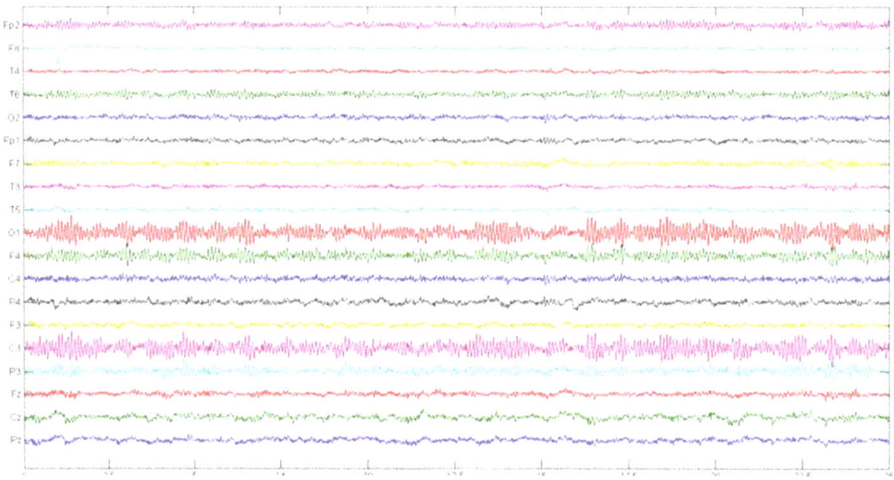

(a)

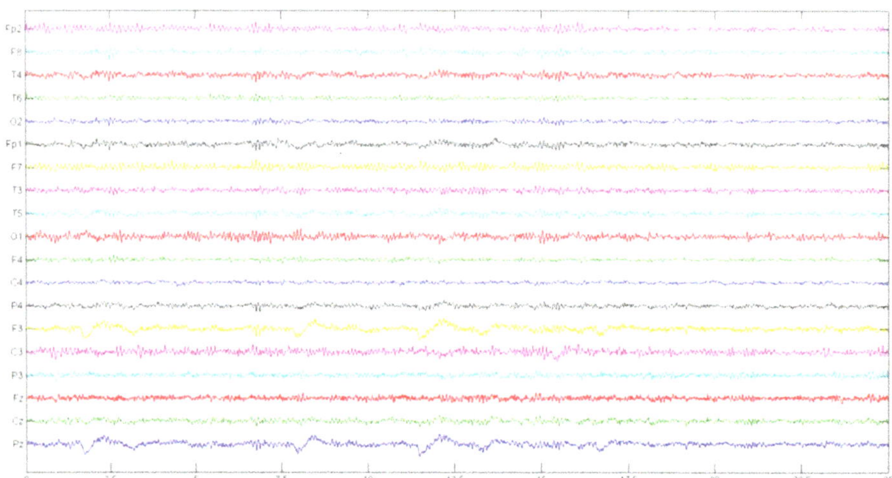

(b)

Figure 9.2. Pre-processed EEG signal with a frame size of 25 s (6250 sample points). (a) Normal case, and (b) schizophrenic case.

Table 9.1. Total number of EEG patterns considered in this study.

Type	Number of EEG segments
Normal	516
Schizophrenia	626
Total	1142

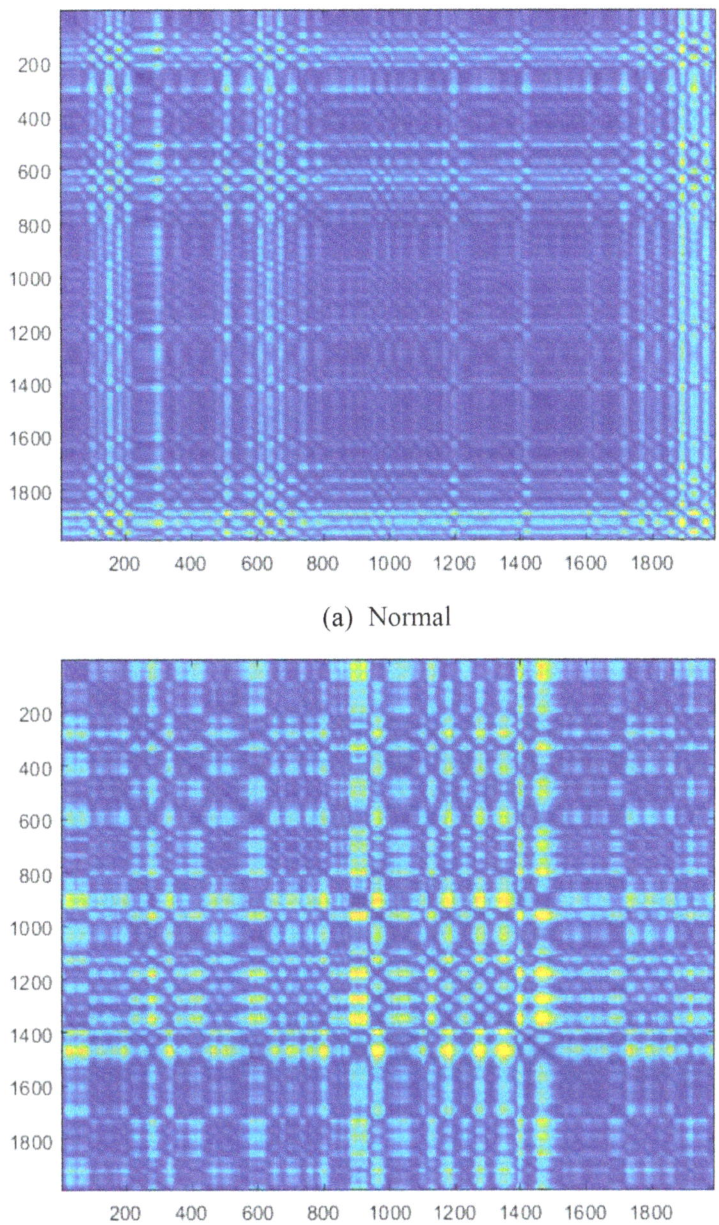

(a) Normal

(b) Schizophrenia

Figure 9.3. Gramian angular summation field image of EEG signal. (a) Normal case, and (b) schizophrenic case.

maximum (16) of selected features. The performance of the DT is then assessed by computing the essential similarity measures, such as TR, TN, FP, FN, ACC, PPV, SEN, and SPE, as shown in table 9.3. From this table, it can be noted that when the feature size is 13, the DT offers better performance than other values of features. A

Table 9.2. Principal features chosen using Student's *t*-test.

	Normal		Schizophrenia			
Selected Features	Mean	SD	Mean	SD	*p*-value	*t*-value
Hjorth complexity	1.1985	0.1802	0.8922	0.3012	2.83E−48	16.5573
H3	381.4749	72.9306	457.9451	99.7012	6.37E−44	14.5133
H2	50.1034	7.6933	57.2959	9.9305	3.41E−38	14.1773
Kolmogorov complexity	6.0053	0.3006	6.1007	0.4012	2.55E−37	13.3766
Hjorth mobility	0.4114	0.1005	0.6036	0.3163	2.11E−35	12.9826
Permutation entropy	1.7048	0.1104	1.5527	0.1055	2.09E−35	11.9905
Renyi entropy	−14.3844	0.7994	−15.1274	0.8786	8.16E−31	11.2115
H1	664.9682	121.2538	757.4083	157.32	1.54E−26	10.9357
Largest Lyapunov exponent	3.2315	0.7140	3.6562	0.9278	4.83E−17	8.5240
H4	8834452	8481768	13995401	16189034	9.32E−11	6.5392
Ent2	0.2533	0.0699	0.2789	0.0843	4.69E−08	5.5000
Lempel–Ziv complexity	2	0	9.0404	30.1197	1.32E−07	5.3093
Ent1	0.5727	0.0831	0.6001	0.0923	2.02E−07	5.2295
Kolmogorov–Smirnov entropy	0.0405	0.0363	0.0303	0.0383	5.31E−06	4.5740
Ent3	0.1567	0.0541	0.1726	0.0654	1.13E−05	4.4110
Approximate entropy	2.0777	0.1908	2200.3610	11809.2000	2.54E−05	4.2282

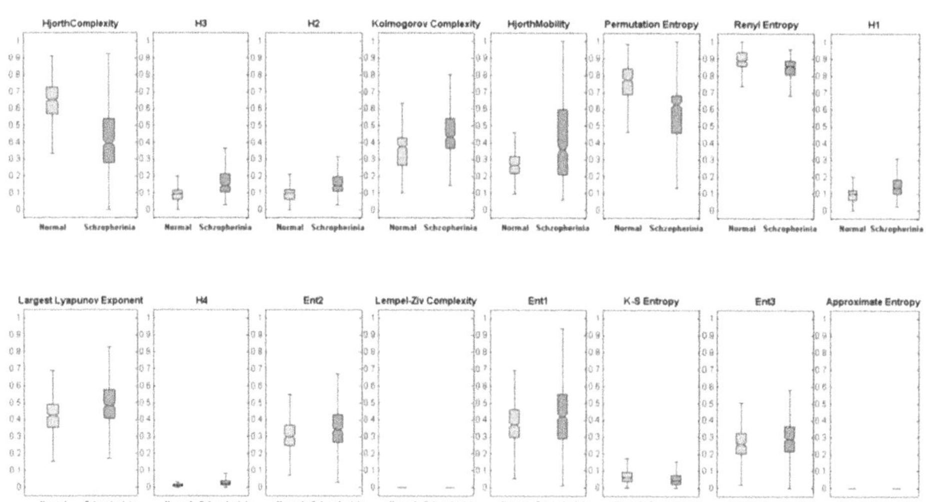

Figure 9.4. Performance of chosen features on the normal/schizophrenic EEG signals.

similar procedure is followed for the other classifiers adopted in this work. Their accuracy values and the dominant feature sizes are shown in figure 9.5.

Figure 9.5(a) presents the accuracy value and the dominant feature number for the DT classifier [57, 58]. This figure confirms that enhanced classifier accuracy can

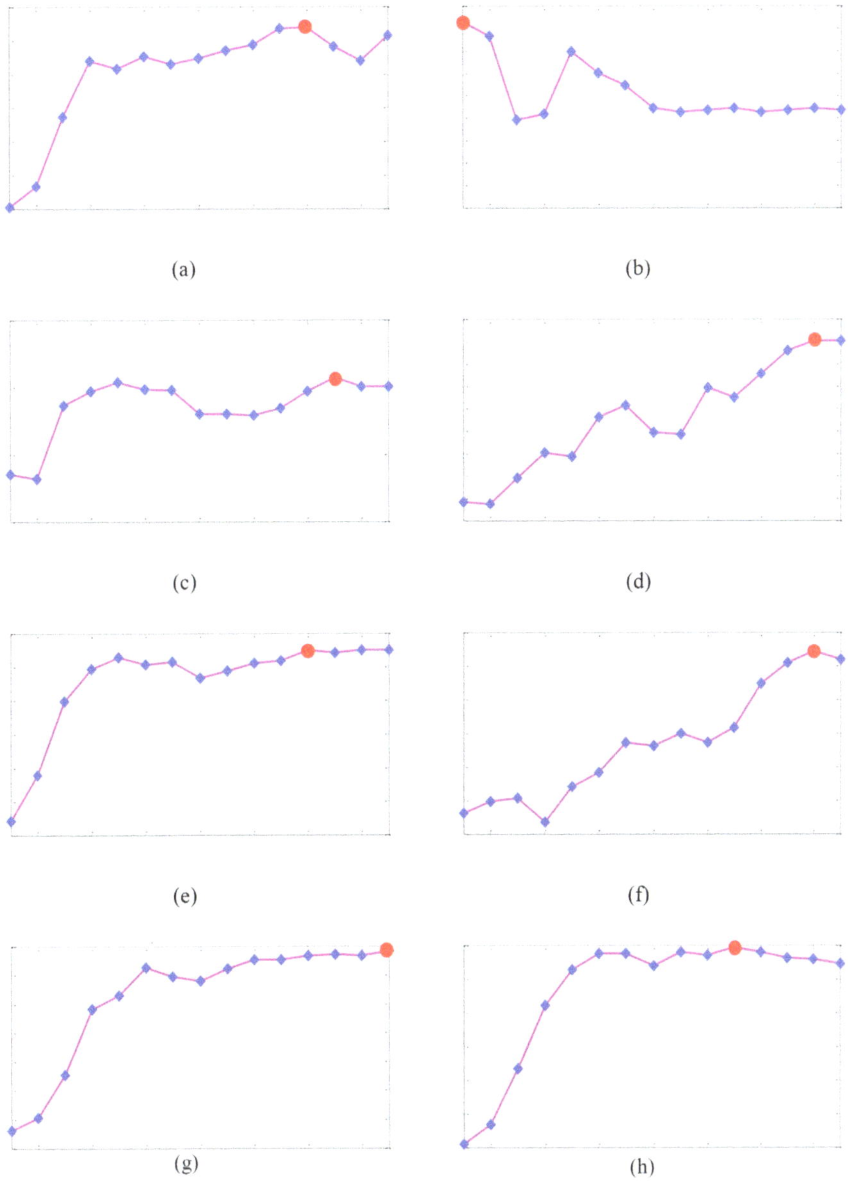

Figure 9.5. Classification accuracy of chosen classifiers with different features. (a) DT classifier, (b) LDA classifier, (c) k-NN classifier, (d) PNN classifier, (e) SVM classifier, (f)–(h) SVM with polynomial kernels (SVM1, SVM2, and SVM3, respectively).

be attained when the chosen feature size is 13. Figure 9.5(b) presents the accuracy of LDA when the feature size is two. Figure 9.5(c) depicts the accuracy value of the *k*-NN classifier; the *k*-NN presents enhanced results when the chosen features are set to 14. The accuracy of PNN is presented in figure 9.5(d), and this confirms that PNN

Table 9.3. Performance assessment with decision-tree classifier.

No. of Features	TP	TN	FP	FN	ACC	PPV	SEN	SPE
2	511	381	135	115	0.7811	0.7910	0.8163	0.7384
3	519	387	129	107	0.7933	0.8009	0.8291	0.7500
4	536	417	99	90	0.8345	0.8441	0.8562	0.8081
5	545	446	70	81	0.8678	0.8862	0.8706	0.8643
6	545	441	75	81	0.8634	0.8790	0.8706	0.8547
7	548	446	70	78	0.8704	0.8861	0.8754	0.8643
8	547	442	74	79	0.8660	0.8808	0.8738	0.8566
9	552	441	75	74	0.8695	0.8804	0.8818	0.8547
10	554	444	72	72	0.8739	0.8850	0.8850	0.8605
11	552	450	66	74	0.8774	0.8932	0.8818	0.8721
12	561	452	64	65	0.8870	0.8976	0.8962	0.8760
13	**566**	**448**	**68**	**60**	**0.8879**	**0.8927**	**0.9042**	**0.8682**
14	566	435	81	60	0.8765	0.8748	0.9042	0.8430
15	559	432	84	67	0.8677	0.8693	0.8929	0.8372
16	563	445	71	63	0.8827	0.8880	0.8994	0.8624

offers superior results when the feature size is 15. Similarly, the SVM-assisted classification provided a good result for 13 features (figure 9.5(e)). Further, the additional results attained with the SVM with polynomial kernels (SVM1, SVM2, and SVM3) are presented in figures 9.5(f)–(h), respectively. From these figures, it can be confirmed that the SVM technique offers better overall results compared to other techniques considered in this work.

Table 9.4 presents the outcomes attained with the SVM classifier for various numbers of features. This table also confirms that when the feature size is 13, the ACC, PPV, SEN, and SPE attained with the SVM are greater than with the other methods considered in this research.

From the literature, it can be noted that performance values such as ACC, PPV, SEN, and SPE are used to appraise the classification techniques [2, 3, 47]. Table 9.5 and figure 9.6 depict the overall performance indexes of the considered classifiers. The table and figure confirm that the SVM classifier helps to attain better values of ACC (92.99%), PPV (94.46%), SEN (92.65%), and SPE (93.41%) compared to DT, LDA, *k*-NN, PNN, SVM1, SVM2, and SVM3. From these results, it can be validated that the proposed automated tool with a SVM classifier offers superior results on both normal and schizophrenic case EEG signals.

In the future, the evaluation of normal/schizophrenic case EEG signals may be performed by converting the signal pattern into RGB scale pictures using the GASF, upon which the feature extraction and classification scheme can be implemented.

Table 9.4. Performance appraisal of SVM with different feature dimensions.

No. of Features	TP	TN	FP	FN	ACC	PPV	SEN	SPE
2	536	410	106	90	0.8284	0.8349	0.8562	0.7946
3	549	428	88	77	0.8555	0.8619	0.8770	0.8295
4	567	460	56	59	0.8993	0.9101	0.9057	0.8915
5	582	467	49	44	0.9186	0.9223	0.9297	0.9050
6	587	470	46	39	0.9256	0.9273	0.9377	0.9108
7	583	469	47	43	0.9212	0.9254	0.9313	0.9089
8	582	472	44	44	0.9229	0.9294	0.9297	0.9147
9	581	462	54	45	0.9133	0.9149	0.9281	0.8954
10	583	465	51	43	0.9177	0.9196	0.9313	0.9012
11	579	474	42	47	0.9221	0.9324	0.92492	0.9186
12	576	479	37	50	0.9238	0.9396	0.9201	0.9283
13	**580**	**482**	**34**	**46**	**0.9299**	**0.9446**	**0.9265**	**0.9341**
14	576	484	32	50	0.9282	0.9474	0.9201	0.9380
15	580	482	34	46	0.9299	0.9446	0.9265	0.9341
16	580	482	34	46	0.9299	0.9446	0.9265	0.9341

Table 9.5. Performance evaluation of the feature-extraction techniques.

Classifier	No. of dominant features	TP	TN	FP	FN	ACC (%)	PPV (%)	SEN (%)	SPE (%)
DT	13	566	448	68	60	88.79	89.27	90.41	86.82
LDA	2	493	401	115	133	78.28	81.09	78.75	77.71
k-NN	14	557	479	37	69	90.72	93.77	88.98	92.83
PNN	15	531	463	53	95	87.04	90.92	84.82	89.73
SVM	**13**	**580**	**482**	**34**	**46**	**92.99**	**94.46**	**92.65**	**93.41**
SVM1	15	483	447	69	143	81.44	87.50	77.16	86.63
SVM2	16	559	488	28	67	91.68	95.23	89.30	94.57
SVM3	12	563	486	30	63	91.86	94.94	89.94	94.19

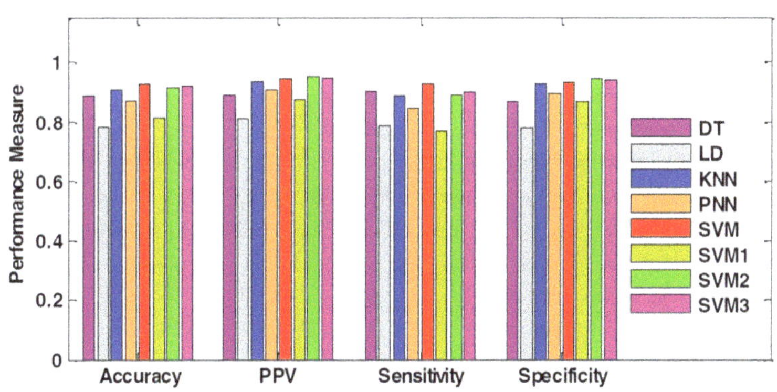

Figure 9.6. Performance evaluation of various classifiers adopted in this work.

9.5 Conclusion

This research aimed to develop an automated tool to classify normal/schizophrenic class EEG signals. The proposed tool employed a sequence of procedures, such as segmentation of the EEG frame, nonlinear feature extraction, Student's t-test-based feature selection, training and testing of classifiers, and performance validation. Initially, a segmentation technique was employed to split the extant 19-channel EEG sequence into various sectors with a sequence time of 25 s to minimize the complexity of evaluation; the nonlinear feature extraction was then implemented to extract around 157 features, and the t-test was then implemented to choose 16 dominant features from the 157 extracted features. Finally, a classification procedure was implemented for various feature values. The resultant performance values were then computed for various features and various classifiers. The outcome of the experimental work confirms that the SVM classifier offers superior results compared to the other classifiers adopted in this work. Furthermore, the outcome of the proposed tool also confirms that the proposed technique works well on the EEG database considered, and offers improved results for the classification of normal/schizophrenic cases.

References

[1] Gudigar A *et al* 2019 Automated categorization of multi-class brain abnormalities using decomposition techniques with MRI images: a comparative study *IEEE Access* **7** 28498–509

[2] Rajinikanth V, Satapathy S C, Fernandes S L and Nachiappan S 2017 Entropy based segmentation of tumor from brain MR images—a study with teaching learning based optimization *Pattern Recognit. Lett.* **94** 87–95

[3] Raja N S M, Fernandes S L, Dey N, Satapathy S C and Rajinikanth V 2018 Contrast enhanced medical MRI evaluation using Tsallis entropy and region growing segmentation *J. Ambient Intel. Humanized Comput.* https://doi.org/10.1007/S12652-018-0854-8

[4] Subudhi U R, Acharya M, Dash S, Jena and Sabut S 2018 Automated approach for detection of ischemic stroke using Delaunay triangulation in brain MRI images *Comput. Biol. Med.* **103** 116–29

[5] Talo M, Baloglu U B, Yıldırım Ö and Acharya U R 2019 Application of deep transfer learning for automated brain abnormality classification using MR images *Cognitive Systems Research* **54** 176–88

[6] Lin H and Rajinikanth V 2018 Normality evaluation of EEG signals based on amplitude level and entropy values *Int. J. Signal Processing Systems* **6** 22–6

[7] Gudigar A, Raghavendra U, San T R, Ciaccio E J and Acharya U R 2019 Application of multiresolution analysis for automated detection of brain abnormality using MR images: a comparative study *Future Gener. Comput. Syst.* **90** 359–67

[8] Acharya U R, Sree S V, Ang P C A, Yanti R and Suri J S 2012 Application of non-linear and wavelet based features for the automated identification of epileptic EEG signals *Int. J. Neural Syst.* **22** 1250002

[9] Acharya U R, Oh S L, Hagiwara Y, Tan J H and Adeli H 2018 Deep convolutional neural network for the automated detection and diagnosis of seizure using EEG signals *Comput. Biol. Med.* **100** 270–8

[10] Yuvaraj R, Acharya U R and Hagiwara Y 2018 A novel Parkinson's disease diagnosis index using higher-order spectra features in EEG signals *Neural Comput. Appl.* **30** 1225–35
[11] Acharya U R *et al* 2019 Characterization of focal EEG signals: a review *Future Gener. Comput. Syst.* **91** 290–99
[12] Oh S L *et al* 2018 A deep learning approach for Parkinson's disease diagnosis from EEG signals *Neural Comput. Appl.* **32** 10927–33
[13] Michielli N, Acharya U R and Molinari F 2019 Cascaded LSTM recurrent neural network for automated sleep stage classification using single-channel EEG signals *Comput. Biol. Med.* **106** 71–81
[14] Sharma M, Achuth P V, Deb D, Puthankattil S D and Acharya U R 2018 An automated diagnosis of depression using three-channel bandwidth-duration localized wavelet filter bank with EEG signals *Cognitive Syst. Res.* **52** 508–20
[15] Acharya U R, Oh S H, Hagiwara Y, Tan J H, Adeli H and Subha D P 2018 Automated EEG-based screening of depression using deep convolutional neural network *Comput. Methods Programs Biomed.* **161** 103–13
[16] Sharma M, Deb D and Acharya U R 2018 A novel three-band orthogonal wavelet filter bank method for an automated identification of alcoholic EEG signals *Appl. Intell.* **48** 1368–78
[17] Bhattacharyya A, Sharma M, Pachori R B, Sircar P and Acharya U R 2018 A novel approach for automated detection of focal EEG signals using empirical wavelet transform *Neural Comput. Appl.* **29** 47–57
[18] Yıldırım Ö, Baloglu U B and Acharya U R 2018 A deep convolutional neural network model for automated identification of abnormal EEG signals *Neural Comput. Appl.* **32** 15857–68
[19] Tripathy R K and Acharya U R 2018 Use of features from RR-time series and EEG signals for automated classification of sleep stages in deep neural network framework *Biocyber. Biomed. Eng.* **38** 890–902
[20] Gupta V, Priya T, Yadav A K, Pachori R B and Acharya U R 2017 Automated detection of focal EEG signals using features extracted from flexible analytic wavelet transform *Pattern Recognit. Lett.* **94** 180–8
[21] Sharma R, Kumar M, Pachori R B and Acharya U R 2017 Decision support system for focal EEG signals using tunable-Q wavelet transform *J. Computational Sci.* **20** 52–60
[22] Bhattacharyya A, Pachori R, Upadhyay A and Acharya U 2017 Tunable-Q wavelet transform based multiscale entropy measure for automated classification of epileptic EEG signals *Appl. Sci.* **7** 385
[23] Ibáñez-Molina A J *et al* 2018 EEG multiscale complexity in schizophrenia during picture naming *Front. Physiol.* **9** 1213
[24] Li Y *et al* 2018 Abnormal EEG complexity in patients with schizophrenia and depression *Clin. Neurophysiol.* **119** 1232–241
[25] Jauhar S, McKenna P J, Radua J, Fung E, Salvador R and Laws K R 2014 Cognitive–behavioural therapy for the symptoms of schizophrenia: systematic review and meta-analysis with examination of potential bias *Br. J. Psychiatry* **204** 20–9
[26] Saha S, Chant D and McGrath J 2007 A systematic review of mortality in schizophrenia: is the differential mortality gap worsening over time? *Arch. Gen. Psychiatry* **64** 1123–31
[27] Kirsch P, Besthorn C, Klein S, Rindfleisch J and Olbrich R 2000 The dimensional complexity of the EEG during cognitive tasks reflects the impaired information processing in schizophrenic patients *Int. J. Psychophysiol* **36** 237–46

[28] Elvevåg B, Foltz P W, Rosenstein M and DeLisi L E 2010 An automated method to analyze language use in patients with schizophrenia and their first-degree relatives *J. Neurolinguistics* **23** 270–84

[29] Strous R D *et al* 2009 Automated characterization and identification of schizophrenia in writing *J. Nerv. Ment. Dis.* **197** 585–8

[30] Olejarczyk E and Jernajczyk W 2017 Graph-based analysis of brain connectivity in schizophrenia *PLoS One* **12** e0188629

[31] Wang Z and Oates T 2015 Imaging time-series to improve classification and imputation arXiv:1506.00327v1

[32] Olejarczyk E and Jernajczyk W 2017 EEG in schizophrenia *Data set* https://doi.org/10.18150/repod.0107441

[33] Bhattacharyya A, Pachori R and Acharya U 2017 Tunable-Q wavelet transform based multivariate sub-band fuzzy entropy with application to focal EEG signal analysis *Entropy* **19** 99

[34] Sharma M, Dhere A, Pachori R B and Acharya U R 2017 An automatic detection of focal EEG signals using new class of time–frequency localized orthogonal wavelet filter banks *Knowl.-Based Syst.* **118** 217–27

[35] Patidar S, Pachori R B, Upadhyay A and Acharya U R 2017 An integrated alcoholic index using tunable-Q wavelet transform based features extracted from EEG signals for diagnosis of alcoholism *Appl. Soft Comput.* **50** 71–8

[36] Acharya U R, Fujita H, Sudarshan V K, Bhat S and Koh J E W 2015 Application of entropies for automated diagnosis of epilepsy using EEG signals: a review *Knowl.-Based Syst.* **88** 85–96

[37] Bhurane A A, Sharma M, San-Tan R and Acharya U R 2019 An efficient detection of congestive heart failure using frequency localized filter banks for the diagnosis with ECG signals *Cognitive Syst. Res.* **55** 82–94

[38] Baloglu U B, Talo M, Yildirim O, San-Tan R and Acharya U R 2019 Classification of myocardial infarction with multi-lead ECG signals and deep CNN *Pattern Recognit. Lett.* **122** 23–30

[39] Sharma M, Raval M and Acharya U R 2019 A new approach to identify obstructive sleep apnea using an optimal orthogonal wavelet filter bank with ECG signals *Informatics in Medicine Unlocked* **16** 100170

[40] Gudigar A *et al* 2019 Global weighted LBP based entropy features for the assessment of pulmonary hypertension *Pattern Recognit. Lett.* **125** 35–41

[41] Viswabhargav C S S S, Tripathy R K and Acharya U R 2019 Automated detection of sleep apnea using sparse residual entropy features with various dictionaries extracted from heart rate and EDR signals *Comput. Biol. Med.* **108** 20–30

[42] Sharma R R, Kumar A, Pachori R B and Acharya U R 2019 Accurate automated detection of congestive heart failure using eigenvalue decomposition based features extracted from HRV signals *Biocyber. Biomed. Eng.* **39** 312–27

[43] Acharya U R *et al* 2016 Automated detection and localization of myocardial infarction using electrocardiogram: a comparative study of different leads *Knowl.-Based Syst.* **99** 146–56

[44] Bakiya A, Kamalanand K, Rajinikanth V, Nayak R S and Kadry S 2018 Deep neural network assisted diagnosis of time-frequency transformed electromyograms *Multimedia Tools Appl.* **79** 11051–67

[45] Bakiya A, Kamalanand K and Rajinikanth V 2018 Assessment of electromyograms using genetic algorithm and artificial neural networks *Evo. Intel.* **14** 261–71

[46] Zhou N and Wang L 2007 A modified *t*-test feature selection method and Its application on the HapMap genotype data *Genomics Proteomics Bioinformatics* **5** 242–49
[47] Chandra B and Gupta M 2011 An efficient statistical feature selection approach for classification of gene expression data *J. Biomedical Informatics* **44** 529–35
[48] Bousseta R *et al* 2016 EEG efficient classification of imagined hand movement using RBF kernel SVM *11th Int. Conf. on Intelligent Systems: Theories and Applications (SITA)* pp 1–6
[49] Li X *et al* 2014 Classification of EEG signals using a multiple kernel learning support vector machine *Sensors* **14** 12784–2802
[50] Neto E, Biessmann F, Aurlien H, Nordby H and Eichele T 2016 Regularized linear discriminant analysis of EEG features in dementia patients *Front Aging Neurosci.* **8** 273
[51] Aydemir O and Kayikcioglu T 2014 Decision tree structure based classification of EEG signals recorded during two dimensional cursor movement imagery *J. Neurosci. Methods* **229** 68–75
[52] Hasan M R, Ibrahimy M I, Motakabber S M A and Shahid S 2015 Classification of multichannel EEG signal by linear discriminant analysis *Adv. Intel. Syst. Comput.* **366** 279–82
[53] Aboalayon K A I, Faezipour M, Almuhammadi W S and Moslehpour S 2016 Sleep stage classification using EEG signal analysis: a comprehensive survey and new investigation *Entropy* **18** 272
[54] Mathew N A, Vivek R and Anurenjan P 2018 Early diagnosis of Alzheimer's disease from MRI images using PNN *Int. CET Conf. on Control, Communication, and Computing (IC4)* pp 161–4
[55] Rachman N T, Tjandrasa H and Fatichah C 2016 Alcoholism classification based on EEG data using independent component analysis (ICA), wavelet de-noising and probabilistic neural network (PNN) *Int. Seminar on Intelligent Technology and Its Application* pp 17–20
[56] Estrela V V, Monteiro A C B, França R P, Iano Y, Khelassi A and Razmjooy N 2018 Health 4.0: applications, management, technologies and review *Med. Tech. J.* **2** 262–76
[57] Estrela V V, Khelassi A, Monteiro A C B, Iano Y, Razmjooy N, Martins D and Rocha D T 2019 Why software-defined radio (SDR) matters in healthcare? *Med. Tech. J.* **3** 421–29
[58] Abreu L M, Hora H R M D, Rangel J J A, Erthal M, Navid, Estrela V V and Iano Y 2020 A multi-criteria modelling for ranking CO_2 emitting G20 countries from the Kaya identity and their impacts on elderly health *Brazilian Technology Symp.* pp 477–87
[59] Alferaidi A, Yadav K, Alharbi Y, Navid R, Viriyasitavat W, Gulati K and Dhiman G 2022 Distributed deep CNN-LSTM model for intrusion detection method in IoT-based vehicles *Math. Problems Eng.* **2022** 3424819
[60] Ranjbarzadeh R, Dorosti S, Jafarzadeh Ghoushchi S, Safavi S, Razmjooy N, Tataei Sarshar N and Bendechache M 2022 Nerve optic segmentation in CT images using a deep learning model and a texture descriptor *Complex Intell. Syst.* **8** 3543–57

IOP Publishing

Frontiers of Artificial Intelligence in Medical Imaging

Navid Razmjooy and Venkatesan Rajinikanth

Chapter 10

Computerized classification of multichannel EEG signals into normal/autistic classes using image-to-signal transformation

Venkatesan Rajinikanth and Seifedine Kadry

Autism spectrum disorder (ASD) is one of the considerable diseases among children. Left unrecognized, ASD can create problems in their personal and social life as they grow and develop. The proposed work aims to develop a clinically significant computer-assisted technique to detect ASD with the help of multichannel electro-encephalogram (MC-EEG) signals obtained using a 64-channel electrode system. This study considered 77 (37 normal and 40 autistic) MC-EEG signals for the experimental investigation. The proposed work initially implements a Morse continuous wavelet transform to convert the attained MC-EEG signals into red-green-blue images. Later, the essential nonlinear features (18 in number) are mined. The feature set is then reduced to three using locality-sensitive discriminant analysis based on the *p*-values. Finally, a chosen classifier system is implemented to classify the MC-EEG into normal/autistic classes. Tenfold cross-validation is executed to confirm the performance of the classifiers. The outcome of the proposed research confirms that a two-class classifier implemented with a probabilistic neural network offered better accuracy (98.7%) compared to other classifiers, such as decision tree (96.10%), linear discriminant analysis (96.10%), quadratic discriminate analysis (89.61%), support vector machine (SVM)-linear (<97%), SVM-radial basis function (97.40%), and *k*-nearest neighbor (96.10%). The outcome of the proposed research confirms its clinical significance.

10.1 Introduction

The availability of modern medical facilities helps the human community to identify various disorders early on, and aids in the implementation of all possible treatment procedures to regulate and cure such diseases [1, 2]. Diseases and disorders in adults and aged people can be easily identified and diagnosed compared to diseases/

disorders in children since the child cannot realize and communicate their problems in a meaningful way. Hence, developing a framework to diagnose diseases/disorders in children with chosen noninvasive diagnostic techniques is essential. If the disorder is diagnosed in its early phases, it may be regulated or cured with a chosen corrective action.

Autism spectrum disorder (ASD), or autism, is one of the brain-related disorders generally found in children. The diagnosis of ASD is essential to provide possible treatment to control its impact. A World Health Organization statement confirmed that one in 160 children has ASD worldwide. Untreated ASD will lead to related brain disorders, such as epilepsy, hopelessness, nervousness, and attention deficit hyperactivity disorder (ADHD) [3]. Further, research has also confirmed that the occurrence rate of ASD has rapidly increased due to causes such as genetics and the lining circumferences [4, 5]. A report has also verifiesd that the incidence rate of ASD is augmented in the USA (one in 59) [6] as well as in the UK (one in 100) [7]. In other parts of the world, the awareness of autism diagnosis is slowly growing. The same report also confirmed that untreated ASD could lead to consequences for the patient ranging from mild difficulty (speech and language impairments) to severe complications (philosophical problems and cerebral palsy).

Various studies conducted over the past 50 years worldwide have confirmed that the prevalence rate of autism is swiftly increasing irrespective of race and locality. The incidence rate in boys is greater compared to girls. Early ASD can be seen and diagnosed in children in the 2–5 age group. In recent years, many handling procedures have been developed to improve the communication and social behavior of children with ASD [7, 8].

Due to its social impacts, several ASD detection procedures have been developed by experts (pediatricians, psychiatrists, and other professionals) to observe the incipient behavioral changes in children in both controlled and other environments. In addition, ASD in adults is diagnosed with proven tests to identify intellectual disability [9, 10]. These tests comprise the initial level tests to identify the occurrence and the level (mild/severe) of ASD among children and adults.

Clinical-level diagnosis of ASD has played a vital role in recent years. The availability of modern therapeutic instruments helps diagnose the presence and level of autism using brain-signal-based [11, 12] and brain-image-based [13–15] techniques. However, image-based methods are difficult to examine since the attained image is in three-dimensional (3D) form, and requires more computational effort compared to the two-dimensional (2D) slices. Further, identification of autism from brain imagery requires more approximations. Hence, brain-signal-based assessment procedures have been widely preferred aup to now, followed by a physical examination of any child suspected of having autism. In signal-assisted techniques, a multichannel electroencephalogram (MC-EEG), collected using a surface electrode array, is sufficient to diagnose ASD with good accuracy. Further, it is a noninvasive procedure, does not incur any side effects, and can be implemented using wearable electrodes.

The proposed research implements EEG-assisted analysis and detection of ASD in children aged 4–13 years. This work considers an EEG-cap system with 64 channels to collect the necessary EEG signals from volunteers (both normal/autistic classes). Then, the collected EEG signals are segmented to acquire essential signals within the required spectrum. The collected MC-EEG is then automatically assessed using a computer-assisted technique (CAT), which involves a Morse continuous wavelet transform (CWT-Morse) converting the MC-EEG into an image, nonlinear feature extraction, and linear sequence discriminate analysis (LSDA) feature reduction, as well as bi-level classification using a chosen classifier system. The outcome of the proposed system confirms that the detection accuracy of CAT is maximized with a probabilistic neural network (PNN) classifier (98.7%) compared to the other classifiers considered in this research work. The outcome of this study also confirms that the proposed method is clinically significant. Therefore, it can be used to diagnose clinical-grade autistic class MC-EEG signals in the future.

10.2 Context

In neuropathology, many brain-image-based and brain-signal-based methods are implemented to detect ASD using a computer-based approach. Image-based practices consider brain sections recorded with magnetic resonance imaging (MRI), a proven procedure in which the brain sections are recorded with a chosen MRI modality. These can be used for diagnostics in 3D or 2D form [80]. This work provides promising results with various brain abnormality assessment tasks [16–20]. Recently, brain-signal-based (i.e. EEG) assessment procedures have been widely implemented by researchers to examine ASD with better accuracy. Earlier works related to MC-EEG-based autism detection can be found in [21–24].

A summary of the chosen ASD detection procedures extant in the literature is presented in table 10.1.

Other recent works existing in the literature are summarized in the recent work of Ibrahim *et al* [22], in which 46 volunteers were examined using a MC-EEG, and well-known classifiers, such as *k*-nearest neighbors (*k*-NNs), artificial neural networks (ANNs), support vector machines (SVMs), and linear discriminant analyses (LDAs) were implemented. The outcome attained with the *k*-NN helped achieve an accuracy of 94.6% with a wavelet and entropy-based features. This work also evaluated the correlation between epileptic and autistic EEG signals.

From the above discussion, it can be noted that the evaluation of autism in its premature stages is highly significant when using a suitable detection technique.

10.3 Problem formulation

The proposed research aims to implement a clinically significant CAT to detect ASD using MC-EEG signals. Recording and analyzing the MC-EEG is a complex task due to the signal strength and complexity. In the proposed work, clinical-level research is conducted to collect 77 MC-EEG patterns (37 of regular class and 40 of autistic class) using a noninvasive approach. Throughout this research, a 64-channel EEG-cap electrode system is considered to collect the signals from the volunteers, and all the experiments are conducted in a controlled environment. The collected

Table 10.1. Summary of some well-known ASD detection techniques.

Reference	Database	Methodology	Outcome
Bosl *et al* [12]	EEG (33 normal and 46 ASD subjects)	Modified multi-scale entropy.	SVM classifier with a classification accuracy ranging from 70% to 100%.
Bhat *et al* [25]	EEG (1 normal and 1 ASD subjects)	Analysis of EEG with features such as time domain, frequency domain, time-frequency domain, and nonlinear features.	Nonlinear features can be used as the indicators to identify normal/autistic EEG.
Lushchekina *et al* [26]	EEG (24 normal and 27 ASD subjects)	Evaluation with spectral characteristics computed by fast Fourier transformation.	Generally visible decrease in spectral strength was in occipital and parietal sections.
Eldridge *et al* [27]	EEG (30 normal and 19 ASD subjects)	Modified multi-scale entropy features and bi-level classification.	Achieved an accuracy of 79% with naïve Bayes technique.
Grobekathofer *et al* [28]	EEG (6 ASD subjects)	Nonlinear feature extraction and classifier implementation.	Accomplished a classification accuracy of 83% (decision tree), 86% (SVM), and >86% (random forest).
Djemal *et al* [29]	EEG (10 normal and 9 ASD subjects)	Discrete wavelet transform (DWT), entropy and statistical features. Artificial neural network (ANN) classifier.	Accuracy of 99.71% was achieved with DWT +Shannon's entropy and ANN.
Heunis *et al* [30]	EEG (46 normal and 16 ASD subjects)	Recurrence quantification analysis features, principal-component-analysis-based reduction, linear and nonlinear classifier implementation.	SVM with leave-one-out helped to achieve an accuracy of 92.9%.
Ahmadlou *et al* [31]	EEG (8 normal and 9 ASD subjects)	Higuchi's and Katz's fractal dimensions with wavelet-chaos neural network for automated EEG detection.	Categorization accuracy of 90% with radial basis function classifier.
Ahmadlou *et al* [32]		Wavelet and visibility graph technique.	Achieved an accuracy of 95.5% with ensemble PNN (EPNN).
Ahmadlou *et al* [33]		Wavelet and fuzzy technique.	Achieved an accuracy of 95.5% with EPNN.

MC-EEG signals are then segmented into 5519 samples, which are then analyzed with the CAT to detect autistic class EEG signals with improved accuracy.

10.4 Methodology

The work proposed in this chapter aims to implement a CAT to diagnose MC-EEF signals with better accuracy. The procedures implemented in the proposed work can be found in figure 10.1.

Initially, a clinical experiment is conducted to collect the volunteers' MC-EEG (64 channels). The collected signals are then segmented into 5519 samples (continual patterns) to select the EEG section to be examined. However, the complexity of the

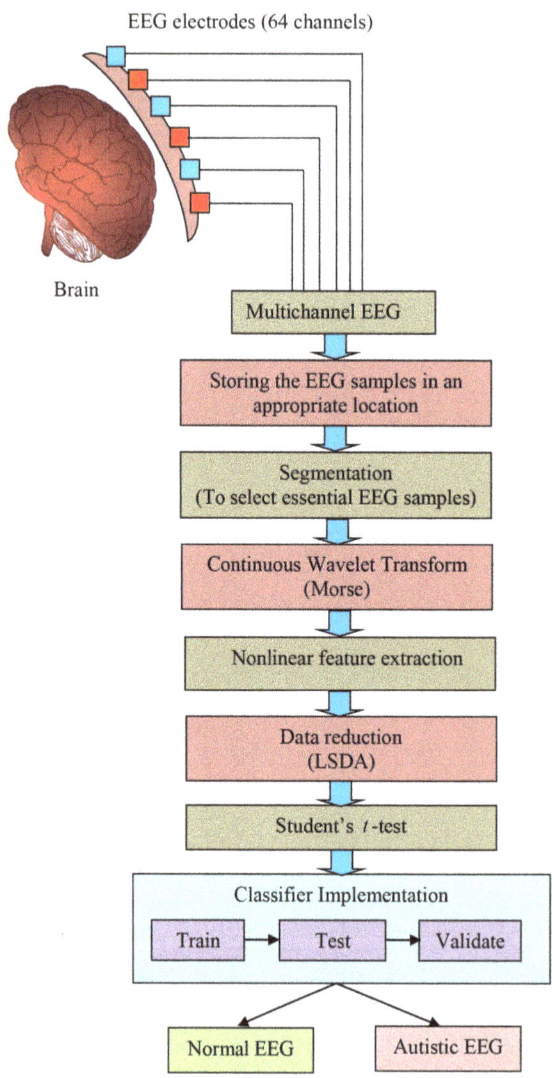

Figure 10.1. Various phases involved in the computer-assisted technique.

signal is significant, and evaluation of the signal patterns for all 64 channels is quite tricky and time consuming. Hence, the existing signals are converted into an equivalent image using a CWT in the proposed work. The CWT-Morse helps achieve a basic image pattern based on the MC-EEG signals. Using a nonlinear feature-extraction technique, the essential information from the CWT-Morse is then extracted for the normal/autistic class signals. This technique helped to extract 18 such features, such as energy, entropies (Kapoor, Max, Renyi, Shannon, Vajda, and Yager), run percentage, nonuniformity (gray-level and run length), and emphasis (short run, long run, low gray-level run, high gray-level run, short-run low gray-level run, short-run high gray-level run, long-run low gray-level run, and long-run high gray-level run). After collecting all the essential features from the 77 CWT-Morse samples, the dominant feature selection process is then implemented using LSDA. Then a statistical evaluation based on Student's t-test is executed for the normal/autistic features sets to sort all the 18 nonlinear features based on their t-test rank. During this process, features with a p-value >0.05 were discarded. The remaining features (LSDA6, LSDA4, and LSDA3) were considered to train, test, and validate the classifier systems utilized in this study.

In this work, a detailed assessment of various well-known classifiers is executed. After constructing a confusion matrix, its classification performance on the considered MC-EEG database is then confirmed. This study confirms that the proposed technique is efficient in detecting autistic class EEGs with better performance measure (PM) values. The overall result attained with the PNN classifier is better than other classifiers implemented in the proposed study.

10.4.1 Electroencephalogram database

This research considered the clinically obtained MC-EEG signals contained in a recent work [79]. This data set consists of 77 children's EEG signals, including 40 ASD volunteers from special education centers and 37 normal volunteers from schools operating in Jordan. The experimental procedure was executed in a controlled environment. From every child, 20 min of brain signals were collected using a noninvasive EEG-cap system with 64 electrodes, based on 10–20 international standards. The signal of each channel was sampled at 500 Hz, and a frequency band of 0.3 Hz to 40 Hz was considered during the data acquisition. These collection processes were achieved using a 6-EEGO amplifier and a workstation with MATLAB®, EEGO, and LA-106 ERP softwares. The raw MC-EEG signals are segmented for the experimental investigation to acquire a signal with 5519 samples.

10.4.2 Signal-to-image conversion with continuous wavelet transform

Most physiological signals are complex, and thus evaluating the information existing in these signals is also quite complex compared to image-based methods. Hence, in recent years existing single/multichannel signals have been efficiently evaluated with the help of transformed images [34–36]. The signal-to-image conversion process is widely implemented in the literature, particularly in CAT-based analysis of physiological signals [37–39].

In this research, a Morse-assisted CWT (i.e. CWT-Morse) is used to translate the existing MC-EEG into a red-green-blue (RGB) scale picture with a chosen dimension. The CWT denotes the sample–frequency space in a matrix whose scale can be readily visualized as a picture to expose significant features, transients, and irregularities. Further, CWTs of several signals can be engaged to evaluate the associations of their frequency stuffing over samples throughout the cross-wavelet transform and to approximate the association among sample–frequency features during wavelet and phase coherence [40]. This present work employed CWT-Morse to analyze the MC-EEGs collected from the volunteers. Details of the signal conversion to image using CWT-Morse can be found in [41–44].

10.4.3 Nonlinear feature extraction

In the proposed work, the RGB scaled image is converted into grayscale. The essential nonlinear features (18 in number), such as energy, entropy (Kapur, Max, Renyi, Shannon, Vajda, and Yager), run percentage, nonuniformity (gray-level and run length), and emphasis (short run, long run, low gray-level run, high gray-level run, short-run low gray-level run, short-run high gray-level run, long-run low gray-level run, and long-run high gray-level run) are extracted. The mathematical expression of these features can be found in [45–50].

For a given image, let, x, y denote the coefficients of the cooccurrence matrix $M(x,y)$. Let, x and y vary from 0, 1, 2, …, $N - 1$; then, the values are as follows:

$$\text{Energy} = \sqrt{\sum_{x=0}^{N-1}\sum_{y=0}^{N-1} M(x, y)}, \tag{10.1}$$

$$\text{Energy} = \sum_{x=0}^{N-1}\sum_{y=0}^{N-1} M(x, y)(-\ln(M(x, y))). \tag{10.2}$$

A gray-level run length matrix (GLRLM) is one of the feature-extraction methodologies used to extract various nonlinear features from the considered image [51–54].

A classical GLRLM consists of the following parameters for the chosen image: G_g is the total number of gray-levels, G_r is the total number of run lengths, G_v is the total number of voxels, G_c is the number of runs in a chosen direction, and $R(x,y)$ is the run length matrix in a chosen direction:

$$\text{Short Run Emphasis} = \frac{\sum_{x=1}^{G_g}\sum_{y=1}^{G_r} \cdot \frac{R(x, y)}{y^2}}{G_c}, \tag{10.3}$$

$$\text{Long Run Emphasis} = \frac{\sum_{x=1}^{G_g}\sum_{y=1}^{G_r} R(x, y)y^2}{G_c}, \tag{10.4}$$

$$\text{Gray level non-uniformity} = \frac{\sum_{x=1}^{G_g}\left(\sum_{y=1}^{G_r} R(x, y)\right)^2}{G_c}, \tag{10.5}$$

$$\text{Run length non-uniformity} = \frac{\sum_{x=1}^{G_r}\left(\sum_{y=1}^{G_g} R(x, y)\right)^2}{G_c}, \tag{10.6}$$

$$\text{Run Percentage} = \frac{G_c}{G_v}, \tag{10.7}$$

$$\text{Low Gray–Level Run Emphasis} = \frac{\sum_{x=1}^{G_g}\sum_{y=1}^{G_r} \cdot \frac{R(x, y)}{x^2}}{G_c}, \tag{10.8}$$

$$\text{High Gray–Level Run Emphasis} = \frac{\sum_{x=1}^{G_g}\sum_{y=1}^{G_r} R(x, y)x^2}{G_c}, \tag{10.9}$$

$$\text{Short Run Low Gray–Level Run Emphasis} = \frac{\sum_{x=1}^{G_g}\sum_{y=1}^{G_r} \frac{R(x, y)}{x^2 y^2}}{G_c}, \tag{10.10}$$

$$\text{Short Run High Gray–Level Run Emphasis} = \frac{\sum_{x=1}^{G_g}\sum_{y=1}^{G_r} \frac{R(x, y)x^2}{y^2}}{G_c}, \tag{10.11}$$

$$\text{Long Run Low Gray–Level Run Emphasis} = \frac{\sum_{x=1}^{G_g}\sum_{y=1}^{G_r} \frac{R(x, y)y^2}{x^2}}{G_c}, \tag{10.12}$$

$$\text{Long Run High Gray–Level Run Emphasis} = \frac{\sum_{x=1}^{G_g}\sum_{y=1}^{G_r} R(x, y)x^2y^2}{G_c}. \tag{10.13}$$

10.4.4 Locality-sensitive discriminant-analysis-based data reduction

LSDA was first proposed by Cai *et al* to reduce the data size by exploiting the geometry of the data manifold [55]. The LSDA initially builds a nearest-neighbor graph to model the neighboring geometrical formation of the fundamental manifold. This approach then segregates the graph into within and between-class and structures the existing data points according to the within and between-class groups. Finally, a classical evaluation approach is implemented to conserve the local neighborhood and discriminant data. In this way, the existing data points are grouped [81–83]. The dimensions of the existing data are reduced by discarding particular information based on a chosen guideline. Due to its merit, many research works have adopted the LSDA technique to reduce feature sets considered for classifier training, testing, and validation. Other information and related applications of LSDA can be found in [56, 57].

10.4.5 Classifier implementation

Classification of medical data is a necessary process that helps to reduce the diagnosis burden. In machine-learning and deep-learning assessments, two-level and multilevel classification is widely implemented to separate the abnormal data from normal data [58–60]. This work similarly employs a two-class classifier. The performance of these classifiers is confirmed based on PMs and a confusion matrix. To authenticate the performance of each classifier, a tenfold class validation with two and three feature sets is performed, and the best value among the trial is considered as the classification result.

This work employs the following classifiers to segregate the existing MC-EEG into normal/autistic classes:

- *Decision tree(DT).*

One of the most commonly considered classifiers to categorize linear and nonlinear data using a series of a testing scheme, which evolves in a tree-resembling formation [61, 62]. A DT utilizes a quality exploration setting as the root and interior nodes and the class labels form terminal nodes. Once a DT has been formed, categorization is achieved based on the decision taken in every tree limb. Other essential information regarding DTs when considered for classifying MC-EEG signals can be found in [63].

- *Discriminant analysis (DA).*

DA is one of the canonical classifiers widely implemented to execute two-class categorization problems. Based on the implementation, a DA can be classified as either a linear/quadratic DA obtained from effortless probabilistic models.

Let $P(A \mid b = \alpha)$ denote the data distribution for every class α.

The forecast of the DA then can be expressed with Bayes' rule as follows:

$$P(b = \alpha \mid A) = \frac{P(A \mid b = \alpha) \mid P(b = \alpha)}{P(A)} = \frac{P(A \mid b = \alpha) \mid P(b = \alpha)}{\sum_l P(A \mid b = l) \mid . \;\; P(b = l)}, \quad (10.14)$$

where α denotes the class to attain the maximized conditional probability.

In a linear/quadratic DA, $P(A \mid b)$ is formed as a multivariate Gaussian distribution with density

$$P(A \mid b = \alpha) = \frac{1}{(2\pi)^{D/2}} \exp\left(-\frac{1}{2}(A - \mu_\alpha)^n \sum\nolimits_\alpha^{-1} (A - \mu_\alpha) \right), \quad (10.15)$$

where D denotes the dimension of the features. Other details on linear/quadratic DA can be found in [64, 65]. The linear DA distinguishes matching data groups according to constraints or results concerning the detection of a finest linear renovation, which maximizes the group reparability. A similar approach is followed in quadratic DA. No assumptions are made for the Gaussian, which leads to a quadratic decision exterior.

• *Support vector machine (SVM).*
This classification is based on a hyperplane that categorizes the information according to the guiding features used during the two and multiclass classification tasks [66]. Earlier works have confirmed the implementation of SVM to classify MC-EEGs based on the considered features [67–70]. The proposed work considers a SVM with linear/radial basis function (RBF) kernels. A multiclass-like technique, known as one against all (OAA), is implemented to classify the MC-EEGs with chosen kernels. In the RBF, the kernel is controlled by a scaling factor σ. In this work, σ is chosen from 0.2 to 1.9 with a step level of 0.1. Further, SVMs with other kernels, such as 1st order (OAA1), 2nd order (OAA2), and 3rd order (OAA3), along with RBF (RBF_OAA), are adopted to classify the MC-EEGs into normal/autistic groups.

• *The k-nearest neighbor (k-NN) classifier.*
This evaluates the space among new features to each training feature and discovers the best neighbor. Earlier work on k-NN classification can be found in [71]. A k-NN classifies therapeutic information based on feature sets. In this work, the k-NN is executed to categorize the MC-EEG. The k-NN also needs the training and testing phases based on chosen features like other classifiers.

• *A probabilistic neural network (PNN).*
A PNN is one of the most widely used classifiers in machine-learning-based approaches, which has various stages, such as an input, hidden, and output layers with predefined neurons in each stage. In a PNN, the hidden layer calculates a probability density value and the summing layer accumulates the result. According to the implemented training process, the output layer then produces a result class [72]. In the proposed work, a PNN is considered to implement a two-class classification task with the help of a chosen input feature with a size of two or three. The PNN is one of the widely used approaches in classification and pattern detection tasks, which operates based on a parent probability distribution function of each class guided by a Parzen window [73]. Our PNN also utilizes the Bayes' rule discussed in equation (10.1) to allocate the class for the new data. The essential details on the PNN considered for the MC-EEG classification task can be found in [74].

10.4.6 Performance measure and validation

To appraise the classifiers' prominence, essential PMs are computed by considering the entire MC-EEG data set. Based on these PMs, the dominance of the classifier system is validated. Initially, the following indices are considered: true positive (TP), false positive (FP), false negative (FN), and true negative (TN). Along with these, associated measures, such as TP rate (TPR), FP rate (FPR), TN rate (TNR), and FN rate (FNR), are computed. From these values, other PMs, such as accuracy (ACC), precision (PRE), sensitivity (SEN), specificity (SPE), negative predictive value (NPV), and F1 Score (F1S) are computed. For a good classifier, PMs such as ACC, PRE, SEN, SPE, NPV, and F1S should be maximum (i.e. close to unity).

The arithmetical expressions of these values are as follows [75, 76]:

$$\mathrm{TPR} = \mathrm{SEN} = \frac{\mathrm{TP}}{\mathrm{TP} + \mathrm{FN}}, \tag{10.16}$$

$$\mathrm{TNR} = \mathrm{SPE} = \frac{\mathrm{TN}}{\mathrm{TN} + \mathrm{FP}}, \tag{10.17}$$

$$\mathrm{FNR} = \frac{\mathrm{FN}}{\mathrm{FN} + \mathrm{TP}}, \tag{10.18}$$

$$\mathrm{FPR} = \frac{\mathrm{FP}}{\mathrm{FP} + \mathrm{TN}}, \tag{10.19}$$

$$\mathrm{ACC} = \frac{\mathrm{TP} + \mathrm{TN}}{\mathrm{TP} + \mathrm{TN} + \mathrm{FP} + \mathrm{FN}}, \tag{10.20}$$

$$PRE = \frac{\mathrm{TP}}{\mathrm{TP} + \mathrm{FP}}, \tag{10.21}$$

$$\mathrm{F1S} = \frac{2\mathrm{TP}}{2\mathrm{TP} + \mathrm{FN} + \mathrm{FP}}, \tag{10.22}$$

$$\mathrm{NPV} = \frac{\mathrm{TN}}{\mathrm{TN} + \mathrm{FN}}. \tag{10.23}$$

10.5 Results and discussion

This section presents the attained results of the proposed research. This research work aims to analyze and detect autistic class EEG signals using the proposed CAT. As aforementioned, it considers an MC-EEG signal of 64 channels, which is very difficult to evaluate with a conventional approach due to its multichannel complexity. Further, the complexity will accumulate according to the number of samples considered for the evaluation [83]. The literature on this topic evidences that signal-to-image conversion is one viable approach to reduce the complexity. Hence, this work considered a CWT-Morse transform to convert MC-EEG signals into RGB scale pictures.

The CWT-Morse is then implemented on all the 77 MC-EEG signals to convert them into an understandable image with implanted features. A sample CWT-Morse image is presented in figure 10.2, in which figure 10.2(a) presents the autistic class Morse and figure 10.2(b) shows the normal class Morse. These images show identifiable differences between the normal/autistic classes.

Subsequently, the essential image features from these images are mined using a nonlinear feature-extraction process. A feature set is then created with 18 vital nonlinear features. The dimension of the raw features is very large, which may introduce some unwanted complications during the classification task, including an overfitting problem [84]. Hence, a feature dimension-reduction process based on LSDA is implemented to avoid said complexity and overfitting. The correctness of these features is then validated using a statistical evaluation. The attained statistical measure values, such as mean, standard deviation (SD), *p*-values, and Student's *t*-values, are recorded for further evaluation. Finally, all these essential features are then sorted in sliding order according to their *t*-value, and the LSDAs that displayed a *p*-value of >0.05 are then eliminated.

The outcome of this process is depicted in table 10.2; the highlighted feature sets (LSDA6, LSDA3, and LSDA4) are then considered to train, test, and validate the classifiers. The range of selected features for the normal/autistic classes is also depicted in figure 10.3 with a box plot.

Finally, a two-class classifier system is then implemented to categorize the considered MC-EEG data set into normal/autistic classes with the chosen classifiers. Tenfold cross-validation is then implemented to authenticate the performance of the classifiers on the CWT-Morse image of the MC-EEG. Each classifier system is tested with the two and three selected features during the classifier implementation. The best result attained with the considered classifier and the selected feature is depicted in tables 10.3 and 10.4. The outcome of the classifier validation process confirms that the result attained with the PNN is superior compared to other classifiers considered in this proposed approach. Table 10.2 presents the preliminary outcome of the validation process, and table 10.3 depicts the outcome. These tables confirm that the proposed CAT with the PNN classifier helped attain an accuracy of 98.7% when the number of features was taken as 3 (LADA6, LADA3, and LSDA4).

Figure 10.4 depicts the accuracy (TPR %) attained with the PNN with two and three features. This figure confirms that the accuracy level is $<97.5\%$ when two features are considered. Supposing the classification is implemented with three features, the accuracy is then improved to $>98\%$. This confirms that the CAT and PNN work well when the number of LSDA features is three.

Figure 10.5 presents a confusion matrix generated with the PNN classifier. A similar result is achieved for the other classifiers considered in this research work. This figure confirms that, along with its accuracy, the other PMs such as precision, negative predictive value, sensitivity, and specificity attained with the PNN is superior compared to the DT, DA(L), DA(Q), *k*-NN, and SVM with various kernel values.

The pictorial analysis is easily comprehensible compared to the number-based assessment. Figure 10.6 shows glyph plots [77, 78] of table 10.4, in which the

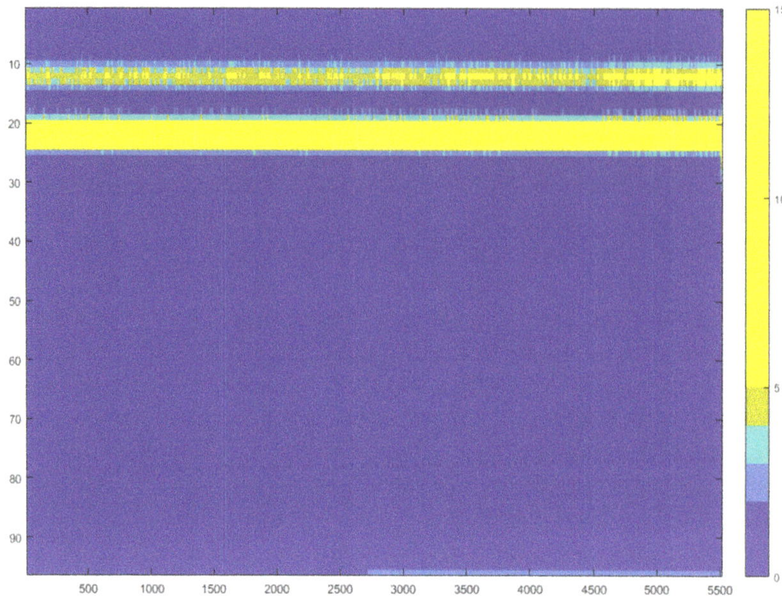

(a) Autistic class MC-EEG (X axis-Samples, Y axis-Frequency)

(b) Normal class MC-EEG (X axis-Samples, Y axis-Frequency)

Figure 10.2. Signal-to-image conversion using CWT-Morse.

Table 10.2. Selected features using LSDA and its statistical measures.

	Normal class		Autistic class			
Nonlinear features	Mean	Standard deviation	Mean	Standard deviation	*p*-Value	*t*-Value
LSDA6	**−3795.83**	**16790.04**	**18375.71**	**20598.3**	**1.76E-06**	**5.193336**
LSDA3	**80076.3**	**4108.905**	**74969.09**	**4587.318**	**2.02E-06**	**5.152786**
LSDA4	**−78218.5**	**6002.346**	**−61794.3**	**26193.27**	**0.000375**	**3.857748**
LSDA2	−26104.4	77236.37	−886.876	9878.242	0.056202	1.971156
LSDA1	82019.75	2259.519	76672.51	27098.59	0.221059	1.243333
LSDA9	32803.5	3977.13	33949.47	4487.939	0.238726	1.187648
LSDA5	4119.027	2432.066	3381.048	3298.4	0.265194	1.122996
LSDA7	104920.6	46175.2	94821.98	51442.44	0.366961	0.907673
LSDA8	−45969.4	26557.89	−50049.7	8396.997	0.376283	0.89411
LSDA21	28292.58	7539.062	28974.49	2954.539	0.609129	0.514834
LSDA14	5238.821	5360.613	5830.407	7063.465	0.678766	0.41583
LSDA12	−14787.5	4606.585	−13705.8	15838.39	0.681179	0.413474
LSDA30	−51322.9	3540.896	−53239.4	30254.44	0.692969	0.397684
LSDA27	36542.07	38806.28	31728.39	77928.14	0.729897	0.346928
LSDA11	454.3063	3150.872	253.5354	1797.068	0.735257	0.339821
LSDA23	−96793.9	13251.22	−98345	28953.86	0.760788	0.305947
LSDA26	82303.89	27019.06	83536.76	5813.962	0.787209	0.271797
LSDA29	48790.78	28898.37	49899.21	2717.882	0.817551	0.232362
LSDA15	61370.22	25650.79	62234.83	4011.783	0.840422	0.20275
LSDA28	34794.56	57111.16	33003.5	15787.21	0.854641	0.184357
LSDA17	40431.75	21159.9	41179.15	18420.12	0.869615	0.164737
LSDA18	−34494.1	13696.07	−34917.9	9340.115	0.875449	0.157381
LSDA19	128824.8	19826.42	128285.8	8145.91	0.878436	0.153786
LSDA16	31527.38	20399.21	30801.71	23765.7	0.885825	0.144081
LSDA25	1589.16	18450.43	1106.522	9643.533	0.887485	0.142165
LSDA22	−84988.2	8581.58	−84685.1	16905.09	0.920454	0.100292
LSDA20	51140.14	7912.016	51334.37	12385.89	0.934403	0.082616
LSDA13	−8785.5	6870.172	−8343.29	35579.44	0.938935	0.077067
LSDA24	−69071	13679.01	−69026.2	32250.76	0.993615	0.00804
LSDA10	−34464.5	3271.61	−34469.2	2362.655	0.994307	0.007163

dimensions of the plots are proportional to superior performance. The DA (Q) presented a poor performance, whereas the PNN showed a better performance than other classifiers on the considered MC-EEG data set.

The above results confirm that the proposed CAT works well on the considered EEG data set and helps achieve a better classification rate on normal/autistic class signals. The merit of the proposed investigation is the development of a CAT to support automated detection of ASD from MC-EEGs with better accuracy with a minimal number of nonlinear features. The inconvenience of this approach is that it

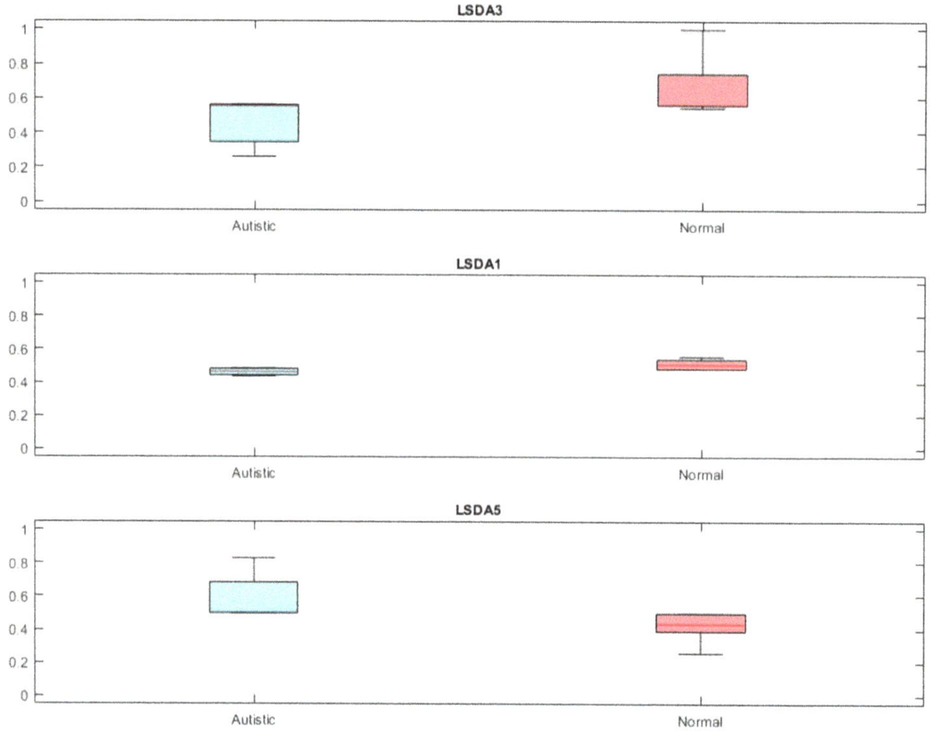

Figure 10.3. Box plots of the reduced feature sets of normal/autistic classes with LSDA.

Table 10.3. Performance measures attained with various classifiers based on the chosen features.

Classifier system	Selected features	TP	TN	FP	FN	TPR	FNR	TNR	FPR
Decision tree	3	39	35	2	1	0.9750	0.0250	0.9459	0.0541
Discriminant analysis (L)	3	39	35	2	1	0.9750	0.0250	0.9459	0.0541
Discriminant analysis (Q)	2	34	35	2	6	0.8500	0.1500	0.9459	0.0541
SVM (OAA_1)	3	39	35	2	1	0.9750	0.0250	0.9459	0.0541
SVM (OAA_2)	3	39	36	1	1	0.9750	0.0250	0.9730	0.0270
SVM (OAA_3)	3	38	37	0	2	0.9500	0.0500	1	0
k-NNs	3	39	35	2	1	0.9750	0.0250	0.9459	0.0541
Probabilistic neural network	3	**39**	**37**	**0**	**1**	**0.9750**	**0.0250**	**1**	**0**
SVM (RBF_OAA)	2	39	36	1	1	0.9750	0.0250	0.9730	0.0270

employs a series of techniques ranging from the segmentation of an EEG sequence to classification and validation. In future work, the dimensions of the MC-EEG samples may be reduced by excluding the channels that have limited information, and the CWT-Morse can be further developed using a novel deep-learning architecture to improve the detection accuracy.

Table 10.4. Essential performance measures achieved in the developed CAT based on chosen features and classifiers.

Classifier system	F1S (%)	NPV (%)	SEN (%)	SPE (%)	ACC (%)	PRE (%)
Decision tree	96.30	97.22	97.50	94.59	96.10	95.12
Discriminant analysis (L)	96.30	97.22	97.50	94.59	96.10	95.12
Discriminant analysis (Q)	89.47	85.37	85.00	94.59	89.61	94.44
SVM (OAA_1)	96.30	97.22	97.50	94.59	96.10	95.12
SVM (OAA_2)	97.50	97.30	97.50	97.30	97.40	97.50
SVM (OAA_3)	97.44	94.87	95.00	100	97.40	100
k-NNs	96.30	97.22	97.50	94.59	96.10	95.12
Probabilistic neural network	**98.73**	**97.37**	**97.50**	**100**	**98.70**	**100**
SVM (RBF_OAA)	97.50	97.30	97.50	97.30	97.40	97.50

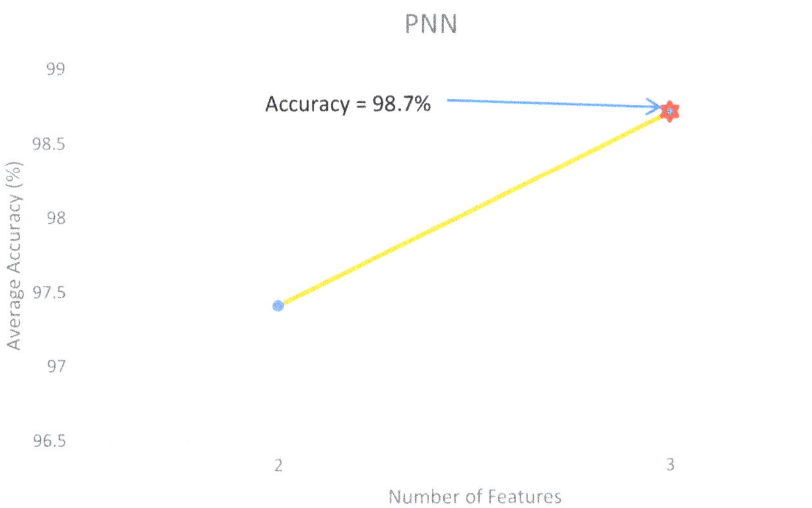

Figure 10.4. Variation in PNN accuracy with respect to selected features.

Identified

Actual		**Normal class**	**Autistic class**	
	Normal class	TP=39	FN=1	SEN=97.50%
	Autistic class	FP=0	TN=37	SPE=100%
		PRE=100%	NPV=97.37%	ACC=98.70%

Figure 10.5. Confusion matrix attained with PNN classifier.

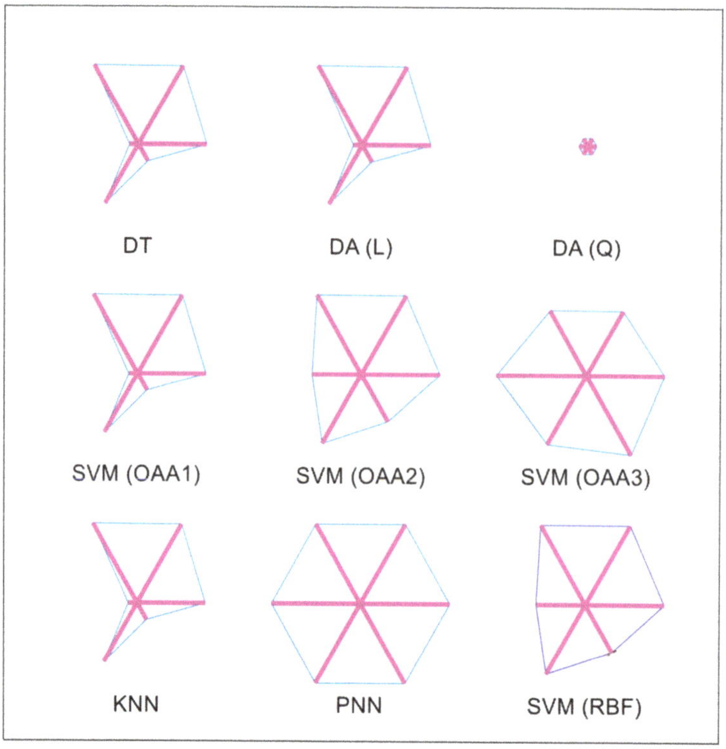

Figure 10.6. Glyph plots of performance measures available in table 10.4.

10.6 Conclusion

The proposed research aimed to develop a CAT to detect autism from MC-EEG signals. This research considered clinical-grade EEG signals obtained from 77 volunteers (37 normal cases and 40 autistic cases) using a 64-channel electrode array. Initially, a segmentation task was implemented to extract the MC-EEG into 5519 samples. Later, a CWT-Morse was implemented to convert the existing MC-EEG into an RGB scale picture using the time-frequency transformation. After acquiring the essential images, 18 nonlinear features were then extracted. Then, a dimension-reduction task was implemented to select three vital features using a LSDA. The chosen features were then considered to train, test, and validate the two-class classifiers employed in the proposed research. The experimental outcome confirmed that the PNN classifier offered superior results (classification accuracy 98.7%) compared to the other related classifiers considered in this study. The overall results of this experiment confirmed that the proposed technique works well on clinically obtained MC-EEG signals, and this approach promises great significance in diagnosing autistic signals.

References

[1] Acharya U R, Sree S V, Swapna G, Martis R J and Suri J S 2013 Automated EEG analysis of epilepsy: a review *Knowl.-Based Syst.* **45** 147–65

[2] Kannathal N, Acharya U R, Lim C M and Sadasivan P K 2005 Characterization of EEG-A comparative study *Comput. Methods Programs Biomed.* **80** 17–23

[3] Elsabbagh M *et al* 2012 Global prevalence of autism and other pervasive developmental disorders *Autism Res. Jun.* **5** 160–79

[4] Lord C, Elsabbagh M, Baird G and Veenstra-Vanderweele 2018 Autism spectrum disorder *Lancet* **392** 508–20

[5] WHO 2022 Fact sheet: autism https://who.int/news-room/fact-sheets/detail/autism-spectrum-disorders

[6] CDC 2022 Autism https://cdc.gov/ncbddd/autism/data.html

[7] Autism.org 2022 The history of autism https://autism.org.uk/about/what-is/myths-facts-stats.aspx

[8] Zecavati N and Spence S J 2009 Neurometabolic disorders and dysfunction in autism spectrum disorders *Curr. Neurol. Neurosci. Rep.* **9** 129–36

[9] Taniai H, Nishiyama T, Miyahci T, Imaeda M and Sumi S 2008 Genetic influences on the board spectrum of autism: study of proband-ascertained twins *Am. J. Med. Genet.* B **147B** 844–49

[10] Ozonoff S *et al* 2015 Diagnostic stability in young children at risk for autism spectrum disorder: a baby siblings research consortium study *J. Child. Psychol. Psychiatry* **56** 988–98

[11] Bosl W J, Teger-Flusberg H and Nelson C A 2018 EEG analytics for early detection of autism spectrum disorder: a data-driven approach *Sci. Rep.* **8** 6828

[12] Bosl W, Tierney A, Tager-Flusberg H and Nelson C 2011 EEG complexity as a biomarker for autism spectrum disorder risk *BMC Med.* **9** 18

[13] Wang L *et al* 2018 Volume-based analysis of 6-month-old infant brain MRI for autism biomarker identification and early diagnosis *Med. Image. Comput. Comput. Assist. Interv.* **11072** 411–19

[14] Chen R, Jiao Y and Herskovits E H 2011 Structural MRI in autism spectrum disorder *Pediatr. Res.* **69** 63R–8R

[15] Li D, Karnath H O and Xu X 2017 Candidate biomarkers in children with autism spectrum disorder: a review of MRI studies *Neurosci. Bull.* **33** 219–37

[16] Talo M, Yildirim O, Baloglu U B, Aydin G and Acharya U R 2019 Convolutional neural networks for multi-class brain disease detection using MRI images *Comput. Med. Imaging Graph.* **78** 101673

[17] Acharya U R *et al* 2019 Automated detection of Alzheimer's disease using brain MRI images—a study with various feature extraction techniques *J. Med. Syst.* **43** 302

[18] Raghavendra U, Acharya U R and Adeli H 2019 Artificial intelligence techniques for automated diagnosis of neurological disorders *Eur. Neurol.* **82** 41–64

[19] Gudigar A *et al* 2019 Brain pathology identification using computer aided diagnostic tool: a systematic review *Comput. Methods Programs Biomed.* **187** 105205

[20] Acharya U R *et al* 2019 Automatic detection of ischemic stroke using higher order spectra features in brain MRI images *Cognitive Systems Research* **58** 134–42

[21] Bhat S, Acharya U R, Adeli H, Bairy G M and Adeli A 2014 Autism: cause factors, early diagnosis and therapies *Rev. Neurosci.* **25** 841–50

[22] Ibrahim S, Djemal R and Alsuwailem A 2018 Electroencephalography (EEG) signal processing for epilepsy and autism spectrum disorder diagnosis *Biocyber. Biomed. Eng.* **38** 16–26

[23] Han J *et al* 2017 Global synchronization of multichannel EEG based on Rényi entropy in children with autism spectrum disorder *Appl. Sci.* **7** 257
[24] Paula C A R *et al* 2017 High-frequency EEG variations in children with autism spectrum disorder during human faces visualization *Biomed. Res. Int.* **2017** 3591914
[25] Bhat S, Acharya U R, Adeli H, Bairy G M and Adeli A 2014 Automated diagnosis of autism: in search of a mathematical marker *Rev. Neurosci.* **25** 851–61
[26] Lushchekina E A, Podreznaya E D, Lushchekin V S, Novototskii-Vlasov V Y and Strelets V B 2014 Comparative studies of EEG theta and gamma rhythms in normal children and children with early childhood autism *Neurosci. Behav. Physiol.* **44** 902–08
[27] Eldridge J, Lane A E, Belkin M and Dennis S 2014 Robust features for the automatic identification of autism spectrum disorder in children *J. Neurodev. Disord.* **6** 1–12
[28] Großekathöfer U *et al* 2017 Automated detection of stereotypical motor movements in autism spectrum disorder using recurrence quantification analysis *Front. Neuroinform.* **11** 9
[29] Djemal R, AlSharabi K, Ibrahim S and Alsuwailem A 2017 EEG-based computer aided diagnosis of autism spectrum disorder using wavelet, entropy, and ANN *BioMed Res. Int.* **2017** 9816591
[30] Heunis T *et al* 2018 Recurrence quantification analysis of resting state EEG signals in autism spectrum disorder—a systematic methodological exploration of technical and demographic confounders in the search for biomarkers *BMC Med.* **16** 101
[31] Ahmadlou M, Adeli H and Adeli A 2010 Fractality and a wavelet chaos-neural network methodology for EEG-based diagnosis of autistic spectrum disorder *J. Clinical Neurophysiology* **27** 328–33
[32] Ahmadlou M, Adeli H and Adeli A 2012 Improved visibility graph fractality with application for the diagnosis of autism spectrum disorder *Physica* A **391** 4720–6
[33] Ahmadlou M, Adeli H and Adeli A 2012 Fuzzy synchronization likelihood-wavelet methodology for diagnosis of autism spectrum disorder *J. Neurosci. Methods* **211** 203–9
[34] Bakiya A, Kamalanand K, Rajinikanth V, Nayak R S and Kadry S 2018 Deep neural network assisted diagnosis of time-frequency transformed electromyograms *Multimedia Tools Appl.* **79** 11051–67
[35] Bakiya A, Kamalanand K and Rajinikanth V 2018 Assessment of electromyograms using genetic algorithm and artificial neural networks *Evolutionary Intelligence* **14** 261–71
[36] Jahmunah V *et al* 2019 Automated detection of schizophrenia using nonlinear signal processing methods *Artif. Intell. Med.* **100** 101698
[37] Acharya U R, Sudarshan V K, Adeli H, Santhosh J and Koh J E W 2015 A novel depression diagnosis index using nonlinear features in EEG signals *Eur. Neurol.* **74** 79–83
[38] Sharma M and Acharya U R 2019 A new method to identify coronary artery disease with ECG signals and time-frequency concentrated antisymmetric biorthogonal wavelet filter bank *Pattern Recognit. Lett.* **125** 235–40
[39] Sharma M, Raval M and Acharya U R 2019 A new approach to identify obstructive sleep apnea using an optimal orthogonal wavelet filter bank with ECG signals *Informatics in Medicine Unlocked* **16** 100170
[40] Acharya U R *et al* 2013 Automated diagnosis of epilepsy using CWT, HOS and texture parameters *Int. J. Neural Syst.* **23** 13500093
[41] Faust O, Acharya U R, Adeli H and Adeli A 2015 Wavelet-based EEG processing for computer-aided seizure detection and epilepsy diagnosis *Seizure* **26** 56–64

[42] Wachowiak M P *et al* 2018 Quantitative feature analysis of continuous analytic wavelet transforms of electrocardiography and electromyography *Philos. Trans. A. Math. Phys. Eng. Sci.* **376** 20170250

[43] Real R G L, Kotchoubey B and Kübler A 2014 Studentized continuous wavelet transform (t-CWT) in the analysis of individual ERPs: real and simulated EEG data *Front. Neurosci.* **8** 279

[44] Turk O and Özerdem M S 2019 Epilepsy detection by using scalogram based convolutional neural network from EEG signals *Brain Sci.* **9** 115

[45] Paul J K *et al* 2019 Characterization of fibromyalgia using sleep EEG signals with nonlinear dynamical features *Comput. Biol. Med.* **111** 103331

[46] Acharya U R *et al* 2019 Application of nonlinear methods to discriminate fractionated electrograms in paroxysmal versus persistent atrial fibrillation *Comput. Methods Programs Biomed.* **175** 163–78

[47] Acharya U R *et al* 2019 Automated diagnosis of celiac disease using DWT and nonlinear features with video capsule endoscopy images *Future Gener. Comput. Syst.* **90** 86–93

[48] Acharya U R *et al* 2018 Automated detection and classification of liver fibrosis stages using contourlet transform and nonlinear features *Comput. Methods Programs Biomed.* **166** 91–8

[49] Adam M *et al* 2018 Automated characterization of cardiovascular diseases using relative wavelet nonlinear features extracted from ECG signals *Comput. Methods Programs Biomed.* **161** 133–43

[50] Adam M *et al* 2018 Automated characterization of diabetic foot using nonlinear features extracted from thermograms *Infrared Phys. Technol.* **89** 325–37

[51] Galloway M M 1975 Texture analysis using gray level run lengths, *Computer Graphics Image Processing* **4** 172–9

[52] Sohail A S M, Bhattacharya P, Mudur S P and Krishnamurthy S 2011 Local relative GLRLM-based texture feature extraction for classifying ultrasound medical images *24th Canadian Conf. on Electrical and Computer Engineering (CCECE)* pp 1092

[53] Chu A, Sehgal C M and Greenleaf J F 1990 Use of gray value distribution of run lengths for texture analysis *Pattern Recogn. Lett.* **11** 415–20

[54] Dasarathy B R and Holder E B 1991 Image characterizations based on joint gray-level run-length distributions *Pattern Recogn. Lett.* **12** 497–502

[55] Cai D, He X, Zhou K, Han J and Bao H 2007 Locality sensitive discriminant analysis *IJCAI'07 Proc. 20th Int. Joint Conf. on Artificial Intelligence* pp 708–13

[56] Khair N M, Hariharan M, Yaacob S and Basah S N 2015 Locality sensitivity discriminant analysis-based feature ranking of human emotion actions recognition *J. Phys. Ther. Sci.* **27** 2649–53

[57] Raghavendra U *et al* 2016 Application of Gabor wavelet and locality sensitive discriminant analysis for automated identification of breast cancer using digitized mammogram images *Appl. Soft Comput.* **46** 151–61

[58] Paul J K *et al* 2019 Characterization of fibromyalgia using sleep EEG signals with nonlinear dynamical features *Comput. Biol. Med.* **111** 103331

[59] Dey N *et al* 2019 Social-group-optimization based tumor evaluation tool for clinical brain MRI of flair/diffusion-weighted modality *Biocyber. Biomed. Eng.* **39** 843–56

[60] Rajinikanth V, Dey N, Satapathy S C and Ashour A S 2018 An approach to examine magnetic resonance angiography based on Tsallis entropy and deformable snake model *Futur. Gener. Comput. Syst.* **85** 160–72

[61] Guan S, Zhao K and Yang S 2019 Motor imagery EEG classification based on decision tree framework and riemannian geometry *Comput. Intell. Neurosci.* **2019** 5627156

[62] Kotsiantis S B 2013 Decision trees: a recent overview *Artif. Intell. Rev.* **39** 261–83

[63] Aboalayo K A I, Faezipour M, Almuhammadi W S and Moslehpour S 2016 Sleep stage classification using EEG signal analysis: a comprehensive survey and new investigation *Entropy* **18** 272

[64] Oka H *et al* 2004 Linear discriminant analysis of dermoscopic parameters for the differentiation of early melanomas from Clark naevi *Melanoma Research* **14** 131–34

[65] Anagnostopoulos C, Tasoulis D K, Adams N M, Pavlidis N G and Hand D J 2012 Online linear and quadratic discriminant analysis with adaptive forgetting for streaming classification *Statistical Analysis and Data Mining* **5** 139–66

[66] Acharya U R, Sree S V, Ang P C A, Yanti R and Suri J S 2012 Application of non-linear and wavelet based features for the automated identification of epileptic EEG signals *Int. J. Neural Syst.* **22** 1250002

[67] Gautam D and Ahmed M 2015 Melanoma detection and classification using SVM based decision support system *Annual IEEE India Conf. (INDICON)* pp 1–6

[68] Sumithra R, Suhil M and Guru D S 2015 Segmentation and classification of skin lesions for disease diagnosis *Procedia Computer Sci.* **45** 76–85

[69] Abe S 2003 Analysis of multiclass support vector machines *Int. Conf. on Computational Intelligence for Modelling Control and Automation (CIMCA 2003)* pp 385–96

[70] Kijsirikul B and Ussivakul N 2002 Multiclass support vector machines using adaptive directed acyclic graph *Proc. Int. Joint Conf. on Neural Networks (IJCNN 2002)* pp 980–5

[71] Dvey-Aharon Z, Fogelson N and Intrator N 2015 Schizophrenia detection and classification by advanced analysis of EEG recordings using a single electrode approach *PLoS One* **10** e0123033

[72] Specht D F 1990 Probabilistic neural networks *Neural Netw.* **3** 109–18

[73] Patel A K and Chatterjee S Computer vision-based limestone rock-type classification using probabilistic neural network *Geoscience Frontiers* **7** 53–60

[74] Wu T, Yang B and Sun H 2010 EEG classification based on artificial neural network in brain computer interface *Commun. Comput. Inform. Sci.* **97** 154–62

[75] Fernandes S L, Rajinikanth V and Kadry S 2019 A hybrid framework to evaluate breast abnormality using infrared thermal images *IEEE Consumer Electronics Magazine* **8** 31–6

[76] Bhandary A *et al* 2019 Deep-learning framework to detect lung abnormality—a study with chest x-ray and lung CT scan images *Pattern Recogn. Lett* **129** 271–8

[77] Ward M O 2008 Multivariate data glyphs: principles and practice *Handbook of Data Visualization* ed C-H Chen, W Härdle and A Unwin (Berlin: Springer) pp 179–98

[78] Maguire E, Rocca-Serra P, Sansone S A, Davies J and Chen M 2012 Taxonomy-based Glyph design—with a case study on visualizing workflows of biological experiments *IEEE Trans. Visual Comput. Graphics* **18** 2603–12

[79] Oh S L, Jahmunah V and Arunkumar N *et al* 2021 A novel automated autism spectrum disorder detection system *Complex Intel. Syst.* **7** 2399–413

[80] Estrela V V *et al* 2018 Health 4.0: applications, management, technologies and review *Med. Tech. J.* **2** 262–76

[81] Estrela V V *et al* 2019 Why software-defined radio (SDR) matters in healthcare? *Med. Tech. J.* **3** 421–9

[82] Abreu L M *et al* 2020 A multi-criteria modelling for ranking CO_2 emitting G20 countries from the Kaya identity and their impacts on elderly health *Brazilian Technology Symp.* pp 477–87
[83] Ranjbarzadeh R *et al* 2022 Nerve optic segmentation in CT images using a deep learning model and a texture descriptor *Complex & Intelligent Systems* **8** 3543–57
[84] Alferaidi A *et al* 2022 Distributed deep CNN-LSTM model for intrusion detection method in IoT-based vehicles *Math. Problems Eng.* **2022** 3424819

www.ingramcontent.com/pod-product-compliance
Ingram Content Group UK Ltd.
Pitfield, Milton Keynes, MK11 3LW, UK
UKHW051857100926
8556IPUK00005B/667

9 780750 340106